PERINATAL AND PEDIATRIC BEREAVEMENT IN NURSING AND OTHER HEALTH PROFESSIONS

Beth Perry Black, PhD, RN, is an associate professor of nursing at the University of North Carolina at Chapel Hill. She teaches a graduate course, Death, Dying, and Care of the Bereaved, for nursing and social work students, an undergraduate course on nursing inquiry and evidence-based practice, and two graduate writing courses. She has published numerous articles, several monographs, and book chapters on perinatal loss; and authored a book on professional nursing practice. Dr. Black has received National Institutes of Health (NIH) funding twice to study perinatal loss and palliative care, and recently completed a study on reproductive loss in lesbian couples.

Patricia Moyle Wright, PhD, RN, ACNS-BC, is an associate professor of nursing at the University of Scranton in Scranton, Pennsylvania. She teaches in the undergraduate and graduate programs and truly loves to share her enthusiasm for the nursing profession with her students. Her clinical expertise is in end-of-life/hospice nursing. Her research is centered on grief and bereavement with a particular emphasis on perinatal loss, and she has published numerous articles on this topic. She continues to work on refining the Pushing On theory of perinatal bereavement, which is included in this book, and is also conducting research on other forms of loss and grief.

Rana Limbo, PhD, RN, CPLC, FAAN, is the associate director of Resolve Through Sharing (RTS), Gundersen Health System, La Crosse, Wisconsin. She was the first coordinator of RTS, the premier international hospital-based perinatal bereavement program, which began in 1981. Dr. Limbo has written numerous articles, book chapters, and two books, and is a frequent speaker on perinatal bereavement, guided participation, and relationship-based care. She is a fellow of the American Academy of Nursing; an elected member of the International Work Group on Death, Dying, and Bereavement; and certified in perinatal loss care.

PERINATAL AND PEDIATRIC BEREAVEMENT IN NURSING AND OTHER HEALTH PROFESSIONS

Beth Perry Black, PhD, RN

Patricia Moyle Wright, PhD, RN, ACNS-BC

Rana Limbo, PhD, RN, CPLC, FAAN

EDITORS

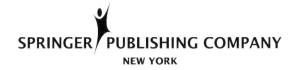

SPRINGER PUBLISHING COMPANY
NEW YORK

Springer Publishing Company, LLC
11 West 42nd Street
New York, NY 10036
www.springerpub.com

Acquisitions Editor: Elizabeth Nieginski
Composition: Exeter Premedia Services Private Ltd.

ISBN: 978-0-8261-2926-0
e-book ISBN: 978-0-8261-2927-7

15 16 17 18 / 5 4 3 2 1

The author and the publisher of this Work have made every effort to use sources believed to be reliable to provide information that is accurate and compatible with the standards generally accepted at the time of publication. Because medical science is continually advancing, our knowledge base continues to expand. Therefore, as new information becomes available, changes in procedures become necessary. We recommend that the reader always consult current research and specific institutional policies before performing any clinical procedure. The author and publisher shall not be liable for any special, consequential, or exemplary damages resulting, in whole or in part, from the readers' use of, or reliance on, the information contained in this book. The publisher has no responsibility for the persistence or accuracy of URLs for external or third-party Internet websites referred to in this publication and does not guarantee that any content on such websites is, or will remain, accurate or appropriate.

Library of Congress Cataloging-in-Publication Data
Black, Beth Perry, author.
  Perinatal and pediatric bereavement in nursing and other health professions / Beth Perry Black,
  Patricia Moyle Wright, and Rana Limbo.
       p. ; cm.
  Includes bibliographical references.
  ISBN 978-0-8261-2926-0 — ISBN 978-0-8261-2927-7 (ebook)
  I. Wright, Patricia Moyle, author.   II. Limbo, Rana K. (Rana Kristina), author.   III. Title.
  [DNLM: 1. Bereavement.   2. Maternal-Child Nursing—methods.   3. Child.   4. Death.
  5. Infant.   6. Perinatal Death. WY 157.3]
  RG631
  618.3'92—dc23
                                                                                    2015017822

Special discounts on bulk quantities of our books are available to corporations, professional associations, pharmaceutical companies, health care organizations, and other qualifying groups. If you are interested in a custom book, including chapters from more than one of our titles, we can provide that service as well.

For details, please contact:
Special Sales Department, Springer Publishing Company, LLC
11 West 42nd Street, 15th Floor, New York, NY 10036-8002
Phone: 877-687-7476 or 212-431-4370; Fax: 212-941-7842
E-mail: sales@springerpub.com

Printed in the United States of America by Gasch Printing.

In memory of my beloved husband Tal, who graced my life with his joyful spirit. —BPB

To my family, with gratitude, for their steadfast love and support. —PMW

In loving memory of my parents, who taught me at an early age to not fear grief. —RKL

Contents

Contributors

Beth Perry Black, PhD, RN Associate Professor, School of Nursing, University of North Carolina at Chapel Hill, Chapel Hill, North Carolina

Joanne Cacciatore, PhD, MSW Associate Professor, School of Social Work, Arizona State University, Tempe, Arizona; Founder/Chairman, MISS Foundation and Center for Loss and Trauma, Phoenix, Arizona

Geoffrey W. Corner Doctoral Student, Department of Psychology, University of Southern California, Los Angeles, California

Denise Côté-Arsenault, PhD, RNC, FNAP, FAAN Eloise R. Lewis Excellence Professor, Chair of Family and Community Nursing, School of Nursing, University of North Carolina—Greensboro, Greensboro, North Carolina

Betty Davies, RN, PhD, CT, FAAN Professor Emerita, Family Health Care Nursing, University of California San Francisco, San Francisco, California; Adjunct Professor and Senior Scholar, School of Nursing, University of Victoria, Victoria, British Columbia, Canada

Dalia El-Khoury, MEd Doctoral Candidate, School of Social Work, Virginia Commonwealth University, Richmond, Virginia

Chris Feudtner, MD, PhD, MPH Steven D. Handler Endowed Chair of Medical Ethics, Pediatric Advanced Care Team and Integrated Care Service, The Children's Hospital of Philadelphia, Philadelphia, Pennsylvania

Jane Heustis, RN, CPLC Resolve Through Sharing National Faculty, New Albany, Indiana; Retired Perinatal Bereavement Coordinator, Indiana University Health Methodist Hospital, Indianapolis, Indiana

Douglas L. Hill, PhD Behavioral Researcher, Pediatric Advanced Care Team, The Children's Hospital of Philadelphia, Philadelphia, Pennsylvania

Rebecca Kabatchnick, BSN, RN Doctor of Nursing Practice Student, University of North Carolina at Chapel Hill, Chapel Hill, North Carolina

Kathie Kobler, MS, APN, PCNS-BC, CHPPN   Pediatric Palliative Care, Center for Fetal Care, Advocate Children's Hospital, Park Ridge, Illinois

Anthony Lathrop, PhD, CNM   Indiana University Health—HealthNet, Indianapolis, Indiana

Wendy G. Lichtenthal, PhD   Assistant Attending Psychologist, Director, Bereavement Clinic, Department of Psychiatry and Behavioral Sciences, Memorial Sloan Kettering Cancer Center, New York, New York

Rana Limbo, PhD, RN, CPLC, FAAN   Associate Director, Resolve Through Sharing, Gundersen Health System, La Crosse, Wisconsin

Andy McNiel, MA   Chief Executive Officer, National Alliance for Grieving Children, Stuart, Florida

Margaret Shandor Miles, PhD, RN, FAAN   Professor Emerita, School of Nursing, University of North Carolina at Chapel Hill, Chapel Hill, North Carolina

Mary Muscari, PhD, MSCr, CPNP, PMHCNS-BC, AFN-BC   Associate Professor, Decker School of Nursing, Binghamton University, The State University of New York, Binghamton, New York

Joann O'Leary, PhD, MPH, MS   Independent Consultant, Minneapolis, Minnesota

Susan Poitras, RN, BScN, MScPsych, CPT   Coordinator Counselling and Bereavement Services, Clinician, Counsellor, Certified Play Therapist, Canuck Place Children's Hospice, Vancouver, British Columbia, Canada

Sarah Kye Price, PhD, MSW, MS   Associate Professor, School of Social Work, Research Scientist in Perinatal Mental Health, Institute for Women's Health, Virginia Commonwealth University, Richmond, Virginia

Kailey E. Roberts, MA   Predoctoral Research Fellow, Department of Psychiatry and Behavioral Sciences, Memorial Sloan Kettering Cancer Center, New York, New York

Donna L. Schuurman, EdD, FT   Chief Executive Officer, The Dougy Center for Grieving Children and Families, Portland, Oregon

Marlene G. S. Sefton, PhD, APN, FNP   Assistant Clinical Professor, University of Illinois at Chicago, College of Nursing, Chicago, Illinois

Rose Steele, PhD, RN   Professor, School of Nursing, Faculty of Health, York University, Toronto, Ontario, Canada

Eric Stephanson, MA, MDiv   Spiritual Care Leader, Canuck Place Children's Hospice, Vancouver, British Columbia, Canada

Kristen M. Swanson, PhD, RN, FAAN   Dean and Professor, College of Nursing, Seattle University, Seattle, Washington

Corinne Sweeney, MA   Doctoral Candidate, Department of Psychology, Fairleigh Dickinson University; Research Study Assistant, Department of Psychiatry and Behavioral Sciences, Memorial Sloan Kettering Cancer Center, New York, New York

Camara van Breemen, MSc, MN, CHPCN   Pediatric Nurse Practitioner and Play Therapist, Canuck Place Children's Hospice, Vancouver, British Columbia, Canada

Sara Rich Wheeler, PhD, RN, PMHCNS-BC, LMHC   Retired National Dean of Nursing Academic Affairs and Online Learning, Education Affiliates, Covington, Indiana

Kimberley Widger, PhD, RN, CHPCN(C)   Assistant Professor, Lawrence S. Bloomberg Faculty of Nursing, University of Toronto, Toronto, Ontario, Canada

Danuta M. Wojnar, PhD, RN, MEd, IBCLC, FAAN   Associate Professor and Chair, Maternal/Child and Family Nursing, College of Nursing, Seattle University, Seattle, Washington

Patricia Moyle Wright, PhD, RN, ACNS-BC   Associate Professor, Department of Nursing, University of Scranton, Scranton, Pennsylvania

Foreword

*T*he idea of losing a child is so overwhelming to all involved—parents, families, professionals, and society—that our natural instinct is avoidance. We wish not to speak of the possibility that a child could die, as if this avoidance would mean it could not happen. But children die. And we now know that the conspiracy of silence only adds to the pain and also keeps health professionals from creating better ways to support children and families.

We have learned over the past 30 years that we must talk about the unspeakable and share stories that make our hearts break with the conviction that, in the telling, we can create a new story. This book on perinatal and pediatric bereavement is really a chapter in a larger "book"; the story the authors will leave for our colleagues and future generations. It is a story of love, hope, and healing. There are 18 chapters in this book covering intimate aspects of a young life ending and how those who remain behind can grieve in such a way that they can go on living. The collective message of these chapters is that there is a better way.

One of the highlights of my professional life has been to be involved in the End-of-Life Nursing Education Consortium (ELNEC) project. ELNEC began in the year 2000 as an educational program to prepare nurses to care for the seriously ill and dying. Soon after, in 2001, we realized the need to create a separate pediatric curriculum to prepare nurses for perinatal and pediatric illness and death. Through the ELNEC pediatric program I have had the honor of learning from pediatric nurses all that can be done to transform the care of children and families.

My commitment to pediatric bereavement goes beyond my profession; it is personal. I have lived it. In 1982, I had a beautiful son, Andrew, who died after 3 months in a neonatal intensive care unit (NICU). He was cared for by wonderful nurses, physicians, and other professionals but very much within a culture of avoidance. There was no discussion about the care of my son relating to any topic written in the pages of this book. My son had been improving and, as we were eagerly preparing for his discharge home, he developed a viral endocarditis and had an acute myocardial infarction. Arriving to the NICU expecting to finalize discharge plans, instead

I witnessed futile resuscitation attempts on my son. When I asked for these efforts to stop, I was told there was no other way, no hospital policy to support my wish that he die in my arms. With my insistence the NICU staff stopped their efforts and many professionals, who had gathered to do all they knew how to do, quickly disappeared. I then stood alone and removed all the tubes, lines, and other equipment from my son's body and held him in my arms until he died. I stood alone with my son in the middle of 30 infants as other parents were guided away. I could sense the sincere angst of the NICU staff but also their intense need for this scene to end. Within moments, my family, including my son's 2-year-old sister, left the hospital with no support, no plan, and certainly no thought of bereavement.

In our ELNEC project we have a mantra: "Nurses can't practice what they don't know." The professionals who cared for my son were some of the smartest, kindest, most dedicated and compassionate people I have known. But they did not know what to do when a child died.

This book is a tribute to all those families like mine, who have sailed on unchartered waters with no map, no guide, and no support through the storm. From these families, the field of pediatric palliative care has been born and now the stories are being transformed.

We know now that, while the pain of losing a child remains, much can be done. We now tell stories of families who are prepared for the death, of siblings who are involved, and of bereavement support that honors the precious life of the child and offers hope for healing for the bereaved. This book is a collection of clinical wisdom, theoretical knowledge, and models of care that can continue to tell the story and change cultures of care. There will soon be a time when the care I experienced when my son died, which was, unfortunately, standard care at that time, would not happen any longer because professionals and families will know there is a better way.

As a palliative care nurse I am honored to write this Foreword and to be included in these pages with the authors who are truly pioneers in perinatal and pediatric bereavement. As a bereaved mother, I am grateful to my colleagues who wrote this book because the memories of the care of a child last a lifetime.

Betty R. Ferrell, PhD, MA, RN, FAAN, FPCN, CHPN
City of Hope National Medical Center
Duarte, California

Preface

*I*n the past few years, the focus of health care has been the development of evidence-based practice; a three-pronged approach to the delivery of the best care possible to our patients or clients. Evidence-based practice requires that interventions be grounded in the best research evidence possible; that patients or clients find the intervention acceptable; and that clinicians have the expertise to carry out interventions appropriately and effectively. In this text, we offer you—providers of care to bereaved families experiencing a perinatal loss or the death of a child—a means of enhancing your practice. First, we offer evidence from research on effective interventions. Second, we provide evidence from the perspective of families regarding what care they need and find acceptable. And third, we provide information to increase your own expertise in caring for families experiencing tragic losses.

In this book, experts in the fields of perinatal and pediatric bereavement contribute their knowledge about the current state of practice and inquiry in their respective fields. Our contributors coalesce findings from research and practice into 18 chapters that we think you will find useful and meaningful. We present theoretical underpinnings of perinatal and pediatric bereavement, chapters on dimensions of perinatal and pediatric loss that have been of interest recently, and clinical interventions derived from research.

We are grateful for Betty R. Ferrell's commitment to bereavement care as her life's work and honored by her generous, thoughtful words in the Foreword. The book is divided into two sections. The first section, "Perinatal Bereavement," has 10 chapters focusing on aspects of perinatal loss. Kristen M. Swanson introduces this section with her perspective on the painful nature of perinatal loss. The second section, "Pediatric Bereavement," has eight chapters focusing on various aspects of caring for families whose children are dying or who have died, and caring for children who are grieving. Mary Muscari introduces this section by describing how this text is "a breath of fresh air that tackles a taboo topic," transforming the discourse around the painful reality of pediatric death.

In the first chapter, Patricia Moyle Wright, Rana Limbo, and Beth Perry Black present background content on various grief theories developed in the past five decades. These theories have expanded our understanding of the processes of death, dying, and bereavement. Although we recognize the widespread acceptance of stage theories of grief, such as that developed by Elisabeth Kübler-Ross, the goal of this chapter is to introduce our readers to other theorists and frameworks to explain grief and bereavement and how these theories may be used in understanding responses to death in perinatal and pediatric settings.

Chapter 2 offers a primer for those seeking to apply theories to empirical work. Authors Sarah Kye Price and Dalia El-Khoury extend the conversation on theory by presenting a review of theories that have been applied to grief studies and offer readers insights into how each theory can be used to frame empirical work. Continuing the focus on theoretical perspectives, Rana Limbo, Anthony Lathrop, and Jane Heustis present an overview of caregiving as a theoretical framework in perinatal palliative care in Chapter 3, beginning with a brief history of social movements that supported the development of perinatal palliative care services in the United States. Chapter 3 contains a review of the current body of literature regarding perinatal palliative care, relates extant research to the theory of caregiving, and ends with a comprehensive overview of clinical guidelines important for the provision of effective perinatal palliative care.

In Chapter 4, Beth Perry Black presents the history of efforts to promote the relationship of mother and infant, first through bonding practices of the 1970s, to the use of ultrasound in the 1980s, and forward. Measures of maternal–fetal attachment are presented and critiqued, and examples from research underscore expectant parents' connections with their babies who are likely to die before or at birth. In Chapter 5, Patricia Moyle Wright presents her Pushing On theory, developed from research interviews with women who have experienced perinatal loss; from finding out about the pregnancy to living with the loss. Wright has recently updated her theory, based on recent research, and describes how to apply Pushing On theory to practice. In Chapter 6, Joanne Cacciatore describes an approach to supporting bereaved parents, noting that normal grief after perinatal loss can be emotionally distressing for parents. She explains mindfulness-based interventions, such as meditation, which are easy to use, low cost, noninvasive, and have no apparent associated negative effect.

Grief reactions in perinatal loss can be quite intense and require special consideration and support. In Chapter 7, Patricia Moyle Wright presents a discussion of the evolving concept of complicated grief, a concept of interest for a few decades that has garnered significant attention. Wright notes the controversy related to whether complicated grief is simply a manifestation of normal grief, presents the literature on what is known about complicated grief in relation to pregnancy loss, and reviews supportive interventions from the literature.

Grief after pregnancy loss can be more complicated for certain groups. In Chapter 8, Danuta M. Wojnar provides a comprehensive overview of perinatal grief among lesbian couples. This topic has yet to be widely explored, despite the circumstances of same-sex childbearing that vary significantly, biologically and socially, from heterosexual couples. Wojnar addresses specific challenges faced by lesbian couples, such as negotiating parenting roles. In Chapter 9, Sara Rich Wheeler and Marlene G. S. Sefton provide an overview of perinatal loss in adolescents, discussing normal adolescent growth and development, and using Sanders's integrated theory of bereavement to discuss the common physical, emotional, social, and cognitive reactions to loss.

Another special circumstance—pregnancy after loss—is addressed in Chapter 10 by Denise Côté-Arsenault and Joann O'Leary, who present theoretical perspectives that underpin understandings of the experience of pregnancy after loss. The authors also discuss parental attachment, and the characteristics of pregnancy after loss in both expectant women and men, offering beneficial interventions for bereaved couples who are experiencing pregnancy after loss.

Section II, "Pediatric Bereavement," begins with Chapter 11 in which Margaret Shandor Miles provides a scholarly review of parental grief, placing it in the context of what is known about grief from a historical perspective. She also reviews psychoanalytic and psychobiological models, crisis models, attachment models, and integrative models, among others. Miles then specifically focuses on parental grief models, with an emphasis on the psychosocial, cognitive, and physical aspects of parental loss and the effects on the family system.

In Chapter 12, Rose Steele and Kimberley Widger address pediatric palliative care, discussing its historical evolution and the development of standards for this specialty. The authors present a comprehensive discourse on various models of pediatric palliative care used in the United States and Canada, ending with a focus on the specialization of pediatric care and support for professionals. Douglas L. Hill and Chris Feudtner offer an excellent discourse in Chapter 13 on the concept of hope and the role of hopeful patterns of thinking in the context of serious pediatric illness and death. They address clinical concerns, such as offering false hope, and present "regoaling" to help parents cope with their child's declining condition. Hope and regoaling provide the platform for parents to cope with the progression of numerous losses that accumulate during a child's illness and eventual death.

Sometimes, the death of a child can occur under traumatic circumstances, setting the stage for very intense psychological responses. In Chapter 14, Wendy G. Lichtenthal, Geoffrey W. Corner, Corinne Sweeney, and Kailey E. Roberts present a comprehensive overview of grief following the traumatic death of a child and review the importance of time in the grief trajectory. The authors then focus on the impact of the cause of the death on posttraumatic stress responses and overall parental health after the traumatic loss of a child and describe supportive interventions for bereaved parents. Suicide is one of the most traumatic losses a family can experience. In Chapter 15, Rebecca Kabatchnick and Beth Perry Black review the literature on sibling survivors after the completed suicide by their brothers or sisters. Little has been written on the "forgotten bereaved"—siblings left behind who are troubled by deep grief made worse by feelings of regret, anger, guilt, and a sense of need to take care of their parents.

The grief of children is the focus of the next two chapters. In Chapter 16, Betty Davies, Camara van Breemen, Susan Poitras, and Eric Stephanson discuss bereavement in young children in pediatric palliative care, providing an overview of theoretical perspectives to frame health care professionals' understanding of bereavement in children. Davies's Shadows in the Sun model is the chapter's centerpiece and provides a platform for understanding responses of bereaved siblings and how to support families effectively. In Chapter 17, Andy McNiel and Donna L. Schuurman discuss how children process death and how the experience of loss affects their mental, social, and emotional well-being. How children make sense out of the death of a loved one and how they express grief are presented, including resources for professionals working with grieving children.

In the final chapter, Rana Limbo and Kathie Kobler present the importance of creating and capturing meaningful moments in the time leading up to and after the death of a child, focusing on the importance of relationships among families and professionals as they prepare for the child's death. Limbo and Kobler describe ritual, photography, creation of keepsakes, and other important ways of creating meaningful moments and, ultimately, creating "ties that bind."

We hope that you find this book to be useful as you seek to improve your practice with bereaved families. We honor your work and are grateful that you have chosen to enter the most vulnerable of spaces in the human experience—those spaces occupied by mothers, fathers, sisters, brothers, grandparents, friends, and others bereft of a child they loved.

Beth Perry Black
Patricia Moyle Wright
Rana Limbo

Perinatal Bereavement

Kristen M. Swanson

Over the past four decades, I have witnessed considerable progress in our understanding of the difficult, sometimes tragic, circumstances that surround the experience of loss during pregnancy and the first year of life. The death of one's longed for daughter or son yields heartache, emptiness, and a lifetime of bittersweet memories. Over time, health care providers have come to recognize that even the earliest miscarriage of the most privately acknowledged pregnancy may hold great significance to the frightened woman who arrives at the emergency department, bleeding and cramping, accompanied by a beleaguered partner clutching a Tupperware container with still warm "scooped up" bloody clots. For some families, loss begins with a prenatally detected serious, life-limiting defect, made all the more unreal by the life-affirming movements of their yet-to-be-born baby. For others, the unexplainable stillbirth of their baby ushers in relentless yearning for answers. Some share their newborn infants with those able to get to the hospital quick enough to say hello and good-bye as they offer witness to a precious short life.

Caring for women and families whose pregnancies end in death challenges providers. They, too, wonder "Why?" "What could I have done differently?" Somewhere in the back of their mind or in the depth of their heart, they know that this pregnancy outcome could have happened to them or to their loved ones. The fear of pregnancy loss looms greater than does the actual threat; however, the very human act of producing our children creates vulnerability as we accept whatever is at stake with each child conceived. Caring—really caring—for women and families experiencing pregnancy loss takes courage, competence, and compassion. It starts with *knowing*, intentional continuous engagement with the other person in order to understand the meaning of what she is going through.

Enhancing practice by seeking out, knowing, and acting on the best evidence available is another form of caring. A nurse, social worker, physician, or another provider whose practice is current and based in evidence is better positioned to provide effective care, to elicit the meaning of the loss for the woman and family, and to create an environment for healing. This text provides the theoretical basis for effective care. It is rooted in years of expertise, research, and the wisdom of the editors and multidisciplined contributors who bring many perspectives to their commitment to caring for families whose lives are touched by perinatal loss. Their words illuminate the dark spaces occupied by families whose babies or children have died, shed light on their experiences, and offer hope for healing.

CHAPTER 1

My Absent Child: Cultural and Theoretical Considerations of Bereavement When a Child Dies

Patricia Moyle Wright, Rana Limbo, and Beth Perry Black

Grief fills the room up of my absent child,
Lies in his bed, walks up and down with me,
Puts on his pretty looks, repeats his words,
Remembers me of all his gracious parts,
Stuffs out his vacant garments with his form;
Then, have I reason to be fond of grief?
Fare you well: had you such a loss as I,
I could give better comfort than you do.
    (Shakespeare, *King John*, Act III, Scene IV)

Shakespeare wrote in the language of maternal bereavement in his play *King John*. In Act III, Lady Constance, mother of Arthur, is so anguished upon learning of his death that Cardinal Pandulph tells her she holds "too heinous a respect of grief," to which Constance responds, "He talks to me that never had a son." King Phillip suggests that she was as fond of grief "as of your child." Constance's response began: *Grief fills the room up of my absent child. . . .*

Secular and sacred texts and musical works alike give witness to the sorrows of bereaved mothers, fathers, sisters, brothers, and friends of children who have died. German poet Friedrich Rückert (1788–1866) penned more than 400 poems in 2 years after the deaths of two of his children to scarlet fever. Austrian composer Gustav Mahler (1860–1911) later set five of these poems, *Kindertotenlieder* (Songs on the Death of Children), to music in an exquisite musical exploration of the grief of a father. In a tragic twist of fate, Mahler's daughter, born about the time he composed the *Kindertotenlieder*, died at age 4 of scarlet fever. Czech composer Antonin Dvořák (1841–1904), best known for his *New World Symphony*, began to compose a cantata based on the ancient Latin hymn *Stabat Mater Dolorosa* (referring to Jesus's mother Mary at his crucifixion) in the aftermath of the death of his infant daughter, who died within days after her birth. Moved by the account of Mary's grief, he recognized his own suffering reflected in the words of the *Stabat Mater Dolorosa*. Dvořák set the work aside, his pain too great to finish it at the time. Two years later, however, he completed it in the aftermath of the deaths of his remaining two young children, a toddler daughter who drank poison and his 3-year-old son who died of smallpox.

These works are among countless in literature and music that remind us of the vulnerability of children historically, and also underscore the universality of profound suffering of parents when their children die. In the developed world today, children are spared deaths by infectious diseases such as scarlet fever and smallpox; stringent attention to safety has reduced their risk of death by poisoning and other accidents. But despite all efforts to make the world safe, children die, rendering their parents, their families, their friends, and their communities heartbroken. For health care providers, scenes surrounding the deaths of children are burned into their memories, even as they struggle to find the professional space to provide consolation to the inconsolable.

Texts on death, dying, and bereavement for health care providers often begin by noting that the death of a child is one of the most traumatic events a person can experience. This text is no different. We honor and respect your work with children and families when death has invaded their lives, acknowledging that persons reading this have scenes of childhood deaths stored among their memories or are willing to enter the tragic spaces where children encounter death. Knowing how to comfort those bereft of any loved one is difficult. Comforting those mourning the death of a child poses a challenge to even the most sensitive and caring clinicians. We also know that being sensitive and caring is not enough, although these are crucial personal and professional attributes in helping families bereft of a child.

Clinical education and training regarding care of the dying and bereaved is often insufficient and may be based on outdated or debunked theoretical understanding of the process of grief. Despite nurses' frequent proximity to dying patients and their families, death and bereavement education in nursing is typically inadequate in both quantity and quality, although nurse educators are increasingly incorporating this content into their curricula (Barrere, Durkin, & LaCoursiere, 2008). In a systematic evaluation of 23 psychiatric nursing textbooks frequently used in undergraduate education, Holman, Perisho, Edwards, and Mlakar (2010) found that 100% contained at least one unsupported myth about grief and 78% had four or more myths and only one finding about coping with loss that was evidence-based. This means that many nurses are inadequately acquainted with evidence that challenges commonly held assumptions about loss and grief. Medicine has similar deficits, with the ongoing—albeit improving—view of hospice and palliative medicine as a "soft specialty" requiring training in advanced communication skills and symptom management, content that lacks importance relative to other specialties (Case, Orrange, & Weissman, 2013).

Throughout this book, various authors expand on theories and concepts that we present in this chapter as fundamental to understanding the development of practice and inquiry related to bereavement. We use the word *bereavement* broadly, recognizing that grief associated with death includes losses in addition to the actual physical death, such as loss of hope, companionship, a future, and a legacy. We first acknowledge that caring for the bereaved occurs within the cultural contexts of the dying person, the family, and the health care providers. Understanding that cultures intersect when a death is near enhances the likelihood of effective care.

ADDRESSING CULTURE: A FIRST STEP IN BEREAVEMENT CARE

Care of the dying and their families occurs within cultural contexts that, unless recognized, may impede sensitive and effective care. Although an extended treatise on culture is beyond the scope of this text, we recognize that any discussion of bereavement must be accompanied by acknowledgment of deeply ingrained cultural aspects of death.

From a macrocultural perspective, there are certain universal elements to the human experience, such as drives to procreate, find food, establish safe shelter, and create social networks. Births are celebrated, deaths are mourned, and the deaths of children are recognized as particularly tragic in light of the universal assumption that children will outlive their parents. One's microculture, however, determines how these events evolve and are lived out. Microculture refers to patterns of shared behaviors and ways of thinking learned in groups by locale, ethnicity, gender, age, religion, nationality, and profession, among many others. In common usage, the word *culture* refers to elements of microculture.

Death practices vary widely across and among microcultures. In their text on ethnic variations in dying, death, and grief, Irish, Lunquist, and Nelsen (1993) referred to "diversity in universality," their description of the variety of death practices that mark the universal human experience of death. Death practices are those rites and rituals that are customary when death is imminent or has occurred. Providers should be aware that cultural practices may influence but not necessarily determine the practices of a family at the time of death. This awareness means that the provider avoids assumptions that any particular family will or should act in any specific manner as the death of their child approaches.

Effective clinicians recognize that they themselves carry out their work in the context of the culture of their profession. Socialization into a profession includes the development of behaviors valued by the profession. These behaviors may become so deeply engrained that clinicians may no longer recognize these behaviors as a function of the professional culture. Language is a characteristic of culture, a manifestation of the need to communicate as social beings. Health care providers' language includes words and acronyms that may be poorly understood by patients and families (Corless et al., 2014). Language surrounding death may contain euphemisms meant to soften the effect of bad news, but in fact may obscure the actual meaning. For example, a woman pregnant for the first time, visiting the United States with her husband and for whom English was a second language, went to a local emergency room (ER) with constant abdominal pain, uterine rigidity, and bleeding in her 30th week of gestation. The obstetrician on call suspected a placental abruption, a severe complication of pregnancy. While doing an ultrasound scan, she noted that the fetus had died.

She conveyed this news to the woman as, "Your baby has passed." In the woman's confusion, pain, and fear, her understanding of English was almost gone. The obstetrician's use of the euphemism "passed" was understood by the woman to mean she had in fact given birth. She pulled back the sheets to search for her baby that she mistakenly understood had been born amid her pain and bleeding. An ER nurse who spoke some French recognized what was happening. He took the frantic woman's hand, established eye contact with her, and explained quietly and in simple words, "Je suis désolé, votre bébé est mort (I am sorry, your baby is dead)." The obstetrician, although attempting to show compassion, did not fully recognize the effect of distress on the ability of the woman to comprehend a euphemism in her limited English fluency. The nurse's words were simple enough to cut through the confusion; delivered in a compassionate way, the words, though heavy with meaning, helped the woman make sense of a situation in which she was culturally disadvantaged in terms of setting, language, and locale.

Theoretical Orientations for Bereavement Care

As demonstrated in the aforementioned example, clinicians working with perinatal or pediatric patients may expect to encounter death infrequently relative to clinicians in specialties such as oncology and gerontology. The language of grief and bereavement is not embedded in the cultures of perinatal and pediatric providers, whose theoretical understanding of bereavement care may be limited to outdated and refuted theories of grief. Theories are particularly useful in explaining very complex human experiences such as grief and bereavement. They are a philosophical lens through which providers make sense of phenomena, offering a unifying framework for evidence that allows providers to anchor interventions in models that can guide clinical decision making. In the remainder of this chapter, we present several basic, current theoretical stances regarding bereavement care. These theories are not specific to perinatal or pediatric settings, but are flexible and robust ways to understand end-of-life care across settings.

Grief Theories Then and Now

Freud and Lindemann: Establishing Norms

Although grief had been studied as early as the 1600s, it was not until the publication of Freud's work "Mourning and Melancholia" (Freud, 1957, as cited in Granek, 2010) in the 20th century that grief was recognized as a legitimate area of scientific inquiry (Granek, 2010). Freud's work set the stage for identification of adverse sequelae after the loss of a loved one, particularly if the bereaved person failed to sever emotional bonds with the deceased (Freud, 1917/1957; see Chapters 2 and 11). Lindemann (1944/1994; see Chapter 11), among others, studied grief responses and further distinguished "normal" from "abnormal" reactions. Lindemann's research has been the basis for the development of clinical guidelines (Wright & Hogan, 2008).

Bowlby, Parkes, and Worden: Stages, Phases, and Tasks

Interest arose in delineating how one moves through the process of grief, resulting in the development of several stage and phase theories aimed to explain how grief unfolds. For example, Bowlby (see also Chapter 11) and Parkes (see also Chapters 4 and 11) offered models that depicted bereavement as a series of emotional reactions to the loss that changed over the course of time (Wright & Hogan, 2008). Bowlby and Parkes suggested four phases (Bowlby, 1969/1982): shock and numbness, searching and yearning, disorganization, and reorganization. They posited that the phases were not linear per se, but provided a framework of an individual's response to the loss of a significant relationship through these four primary categories of experiences. The phases have clinical application; these are used by clinicians to describe for mourners what their grief might be like and provide a framework for follow-up clinical care (Wilke & Limbo, 2012).

The shock and numbness phase is characterized by a sense of unreality, being mentally and emotionally distant from the trauma of the death, and with blunted feelings of disbelief. Most often, searching and yearning, with distinctly different elements of strong emotions (e.g., sobbing, screaming, intense desire for the deceased person's return), oscillate with shock and numbness, which emphasizes the nonlinearity of a phase model. The third phase, disorganization, refers to a time when the mourner accepts that the death occurred, yet remains bereft, with hope, transformation, and growth seeming impossible or far away. The final phase of reorganization denotes a period of moving forward without forgetting, continuing the relationship with the deceased in meaningful ways. In his dissertation work with 1,200 mourners, Davidson (1984) described the phases as peaking and waning, with overlapping of all four phases at times of particular relevance to the mourner, such as the death date anniversary or holidays.

Worden (2009; see also Chapter 11, this text) noted that bereavement involved a series of adjustments to the loss, which he called tasks of mourning. These tasks involved accepting the reality of the loss, processing the pain of grief, adjusting to a world without the deceased, and finding an enduring connection with the deceased in the midst of embarking on a new life. More recently, the grief process is recognized as less linear and predictable than originally conceptualized. Worden (2009) promoted tasks as useful in understanding the process of mourning, as long as one considered mediators such as how the person died, one's own self-esteem and self-efficacy, and social variables (e.g., support).

CONTINUING BONDS: RE-EXAMINING HOW ATTACHMENTS ARE MAINTAINED AFTER DEATH

In contrast to some of the work of the past 100 years postulating that emotional separation from the deceased was necessary for recovery, Silverman and Klass (1996) explored the idea that the continuation of bonds of attachment after death is in fact normal. Continuing bonds has gained a foothold in the grief literature. A continuing emotional attachment to a deceased loved one has been identified as a factor in emotional healing and serves as a way to honor the deceased person and reintegrate him or her into the survivor's life (Bowlby, 1969/1982; Wright & Hogan, 2008). Continuing to maintain an emotional connection with a deceased loved one is now generally considered to be natural and healing. However, some (e.g., Field & Filanosky, 2010) have questioned whether deep, sustained relationships with the deceased might indicate a form of denial. According to Field, it is natural to exhibit protest or denial when faced with a loss. However, prolonged and exaggerated efforts to reject the reality of the loss can indicate maladaptive responses to loss.

Field and Filanosky (2010) described two distinct ways that continuing bonds are expressed: internalized and externalized. Internalized expressions of continuing bonds are based on the bereaved individual's imagined viewpoint of the deceased. For example, a bereaved mother might say that the baby who died would have loved playgrounds or puppies. Such expressions are based solely on the projections of how the deceased is imagined and "may facilitate integration of the loss" (p. 2).

Conversely, external expressions of continuing bonds can indicate that the loss is as yet unresolved for the bereaved individual. External expressions can include hallucinations and other exaggerated manifestations of grief. Such experiences are more closely associated with traumatic losses for which survivors blame themselves (Field & Filanosky, 2010), as is occasionally the case with perinatal death when an expectant mother questions her role in a pregnancy loss. Importantly, externalized expressions of continuing bonds were more closely associated with complicated grief reactions (Field & Filanosky, 2010). There is, however, a fine line drawn in the literature between adaptive and maladaptive forms of continuing bonds. Researchers caution against the overinterpretation of findings and emphasize that expressions of continuing bonds occur on a spectrum, illustrating ways of coping with loss (Boelen, Stroebe, Schut, & Zijerveld, 2006). While maladjustment to loss should be identified as early as possible, some forms of coping such as cherishing items associated with the deceased have been associated with adaptive grief responses (Boelen et al., 2006).

Research on Continuing Bonds in Bereaved Mothers

Twenty-eight bereaved mothers participated in a study of external and internal expressions of continuing bonds (Field et al., 2013). Researchers studied the effects of continuing bonds in affect regulation—whether continuing bonds experiences were comforting to the bereaved mothers or caused them distress. The study is especially relevant to the understanding of continuing bonds as a framework because 15 were mothers of older children (pediatric) and 13 experienced perinatal death: interruption of pregnancy for medical reasons, stillbirth, and newborn death (i.e., within the first 28 days of life). The time since their child's death ranged from 1 month to 4.8 years (Field et al., 2013).

Mothers' narratives demonstrated whether a continuing bonds expression they endorsed was associated with comfort or distress (Field et al., 2013). Significantly more mothers of older children (rather than death in the perinatal period) reported imaginary conversations with their children. Illusions of mistaking sights and sounds for the deceased or hallucinations (e.g., sense of presence through seeing, hearing, smelling, feeling) were endorsed as comforting by some mothers, yet intrusive by others. Otherwise, continuing bonds expression was equally prominent in both groups, suggesting emotion regulation after the death of a child at any age is associated with ongoing connection. Overall, mothers rated continuing bonds experiences as more comforting than distressing, with no significant difference between the early death group (perinatal) and the later (pediatric) (Field et al., 2013).

The Empty Space Phenomenon (McClowry, Davies, May, Kulenkamp, & Martinson, 1987), a concept developed through grounded theory research, provided one of the earliest examples of what is now called *continuing bonds*. The researchers used grounded theory methodology to analyze interview data from members of 49 families whose child or sibling died 7 to 9 years previously. Most family members spoke of an ever-present emptiness resulting from the child being physically absent from the family. The empty space was primarily described in two ways: "filling the emptiness" (p. 365) and "keeping the connection" (p. 367). Those who spoke of "getting over it" (p. 365) did not have an intense grief response; rather, their memories were less vivid and the experience of the child's death less present than those in the two "emptiness" categories. Family members filled the empty space by keeping busy. At times, keeping busy meant filling the space with other tasks or relationships that required energy, in essence, refocusing away from the child's death and toward other events or situations. The researchers cited building a new house, adopting a child, and developing marital distress as examples. The second way family members filled the emptiness was through altruism such as becoming active in bereaved parent groups. Interestingly, most who filled the emptiness with altruism reported a shift in focus at some point, a "need to go beyond where they were as if the emptiness was for the most part filled" (McClowry et al., 1987, p. 366).

The researchers (McClowry et al., 1987) described those who kept the connection as never forgetting, but at the same time, being able to continue the connection with the child who died by remembering and cherishing the relationship. The grief of family members lessened in intensity because they were able to integrate the pain and suffering into their lives in the present. They reserved "a small part of themselves for the loss of a special relationship which they view as irreplaceable" (p. 368). The idea of keeping the connection fits well with the current understanding of continuing bonds.

POSTTRAUMATIC GROWTH IN RESPONSE TO LOSS

Reconstituting a life without the deceased loved one is certainly the most daunting aspect of loss; yet in the midst of profound loss and bereavement, personal growth can occur. Posttraumatic growth (PTG) has been identified, described, and measured most thoroughly by Tedeschi and Calhoun (1996, 2004, 2008). PTG as a result of bereavement has been identified through empiric inquiry in several populations (Schoulte et al., 2012), including bereaved siblings (Hogan & DeSantis, 1992), perinatally bereaved families (Black & Wright, 2012), and bereaved spouses (Hogan, Greenfield, & Schmidt, 2001; Kaunonen, Tarkka, Paunonen, & Laippala, 1999). Several studies have demonstrated that PTG involves tendencies to feel more compassionate, more loving, more tolerant, and more grateful than before a loss (Black & Sandelowski, 2010; Black & Wright, 2012; Hogan, Greenfield, & Schmidt, 2001; Wright, 2010). Early conceptualizations of growth after loss described positive and negative aspects of grief as somewhat dichotomous. For example, Hogan, Greenfield, and Schmidt (2001) found that as the most intense negative aspects of grief passed, aspects of personal growth became more prominent. Yet, following pregnancy loss, aspects of PTG surface even as negative responses to loss persist (Black & Wright, 2012; Schoulte et al., 2012). Authors of a review of studies of PTG after a serious pediatric illness called the area "understudied and inadequately understood" (Picoraro, Womer, Kazak, & Feudtner, 2014, p. 209).

Thus, while PTG indicates awareness of positive aspects of loss, it should not be viewed necessarily as a turning point in the grief process after which negative aspects cease. Rather, personal growth has become recognized as an integral part of myriad responses to the multidimensional process of perinatal loss. Further research is needed to determine triggers for personal growth and factors that inhibit movement toward positive grief outcomes. Personal growth after pregnancy loss is discussed as a component of the Pushing On theory in Chapter 5.

Caring Theory: From Work With Perinatally Bereaved Couples

Caring is a concept central to nursing and other practice disciplines. Swanson developed her theory of caring from three different phenomenological studies of women who experienced miscarriage, neonatal intensive care caregivers, and at-risk mothers. The theory involves five processes that are useful in clinical practice. The first process—knowing— involves the ability to perceive "an event as it has meaning in the life of the other" (Swanson, 1991, p. 163), in which health care providers strive to understand the event through the eyes of the bereaved. The second process identified is "being with" (p. 163), described by Swanson as "being emotionally present to the other" (p. 163). Health care providers who convey a sense of understanding and are emotionally present to their patients provide comfort at a time when families may feel isolated and misunderstood.

The third and fourth processes of Swanson's caring theory entail "doing for" (p. 164), wherein the health care provider does for the patient what the patient would otherwise do but cannot because of physical or emotional distress, and "enabling" (p. 164), which involves efforts to encourage others through difficult life events. Doing for and then enabling self-care is integral in demonstrating professional caring.

The last process in Swanson's theory is "maintaining belief" (p. 165), which involves "sustaining faith in the others' capacity to get through an event or transition and face a future with meaning" (p. 165). In this process, providers determine patients' goals and help them sustain the belief that their goals are achievable despite dire circumstances and may involve support to believe that despite a loss, the future can still hold joy and meaning.

Although Swanson's theory was derived in part from her research with women who had miscarried, caring theory is broadly applicable. Adoption of this theoretical stance in bereavement care provides a framework for conveying genuine human caring within professional boundaries and clarifies roles and expectations of providers when facing the heartbreak of bereaved parents and families.

Williams's Transition Model

An important function of caring as described by Swanson is to determine meaning of losses. In a study of eight women who had an early miscarriage and their 16 health care providers, Murphy and Merrell (2009) found that the emotional response to miscarriage varies (see Chapter 18). Using interviews, review of key documents, and participant observation, the researchers proposed that grief theory may be suitable for describing many women's miscarriage experiences, but not all. For example, one health care professional stated, "Check how they're feeling really. Not everyone is going to be upset after miscarriage" (p. 1587). The researchers suggested that a *transitions model* may also be a relevant framework for understanding women's responses to miscarriage, supporting miscarriage as a significant life event and transition (Murphy & Merrell, 2009). Williams's (1999) transition model is particularly useful and relevant to miscarriage as one assumption is that life events may be perceived as positive or negative. Additionally, the researchers assert that strong emotions such as anxiety, uncertainty, and fear may be associated with the meaning of the event, without the emotions of grief. They remind care providers to offer sensitive, responsive care to all women experiencing miscarriage, staying alert and mindful of each individual woman's symptoms and behaviors (Murphy & Merrell, 2009).

CONCEPTS RELATED TO BEREAVEMENT THEORIES

Theories are fundamentally the organization of concepts (ideas) into a cohesive framework meant to predict outcomes and wholly explain phenomena.

Theories can be difficult to grasp, particularly highly abstract frameworks in which their links to practice may seem obscure. Concepts, however, are often more easily apprehensible and can be used to understand certain dimensions of phenomena. In the following section, we demonstrate how two concepts central to grief studies—*being sure* and *final acts of caregiving*—can help explain certain aspects of the experience of pregnancy loss.

Being Sure

Researchers interviewed 23 women who were diagnosed with an inevitable miscarriage (Limbo, Glasser, & Sundaram, 2014). With three treatment choices (surgical intervention, medical intervention, or watch and wait), women identified that they needed to be sure that their pregnancy was not viable. Most women characterized their pregnancy as a baby; several spoke of tissue or, in one case, "It's for sure there is no life amongst this pregnancy matter" (p. 168). We believe that being sure may be a relevant concept in other decision-making opportunities, one which professionals could engage patients and family members in discussing to determine what decision may best fit their values, goals, and beliefs.

Final Acts of Caregiving

In a study of mothers receiving perinatal hospice care, Limbo and Lathrop (2014) used caregiving theory (Bowlby, 1988) as a framework for analysis of narratives of mothers whose babies were diagnosed prenatally with a life-threatening condition and subsequently died. In addition to nurturing, protecting, and socializing their babies (see Chapter 3, this text; Limbo & Pridham, 2007), the mothers provided numerous examples of the importance of the final tasks of parenting they were able to provide their babies. This frequently meant care given after death, such as choosing just the right flowers for the funeral, bathing the baby, and placing the baby into the casket (Limbo & Lathrop, 2014). Again, we believe that final acts of caregiving may be relevant to all families who are bidding a final farewell to a loved one, whether that be placing a special keepsake in the casket, asking grandchildren to write a special letter, or a sibling to read a book. One woman, who had elected to stop dialysis and prepare for her death, told her daughters she wanted to wear her golden slippers as she passed on to the other side. One of her daughters sensed that death was near, retrieved the slippers from the windowsill, and as she placed them on her mother's feet, her mother took her last breath. The memory of this final act of caregiving (in this case, child to parent) is a lasting memory to the woman's family.

CONCLUSION

This chapter has provided you with foundational information about cultural considerations, theories, and concepts germane to grief and bereavement. Providers in perinatal and pediatric settings may encounter death infrequently and, as a result, often feel inadequately prepared to take care of children, their parents, and families when death occurs. From this chapter, you have a basic understanding of the conceptual development of grief and how it does its healing work from a theoretical perspective. The following chapters expand on current grief theories and research and provide specific clinical interventions.

Although clinicians and researchers today are working to formalize identification of concepts related to bereavement, the universality of profound distress related to the death of children is nothing new. Rückert's poem of his absent children, lost to death, is immortalized by Mahler in the fourth cycle of the *Kindertotenlieder* (Songs on the Death of Children). His words, borne of tragedy, capture parental grief in an intimate and timeless way:

I often think: they have only just gone out,
and now they will be coming back home.
The day is fine, don't be dismayed,
They have just gone for a long walk.
Yes indeed, they have just gone out,
and now they are making their way home.
Don't be dismayed, the day is fine,
they have simply made a journey to yonder heights.
They have just gone out ahead of us,
and will not be thinking of coming home.
We go to meet them on yonder heights
In the sunlight, the day is fine
On yonder heights.

REFERENCES

Barrere, C. C., Durkin, A., & LaCoursiere, S. (2008). The influence of end-of-life education on attitudes of nursing students. *The International Journal of Nursing Education Scholarship, 5*, 1–18.

Black, B., & Sandelowski, M. (2010). Personal growth after severe fetal diagnosis. *Western Journal of Nursing Research, 32*, 1011–1030.

Black, B., & Wright, P. M. (2012). Posttraumatic growth and transformation as outcomes of perinatal loss. *Illness, Crisis, & Loss, 20*(3), 225–237. Retrieved from http://www.baywood.com/journals/previewjournals.asp?id=1054-1373

Boelen, P. A., Stroebe, M. S., Schut, H. A., & Zijerveld, A. M. (2006). Continuing bonds and grief: A prospective analysis. *Death Studies, 30,* 767–776.

Bowlby, J. (1969/1982). *Attachment and loss: Attachment* (Vol. I). New York, NY: Basic Books.

Bowlby, J. (1988). *A secure base: Parent–child attachment and healthy human development.* New York, NY: Basic Books.

Case, A. A., Orrange, S. M., & Weissman, D. E. (2013). Palliative medicine physician education in the United States: A historical review. *Journal of Palliative Medicine, 16*(3), 230–235.

Corless, I. B., Limbo, R., Szylit Bousso, R., Wrenn, R. L., Head, D., Lickiss, N., & Wass, H. (2014). Languages of grief: A model for understanding the expressions of the bereaved. *Health Psychology and Behavioral Medicine: An Open Access Journal, 2*(1), 132–143.

Davidson, G. W. (1984). *Understanding mourning: A guide for those who grieve.* Minneapolis, MN: Augsburg Press.

Field, N., & Filanosky, C. (2010). Continuing bonds, risk factors for complicated grief and adjustment to bereavement. *Death Studies, 34,* 1–29.

Field, N. P., Packman, W., Ronen, R., Pries, A., Davies, B., & Kramer, R. (2013). Types of continuing bonds expression and its comforting versus distressing nature: Implications for adjustment among bereaved mothers. *Death Studies, 37,* 889–912.

Freud, S. (1957). Mourning and melancholia. In J. Strachey (Ed.), *The standard edition of the complete psychological works of Sigmund Freud* (Vol. 14, pp. 237–260). London, England: Hogarth Press and Institute for Psychoanalysis. (Original work published in 1917.)

Granek, L. (2010). Grief as pathology: The evolution of grief theory in psychology from Freud to the present. *History of Psychology, 13*(1), 46–73.

Hogan, N. S., & DeSantis, L. (1992). Adolescent sibling bereavement: An ongoing attachment. *Qualitative Health Research, 2*(2), 159–177.

Hogan, N. S., Greenfield, D. B., & Schmidt, L. A. (2001). Development and validation of the Hogan grief reaction checklist. *Death Studies, 25,* 1–32.

Holman, E. A., Perisho, J., Edwards, A., & Mlakar, N. (2010). The myths of coping with loss in undergraduate psychiatric nursing books. *Research in Nursing & Health, 33,* 486–499.

Irish, D. P., Lundquist, K. F., & Nelsen, V. J. (1993). *Ethnic variations in dying, death, and grief: Diversity and universality.* New York, NY: Routledge.

Kaunonen, M., Tarkka, M. T., Paunonen, M., & Laippala, P. (1999). Grief and social support after the death of a spouse. *Journal of Advanced Nursing, 30*(6), 1304–1311.

Limbo, R., & Lathrop, A. (2014). Caregiving in the mothers' narratives of perinatal hospice. *Illness, Crisis, & Loss, 22*(1), 43–65.

Limbo, R., & Pridham, K. (2007). Mothers' understanding of their infants in the context of an internal working model of caregiving. *Advances in Nursing Science, 30*(2), 139–150.

Limbo, R., Glasser, J. K., & Sundaram, M. E. (2014). Being sure: Women's experience with inevitable miscarriage. *MCN, The American Journal of Maternal/Child Nursing, 39*(3), 165–174.

Lindemann, E. (1994). Symptomatology and management of grief [Special section]. *American Journal of Psychiatry, 151*(6), 155–160. Retrieved from http://ajp.psychia-tryonline.org. (Original work published in 1944.)

McClowry, S. G., Davies, B., May, K. A., Kulenkamp, E. J., & Martinson, I. M. (1987). The empty space phenomenon: The process of grief in the bereaved family. *Death Studies, 11*, 361–374.

Murphy, F., & Merrell, J. (2009). Negotiating the transition: Caring for women through the experience of early miscarriage. *Journal of Clinical Nursing, 18*(11), 1583–1591.

Picoraro, J. A., Womer, J. W., Kazak, A. E., & Feudtner, C. (2014). Posttraumatic growth in parents and pediatric patients. *Journal of Palliative Medicine, 17*(2), 209–218.

Schoulte, J., Sussman, Z., Tallman, B., Deb, M., Cornick, C., & Altmaier, E. (2012). Is there growth in grief: Measuring posttraumatic growth in the grief response. *Open Journal of Medical Psychology, 1*, 38–43.

Silverman, P. R. & Klass, D. (1996) Introduction: What is the problem? In D. Klass, P. R. Silvermanm, & S. L. Nickman (Eds.), *Continuing bonds: New understandings of grief* (pp. 3–30). New York, NY: Routledge.

Swanson, K. M. (1991). Empirical development of a middle range theory of caring. *Nursing Research, 40*(3). 161–166. Retrieved from: http://journals.lww.com/nursingresearchonline/pages/default.aspx

Tedeschi, R. G., & Calhoun, L. G. (1996). The posttraumatic growth inventory: Measuring the positive legacy of trauma. *Journal of Traumatic Stress, 9*, 455–471.

Tedeschi, R. G., & Calhoun, L. G. (2004). Posttraumatic growth: Conceptual foundations and empirical evidence. *Psychological Inquiry, 15*, 1–18.

Tedeschi, R. G., & Calhoun, L. G. (2008). Beyond the concept of recovery: Growth and the experience of loss. *Death Studies, 32*, 27–39.

Wilke, J., & Limbo, R. (2012). *Resolve Through Sharing® bereavement training manual: Perinatal death* (8th ed). La Crosse, WI: Gundersen Lutheran Medical Foundation, Inc.

Williams, D. (1999). Human response to change. *Futures, 31*, 609–616.

Worden, J. W. (2009). *Grief counseling and grief therapy: A handbook for the mental health practitioner.* (4th ed). New York, NY: Springer Publishing Company.

Wright, P. M. (2010). *Pushing On: A grounded theory study of maternal perinatal bereavement* (Doctoral dissertation). Retrieved from ProQuest Dissertations and Theses. (AAT 3404182)

Wright, P. M., & Hogan, N. S. (2008). Grief theories and models: Applications to hospice nursing practice. *Journal of Hospice & Palliative Nursing, 10*(6), 350–356.

CHAPTER 2

Applying Theoretical Frameworks to Research in Perinatal Bereavement

Sarah Kye Price and Dalia El-Khoury

*P*erinatal bereavement researchers, and practitioners who utilize research to guide their practice, should be fully aware of the theoretical frameworks that underscore existing and future research studies. In this chapter, we review a range of theoretical frameworks and approaches that have been applied to research in perinatal bereavement, including attachment theory, psychodynamic theory, interpersonal theory, cognitive stress theory, feminist theory, and the emerging perspectives of strengths-based and trauma-informed approaches to research and practice. In this chapter, we present each theory or approach and discuss its applicability to various research methods (quantitative, qualitative, and/or mixed methods) and how it informs research design, selection of measures, framing of questions, analysis, and implications. At the conclusion of the chapter, the reader should be able to describe the implicit and explicit benefits and challenges of research conducted by applying various theoretical frameworks, and to critically evaluate and/or design research studies that meaningfully inform knowledge of perinatal loss and bereavement.

ATTACHMENT THEORY

Attachment theory (Bowlby, 1980) emphasizes the interrelationships between attachment, affectional bonds, separation, and loss in human relationships. Historically, attachment theory has most often studied the relationship between mother and child (Bowlby, 1977). However, attachment theory is applicable across multiple relationship contexts, such as those among spouses and intimate partners, between parents, and with children (Bowlby, 1977). Attachment theory posits four archetypal attachment styles: secure, avoidant, anxious/ambivalent, and disorganized/disoriented; the latter three collectively may be described as insecure attachment (Bowlby,

1980). Attachment theory can provide a framework for understanding the patterns people elicit when experiencing both grief and bereavement, and how these extend from the pre-existing relational bonds (Stroebe, Schut, & Stroebe, 2005). People exhibiting different attachment patterns or styles have been identified as handling emotions related to loss differently (Fraley & Bonanno, 2004; Parkes, 2001; Shaver & Tancredy, 2001; Wayment & Vierthaler, 2002). Since attachments form differently throughout life, individuals may enlist generalized attachment styles that guide expectations of potential relationships, and also develop specific models of attachment that are unique to each attachment figure (Shear & Shair, 2005).

Understanding Loss and Grief as a Function of Attachment

Broadly speaking, attachment theory is a way to understand how individuals react to loss and grief, whether that is loss due to death, separation, or distance. When a loss is experienced, the individual is theorized to react in a specific manner (based on his or her own attachment style) in order to ameliorate the intensity and pain of that loss, and in order to try to recover a sense of proximity to the attachment figure. When the loss is due to death, the recovery of attachment may prove more challenging, resulting in emotional disequilibrium (Stroebe & Schut, 2001). This attachment-based disequilibrium offers one lens for understanding the internal processes that take place during both normal and complicated grief.

Expanding Bowlby's (1977, 1980) initial conception of attachment theory to perinatal loss, attachment may begin during pregnancy, reflecting a bond between mother and fetus. Therefore, if a pregnancy ends before those bonds of affection are fully actualized, the result can be intense longing and disequilibrium from having to "let go" before full and complete attachment could occur. Medical advances, including certain prenatal diagnostic procedures that allow parents to monitor fetal development, contribute to the growing attachment between mother and fetus (Robinson, Baker, & Nackerud, 1999). Research indicates that attachment can begin as early as the planning and learning of the pregnancy, and is often heightened when fetal movement is felt, which is hypothesized to be related to the mother's ability to conceptualize the infant (Robinson et al., 1999). While prenatal attachment is associated with this awareness of gestational and relational development, the degree of prenatal attachment (and subsequent grieving and bereavement if a loss occurs) cannot be ascertained by gestational age alone (Moulder, 1994; Robinson et al., 1999). Prenatal attachment, just like adult attachment, is highly dependent on life context.

Attachment theory may be applied in research to understand the impact of perinatal loss on the parent's grief, as well as on subsequent pregnancies and parenting. Uren and Wastell (2002) found that mothers who have experienced a perinatal loss continue to have an emotional relationship with the deceased baby; this parallels research conducted on the development of continuing bonds (Stroebe, Schut, & Boerner, 2010). Grief and meaning making with respect for a baby who has died are essential in order to develop a healthy attachment to a future baby (O'Leary, 2004). Research asserts that prior perinatal loss has been associated with higher levels of anxiety with ensuing pregnancies (Côté-Arsenault & Donato, 2007), decreased prenatal attachment to the current baby (Armstrong & Hutti, 1998), and higher levels of depressive symptoms (Armstrong, 2002). Additionally, the unresolved grief parents may exhibit has been shown to predict the development of disorganized attachment patterns in their subsequent children (O'Leary, 2004).

Measures in Attachment and Grief Research

Attachment theory informs much of the research design and measurement instrumentation in studies pertaining to subsequent pregnancy after perinatal loss. There is an inherent assumption in attachment theory that some degree of disequilibrium is normative in bereavement, and that greater emotional stability should begin to take shape over time if one is attentive to the energy it takes to work through a state of grief-induced disequilibrium and emerge into a "new normal" as a result of the grief process. Attachment theory posits that grief resolution is not simply better for the individual griever, but for those who will continue or develop new relationships following the grief event. Therefore, measurement of grief symptoms and impact may need to be longitudinal, or at a minimum, research designs may consider including the length of time since the grief occurred as a part of research models. Research related to subsequent pregnancy in particular often relies on measurement of grief and attachment response in the parent and subsequent child, in order to consider the impact of grieving (and resolution of the intensity of grief) on the development of attachment patterns over time. Applications of attachment theory also seek to identify long-term, generational patterns that exemplify adaptive or complicated bereavement patterns that may impact the family system over time.

In quantitative research solely involving the griever, attachment theory suggests that it is important to consider the differential severity of symptoms present in the time since loss occurred as a part of the analytic plan, and to include variables such as the degree to which parents perceive themselves to have played out roles that may foster attachment (i.e., holding, seeing, bathing, caring for the infant including postmortem care) as adaptive to moving through the disequilibrium of grief. These variables, measured appropriately, reflect an understanding of the intersecting roles that attachment, separation, and loss may play in grief response. Expanding questions in research protocols that include items reflecting parental perceptions of choice in their level of tactile involvement in perinatal end-of-life care will allow for a rich research design that integrates an understanding of the dynamics of the grief process rather than merely the observed outcome or symptoms devoid of the attachment context.

In terms of analysis and interpretation of findings, attachment theory may also help explain why the intensity of emotional expression (or symptoms of grief) during and after a subsequent pregnancy may be heightened. Specifically, attachment theory would suggest that disequilibrium may lessen over time when these affective bonds are able to be adequately expressed at the time of loss. This theoretical underpinning may be important to interpretation of findings and implications for client-centered companioning and choice making throughout the grief process.

PSYCHODYNAMIC THEORY

Psychodynamic (or psychoanalytic) theory, particularly advanced by the work of Freud's "Mourning and Melancholia" (1917/1957), provides an introspective perspective on the process of coping with any loss in an adaptive manner. Freud argued that grief following loss serves a functional purpose in that it allows the individual to detach from the deceased (Stroebe & Schut, 2001). Psychodynamic theories of bereavement conceptualize that the duration and intensity of the grieving process force a psychological restructuring of self. This model indicates that relief will follow as a result of detachment that ensues from the adaptive process of grieving (Shapiro, 2001). In addition, objects relations theory, a subset of psychodynamic theory, conceptualizes one's life as an amalgamation of internalized representations of actual relationships with childhood caretakers (Shapiro, 2001). As a result of a loss, an intrapsychic reorganization takes place in which one's internal object universe is changed.

Psychodynamic Frameworks

Psychodynamic theory posits that intrapsychic meanings attributed to pregnancy, parenting, and death impact the resolution of the grieving process and the ensuing restructuring of one's inner self. Leon (1992) presents four psychodynamic frameworks within which to understand pregnancy, and the personal meaning behind pregnancy as well as perinatal and reproductive loss: developmental, conflictual, object-oriented, and narcissistic frameworks (Leon, 1996). The developmental framework presents perinatal loss as interference within a normal developmental process of adulthood and parenthood. In the conflictual framework, perinatal loss may intensify intrapsychic conflicts, particularly related to the female drive to reproduce that may or may not be realized. The object-oriented framework focuses on the importance of the detachment process of grief following a perinatal loss as essential to a reconceptualization of self. The narcissistic framework presupposes that perinatal loss may result in feelings of narcissistic injury and rage, as the unborn child is seen as an extension of the mother and is therefore tied to her sense of self and self-esteem (Leon, 1992). Perinatal loss may also impact the feeling of immortality and omnipotence associated with continuing a biological or genetic line (Leon, 1996). Upon experiencing a perinatal loss, individuals may react with guilt and self-blame, which may be associated with feelings of helplessness and lack of control over one's own body (Leon, 1996).

Psychodynamic theory may be an important consideration in research that emphasizes the meaning, personal significance, and intrapsychic conflicts of perinatal loss. In both qualitative and quantitative methods, the exploration of personal meaning associated with grief following perinatal bereavement may mirror, or challenge, the lens offered through psychodynamic theory. Research designs that integrate a psychodynamic perspective are often individualized, and frame research questions and exploratory dialogue on the way in which the experience of loss impacts identity, self-worth, and/or conflicts within the person's self-conceptualization. Psychodynamic theory also provides theoretical foundations for interventions such as interpersonal psychotherapy (IPT) that have been applied to perinatal bereavement. In keeping with this theoretical perspective, process and outcome measures used in intervention research using a psychodynamic framework should focus on the individual changes in meaning associated with the loss, as well as resolution of both internal and interpersonal conflicts that may have emerged as a result of the grief process.

INTERPERSONAL THEORY

Interpersonal theory offers a lens to understand the impact prolonged depression (or events that contribute to similar symptomatology) can have on interpersonal relationships, as well as social relations in general (Weissman, Markowitz, & Klerman, 2000). In practice, interpersonal theory (as IPT) advocates for individual change, rather than the mere development of insight. It focuses on addressing the experience of symptoms, as well as social adjustment and interpersonal relations. IPT utilizes time limited and focused treatments that concentrate on current interpersonal relationships (Weissman et al., 2000). Interpersonal theory can be applied to the process of grief (or complicated bereavement), particularly accompanying difficulties associated with the mourning process following the death of a loved one, resulting in experiences of depression (Weissman et al., 2000). The goals of IPT in this situation are to assist the individual through the mourning process, as well as re-establish interpersonal relationships and interests that can begin to take the place of the loss (Weissman et al., 2000). Interpersonal relationships provide a link between one's individual grief experience and bereavement outcomes (Shapiro, 2001). Interventions utilizing the interpersonal theory base of IPT have been shown to be effective in the treatment of postpartum depression (Pearlstein et al., 2006), major depression (Johnson & Zlotnick, 2012), as well as bereavement and mild depression following miscarriage (Neugebauer et al., 2007).

Interpersonal Dynamics of Grief

The interpersonal dynamics of grief impact the parent–child as well as partner and social system dynamics of perinatal bereavement. Interpersonal theory is often combined with psychodynamic and attachment theories as it takes shape in practice. The ensuant perspective takes into account the importance of attachment, and focuses on the resolution of loss through enhancing the interpersonal dynamic surrounding grief. Interpersonal theory views personality as an amalgamation of patterns representing interpersonal relationships, and argues that healthy attachments can serve an adaptive purpose. Interventions utilizing both an interpersonal and psychodynamic perspective assume that the death of a loved one disrupts the unique individual strategies used to self-define interpersonally and to retain control over emotions (Shapiro, 2001). In reproductive loss, as well as the personal, marital, and social stress associated with infertility, the intensity of the grief response may be ameliorated by perceptions of interpersonal and social support (Martins et al., 2013).

Gender Differences in Grief

The grieving process may also reflect gender differences, particularly related to communication styles, incongruent coping strategies, and a propagation of misunderstandings (Wing, Clance, Burge-Callaway, & Armistead, 2001). The experience of men coping with perinatal and reproductive loss is particularly important to consider when applying interpersonal theory, in part because men may play an integral role in the provision of interpersonal and social support (Rinehart & Kiselica, 2010). Men also go through the grieving process following a perinatal or reproductive loss, although the intensity and duration of their grief may differ from that of women (Abboud & Liamputtong, 2003; Rinehart & Kiselica, 2010). Gender-based incongruence, real or perceived, can be challenging to the interpersonal dynamic that implicitly exists within a couple or family.

Sampling and Intervention in Research

In designing perinatal loss research, interpersonal theory may inform the choice of intervention, as well as influence sampling. Most importantly, to fully understand the interpersonal impact of grief and loss requires data gathering from all those who interact with each other in the interpersonal context. Measuring relationship quality and stressors or comparing differential grief expression and responses in a partner dyad requires sampling that includes accessibility to both partners, and therefore requires heightened attention to research ethics, confidentiality, and informed consent both in the conduct of research and in the dissemination of results. This lens of interpersonal theory offers an important manifestation of our value of human relationships and acknowledges that our ability to fully understand and appreciate the impact of grief requires a theoretical and empirical acknowledgement of its relational impact.

COGNITIVE STRESS THEORY

Cognitive stress theory (Lazarus & Folkman, 1984) asserts that any stress-inducing situation warrants a need for cognitive processing and restructuring. Individuals utilize "cognitive schemas" to help make sense of the world, particularly in situations eliciting stress, discomfort, or pain. These schemas guide thoughts, beliefs, and assumptions about the origin and outlook of particular events, and may be either adaptive or maladaptive. Some common schemas we carry, such as "good things happen to good people" or "pregnancy is a time of joyful expectation," can become deeply challenged by perinatal loss. The primary role of cognitive adaptation to a stressful event or situation is a hallmark of this theoretical orientation.

Three Types of Human Responses to Stress

Lazarus (2000) identified three types of human responses to stress: one's appraisal of said event; one's choice of responses (coping strategies); and the ensuing emotions. Coping strategies are cognitive or behavioral responses intended to assist one's external and internal adaptation to a stressful event. The coping strategies chosen, if effective, are hypothesized to be used consistently over time (Lazarus & Folkman, 1984). When applied to bereavement, this theory is predicated on the assumption that coping makes a difference in adjustment and recovery from loss (Folkman, 2001). In addition, Folkman (2001) proposed the inclusion of the personality trait of positive affect to the coping process, particularly related to personal growth within the bereavement experience.

Dual Stresses of Pregnancy and Loss During Pregnancy

The biological and psychological experience of pregnancy is generally considered to be stressful, and a loss within that time period can be perceived as a stress within a stress (Price, 2008). Regarding perinatal and reproductive loss, cognitive stress theory argues that this loss must be processed, a new role must be identified and adapted to (for example, from "expectant" to "grieving"), and the future impact of this loss must be examined for its continuing and changed life expectations (Price, 2008). For example, women experiencing pregnancy after a perinatal loss may view that entire pregnancy as threatening, stressful, and anxiety-inducing (Côté-Arsenault, 2003, 2007), which likely differs from the experience of mothers who have not experienced a perinatal loss.

An individual's response to loss may be polarized: at the same time profoundly sad, but perhaps relieved, which may then be followed by guilt. Additionally, infertility-related stress can be ameliorated through the presence of social support, as well as the use of successful coping strategies (Martins, Peterson, Almeida, & Costa, 2011). One's cognitive schema will guide the way in which he or she processes through a perinatal or reproductive loss. Being able to authentically identify and confront one's thoughts is a key element of this theory, even if those thoughts and beliefs are at times disturbing or differ from one's perception of the norm.

Instrumentation in Perinatal Bereavement Research

In designing perinatal bereavement research, cognitive stress theory guides the selection of instrumentation as well as the inclusion of items and descriptions that are cognitive in nature in addition to typical emotional components of grief response. For example, including stress appraisal measures, coping inventories, and questionnaires that suggest patterns of thought and reflect cognitive schemas may assess coping style in addition to emotional symptomatology of grief. Stress and coping may be measured in cross-sectional as well as longitudinal studies; this offers flexibility in research design. Finally, the integration of cognitive stress measures can occur simultaneously with other relational and emotional measures. Introducing cognitive components into research design and measurement may allow for richer comparisons and theory testing regarding the interface of cognitive, emotional, and relational aspects of grief related to perinatal and pediatric bereavement.

FEMINIST THEORY

Feminist theory is reflective of the diversity of women's perspectives and experiences, and takes into account issues that affect women in a unique manner, including pregnancy and reproductive loss. An inherent assumption within feminist frameworks is that women have historically been suppressed and served in subordinate roles, and that this is no longer acceptable (Valentich, 2011). Feminist theory encompasses a commitment to social justice issues, social change and activism, gender equality, multicultural perspectives, diversity issues, and culturally competent practice (Valentich, 2011). The role of feminist practice is to free women from oppression that has been propagated through societal norms, role expectations, and mores. Feminist theory accounts for and undergirds the complexity and diversity of factors that have an impact on the functioning of women all over the world.

Constructions of Meanings of Perinatal and Reproductive Loss

Perinatal and reproductive loss is an experience that impacts women in a unique manner. Historically, social norms perpetuated silence around experiences of miscarriage and loss, which contributed to a sense of secrecy and shame (Price, 2008). However, in the past few decades, it has become more acceptable for women to speak out about their grief and emotions following experiences of perinatal loss (Reagan, 2003). Women's experiences of perinatal and reproductive loss are neither unique nor universal—they are socially, historically, and culturally constructed (Reagan, 2003). For example, the meaning that women ascribe to miscarriage will depend upon the era in which they live. An emphasis on the notion of "happy endings" related to pregnancy and motherhood renders a negative judgment or social taboo on those pregnancies that end in loss (Layne, 2003). When a pregnancy does not result in the "happy ending" society leads women to expect, the self-blame burgeons, particularly among women (Layne, 2003). Women have historically borne an unequal share of the burden associated with pregnancy loss, including medical risk, shifts in identity, placement of blame, and invalidation of the experience of loss (Layne, 2006). Additionally, within a woman's own lifetime, the meaning she ascribes to a perinatal or reproductive loss may shift. Currently, with feminist theories and frameworks calling for the voices of women to be heard, women have begun to break the silence around perinatal and reproductive loss. An example of the leadership role that women have begun to undertake is the pregnancy and infant loss support movement in the United States, which has been initiated, organized, and led by women (Layne, 2006).

Effects of Research Design on Women's Bereavement Experiences

In designing research around perinatal bereavement, it is important to realize that choices around design, instrumentation, language, and sample all have the potential to affect women's experiences of perinatal bereavement in both explicit and implicit ways. Research that fails to objectively measure capacity as well as challenges or that overlooks social stigma or norms that may impact a woman's sense of self may perpetuate negative stereotypes or reinforce a need for secrecy and silence. Research that attends to the variety of women's experiences using nonjudgmental language and gender attentive descriptors of people and events is the first step to integrating a feminist perspective into research design.

Additionally, attention to selection of instrumentation that has been appropriately applied to women in other studies, and has been validated based on women's grief experiences, avoids a common research pitfall of pathologizing emotional responses, which may be quite normative from a feminist standpoint. Additionally, the prospect of adding open-ended response items to elicit participant's view (which may be possible, even in quantitatively oriented studies) allows for greater participant voice and the possibility of raising an alternative experience or point of view. This, in turn, may widen the lens with which we come to know the range of response to perinatal and pediatric bereavement, furthering our awareness of lived experiences of all people who experience perinatal and pediatric bereavement.

EMERGING PERSPECTIVES: TRAUMA-INFORMED AND STRENGTHS-BASED APPROACHES TO RESEARCH

There are a number of emerging perspectives in recent literature, including several chapters of this text, that can inform approaches to research and practice with perinatal and reproductive loss. Most significantly, these include trauma-informed perspectives and strengths-based approaches to research and practice.

Trauma-Informed Perspective

A trauma-informed perspective endeavors to identify and explain patterns of responses to traumatic events such as the bereavement associated with a perinatal or reproductive loss (Stroebe & Schut, 2001). While the process of bereavement shares some commonalities with general traumas, there are singular differences as well, particularly in that bereavement models do not commonly include a confrontation–avoidance pattern of behavior that may be exhibited consequent to a general trauma (Stroebe & Schut, 2001). A trauma-informed perspective leads with the assumption that an individual has been impacted by a trauma, and the selection of questions, interventions, and exploratory research must attend to its potential to impact the trauma experience. This leads to heightened sensitivity regarding the ethical conduct of research, as well as to considering the potential therapeutic benefit of participation in research as a component of recovery.

The experience of miscarriage has been viewed as a traumatic event, which has implications for interventions aimed at easing emotional adjustment and providing appropriate long-term follow-up care to address any future negative responses that arise (Lee & Slade, 1996). In addition, some of the symptoms women experience following a miscarriage may be ascribed to the trauma. Individuals experiencing trauma tend to show a characteristic set of symptoms, including restlessness, irritability, fatigue, disturbance with sleep, heightened anxiety and startle responses, depression, difficulty concentrating, and denial of the event (Lee & Slade, 1996). Many of these symptoms are present for women who have experienced a perinatal or reproductive loss, strengthening the argument that this experience is in fact a traumatic experience, warranting the use of different interventions.

Strengths-Based Perspective

Given the experience of trauma associated with perinatal and reproductive loss, what characteristics differentiate those individuals who adapt and survive the traumatic experience from those who do not? It is important to note that not all traumas are experienced equally; as such, the nature and duration of the intensity of the reaction will differ, although similarities and patterns in symptom profiles exist (Norman, 2000). One of the factors that has been acknowledged in survival from trauma is personal strength (Norman, 2000).

Specific to the process of bereavement following perinatal loss, Lang, Goulet, Aita, Giguere, Lamarre, and Perreault (2001) argue that the personal characteristic of hardiness will allow individuals to survive, transcend, and grow as a result of the experience of perinatal loss. Hardiness is a personal resource that contributes to one's ability to remain proactive and retain a sense of control during the experience of a trauma, such as a perinatal or reproductive loss, as well as make sense of the experience (Lang et al., 2001). Hardiness implies more than just resilience; hardiness implies the individual grows beyond what he or she would previously have been capable of doing as a result of the experience. This perspective emphasizes the strengths inherent in the individual and the family, rather than focusing solely on the negative consequences or reactions to the perinatal or reproductive loss (Lang & Carr, 2013). Implications of strengths-based research for practice include a goal of fostering the personal characteristic of hardiness among those who have experienced a perinatal loss, concomitantly with reducing the psychosocial distress that so often accompanies bereavement (Lang & Carr, 2013). From a strengths-based framework, grief becomes an opportunity for growth.

Perinatal bereavement research has focused predominantly on the identification and reduction of negative symptoms associated with grief and its psychological sequelae. Inadvertently, this emphasizes the pathological aspects of grief and may even mean that those without a clinically significant level of "symptoms" are not included in research samples. A strengths-based approach could equally include items of personal growth, as well as psychosocial challenge and open research to those with a range of responses to perinatal bereavement. An analysis of secondary data recently suggested that women experiencing both perinatal loss and fertility barriers demonstrated personal growth with more similarity with each other than in the nonbereaved population (Price & McLeod, 2012).

The emotional, cognitive, and relational challenges accompanying the experience of perinatal and pediatric bereavement simultaneously create the opportunity for growth. Attention to inclusion of strengths in quantitative measurement and qualitative interviewing is essential to understanding the wider picture of how perinatal and pediatric bereavement impact the lives of individuals, families, and communities both as a challenge, and as an opportunity for growth.

CONCLUSION

This chapter covered a range of theoretical perspectives on perinatal and pediatric bereavement, and has offered information for the conduct and interpretation of research in the field. To summarize these perspectives, we have included in Table 2.1 the theories and perspectives reviewed with the key points related to research design. In order to advance knowledge of perinatal and pediatric bereavement, attention to the theories that inform research and practice is essential to sensemaking of the data that emerges and the way that data is applied to understanding the grief and growth experiences of individuals, families, and communities.

TABLE 2.1 A Summary of Theoretical Perspectives and Research Applications

THEORETICAL FRAMEWORK	RESEARCH DESIGN	SAMPLE	MEASUREMENT	IMPLICATIONS FOR PRACTICE
Attachment theory	Time series or longitudinal	Dyads	Individual and dyadic interaction	Current and generational relationships
Psychodynamic theory	Retrospective or historical	Individuals	Meaning-focused, internalized experience	Individual insight
Interpersonal theory	Retrospective and prospective	Couples, families, or other interpersonal units	Comparative, relational measures	Current and future interactions and relationships
Cognitive stress theory	Cross-sectional, prospective	Individuals	Cognitive appraisal, coping skills, schemas	Individual decision making, future coping skill development
Feminist theory	Cross-sectional or historical	Individuals, social representatives	Social norms, individual experience, open-ended	Person-centered practice; macro- to microchange
Strengths-based perspective	Retrospective and prospective	Individuals and/or families	Hardiness, strengths assessment, current challenges	Joint focus on alleviating distress and promoting personal growth

CASE STUDY

Mora is a 24-year-old patient who is 28 weeks pregnant. She is seeking care for vaginal bleeding that began a few hours ago. Her partner is present but states that he is not the father of the baby. Mora explains that she met her partner after she became pregnant but wishes he were the father of her baby. The provider advises Mora to be admitted to the hospital for care. Mora agrees, and her partner will drive her to the hospital. Her mother and sister will meet her there. Mora states that her mother is her "rock" and her sister is her "best friend."

FOCUS QUESTIONS

1. Describe the key concepts of each of the theories described in the chapter.
2. Which of the theories or concepts described in the chapter would be most applicable to the case study? Why?
3. Using one of the theoretical frameworks from the chapter, describe how care should be structured for Mora.
4. If you were designing a research study using one of the theories in the chapter, which one would you choose? Why?

REFERENCES

Abboud, L. N., & Liamputtong, P. (2003). Pregnancy loss. What it means to women who miscarry and their partners. *Social Work in Health Care, 36*(3), 37–62.

Armstrong, D. S. (2002). Emotional distress and prenatal attachment in pregnancy after perinatal loss. *Journal of Nursing Scholarship, 34*(4), 339–345. doi:10.1111/j.1547-5069.2002.00339.x

Armstrong, D., & Hutti, M. (1998). Pregnancy after perinatal loss: The relationship between anxiety and prenatal attachment. *Journal of Obstetric, Gynecologic, & Neonatal Nursing, 27*(2), 183–189. doi:10.1111/j.1552-6909.1998.tb02609.x

Bowlby, J. (1977). The making and breaking of affectional bonds: Etiology and psychopathology in the light of attachment theory. *The British Journal of Psychiatry, 130*, 201–210. doi:10.1192/bjp.130.3.201

Bowlby, J. (1980). *Attachment and loss, Vol. 3: Loss*. New York, NY: Basic Books.

Côté-Arsenault, D. (2003). The influence of perinatal loss on anxiety in multigravidas. *Journal of Obstetric, Gynecologic, & Neonatal Nursing, 32*(5), 623–629. doi:10.1177/0884217503257140

Côté-Arsenault, D. (2007). Threat appraisal, coping, and emotions across pregnancy subsequent to perinatal loss. *Nursing Research, 56*(2), 108–116.

Côté-Arsenault, D., & Donato, K. L. (2007). Restrained expectations in late pregnancy following loss. *JOGNN: Journal of Obstetric, Gynecologic & Neonatal Nursing, 36*(6), 550–557. doi:10.1111/j.1552-6909.2007.00185.x

Folkman, S. (2001). Revised coping theory and the process of bereavement. In M. S. Stroebe, R. O. Hansson, W. Stroebe, & H. Schut (Eds.), *Handbook of bereavement research* (pp. 563–584). Washington, DC: American Psychological Association. doi:10.1037/10436-024

Fraley, R. C., & Bonanno, A. (2004). Attachment and loss: A test of three competing models on the association between attachment-related avoidance and adaptation to bereavement. *Personality and Social Psychology Bulletin, 30*, 878–890.

Freud, S. (1957). Mourning and melancholia. In J. Strachey (Ed.), *The standard edition of the complete psychological works of Sigmund Freud* (Vol. 14, pp. 237–260). London, England: Hogarth Press and Institute for Psychoanalysis. (Original work published in 1917.)

Johnson, J. E., & Zlotnick, C. (2012). Pilot study of treatment for major depression among women prisoners with substance use disorder. *Journal of Psychiatric*

Research, 46(9), 1174–1183. doi: http://dx.doi.org.proxy.library.vcu.edu/10.1016/j.jpsychires.2012.05.007

Lang, A., & Carr, T. (2013). Bereavement in the face of perinatal loss: A hardiness perspective. In D. S. Becvar (Ed.), *Handbook of family resilience* (pp. 299–319). New York, NY: Springer Science + Business Media.

Lang, A., Goulet, C., Aita, M., Giguere, V., Lamarre, H., & Perreault, E. (2001). Weathering the storm of perinatal bereavement via hardiness. *Death Studies, 25,* 497–512.

Layne, L. L. (2003). Unhappy endings: A feminist reappraisal of the women's health movement from the vantage of pregnancy loss. *Social Science & Medicine, 56*(9), 1881–1891. doi:http://dx.doi.org.proxy.library.vcu.edu/10.1016/S0277-9536(02)00211-3

Layne, L. L. (2006). Pregnancy and infant loss support: A new, feminist, American, patient movement? *Social Science & Medicine, 62*(3), 602–613. doi:http://dx.doi.org.proxy.library.vcu.edu/10.1016/j.socscimed.2005.06.019

Lazarus, R. S. (2000). Evolution of a model of stress, coping, and discrete emotions. In V. H. Rice (Ed.), *Handbook of stress, coping, and health* (pp. 195–222). Thousand Oaks, CA: Sage.

Lazarus, R. S., & Folkman, S. (1984). *Stress, appraisal, and coping.* New York, NY: Springer.

Lee, C., & Slade, P. (1996). Miscarriage as a traumatic event: A review of the literature and new implications for intervention. *Journal of Psychosomatic Research, 40*(3), 235–244. doi: http://dx.doi.org.proxy.library.vcu.edu/10.1016/0022-3999(95)00579-X

Leon, I. G. (1992). The psychoanalytic conceptualization of perinatal loss: A multidimensional model. *The American Journal of Psychiatry, 149*(11), 1464–1472.

Leon, I. G. (1996). Revising psychoanalytic understandings of perinatal loss. *Psychoanalytic Psychology, 13*(2), 161–176.

Martins, M. V., Peterson, B. D., Almeida, V. M., & Costa, M. E. (2011). Direct and indirect effects of perceived social support on women's infertility-related stress. *Human Reproduction, 26*(8), 2113–2121.

Martins, M. V., Peterson, B. D., Costa, P., Costa, M. E., Lund, R., & Schmidt, L. (2013). Interactive effects of social support and disclosure on fertility-related stress. *Journal of Social and Personal Relationships, 30*(4), 371–388.

Moulder, C. (1994). Towards a preliminary framework for understanding pregnancy loss. *Journal of Reproductive and Infant Psychology, 12*(1), 65–67. doi:10.1080/02646839408408869

Neugebauer, R., Kline, J., Bleiberg, K., Baxi, L., Markowitz, J. C., Rosing, M., . . . & Keith, J. (2007). Preliminary open trial of interpersonal counseling for subsyndromal depression following miscarriage. *Depression and anxiety, 24*(3), 219–222.

Norman, J. (2000). Constructive narrative in arresting the impact of post-traumatic stress disorder. *Clinical Social Work Journal, 28*(3), 303–319. doi:10.1023/A:1005135802159

O'Leary, J. (2004). Grief and its impact on prenatal attachment in the subsequent pregnancy. *Archives of Women's Mental Health, 7*(1), 7–18. doi:10.1007/s00737-003-0037-1

Parkes, C. M. (2001). A historical overview of the scientific study of bereavement. In M. S. Stroebe, R. O. Hansson, W. Stroebe, & H. Schut (Eds.), *Handbook of bereavement research* (pp. 25–45). Washington, DC: American Psychological Association. doi:10.1037/10436-001

Pearlstein, T. B., Zlotnick, C., Battle, C. L., Stuart, S., O'Hara, M. W., Price, A. B., . . . Howard, M. (2006). Patient choice of treatment for postpartum depression: A pilot study. *Archives of Women's Mental Health, 9*(6), 303–308. doi:10.1007/s00737-006-0145-9

Price, S. K. (2008). Women and reproductive loss: Client-worker dialogues designed to break the silence. *Social Work, 53*(4), 367–376. doi:10.1093/sw/53.4.367

Price, S. K., & McLeod, D. A. (2012). Definitional distinctions in response to perinatal loss and fertility barriers. *Illness, Crisis, & Loss, 20* (3), 255–273.

Reagan, L. J. (2003). From hazard to blessing to tragedy: Representations of miscarriage in twentieth century America. *Feminist Studies, 29*(2), 356–378.

Rinehart, M. S., & Kiselica, M. S. (2010). Helping men with the trauma of miscarriage. *Psychotherapy: Theory, Research, Practice, Training, 47*(3), 288–295. doi:10.1037/a0021160

Robinson, M., Baker, L., & Nackerud, L. (1999). The relationship of attachment theory and perinatal loss. *Death Studies, 23*(3), 257–270.

Shapiro, E. R. (2001). Grief in interpersonal perspective: Theories and their implications. In M. S. Stroebe, R. O. Hansson, W. Stroebe, & H. Schut (Eds.), *Handbook of bereavement research* (pp. 301–327). Washington, DC: American Psychological Association. doi:10.1037/10436-013

Shaver, P. R., & Tancredy, C. M. (2001). Emotion, attachment, and bereavement: A conceptual commentary. In M. S. Stroebe, R. O. Hansson, W. Stroebe, & H. Schut (Eds.), *Handbook of bereavement research* (pp. 63–88). Washington, DC: American Psychological Association. doi:10.1037/10436-003

Shear, K., & Shair, H. (2005). Attachment, loss, and complicated grief. *Developmental Psychobiology, 47*(3), 253–267. doi:10.1002/dev.20091

Stroebe, M. S., & Schut, H. (2001). Models of coping with bereavement: A review. In M. S. Stroebe, R. O. Hansson, W. Stroebe, & H. Schut (Eds.), *Handbook of bereavement research* (pp. 375–403). Washington, DC: American Psychological Association. doi:10.1037/10436-016

Stroebe, M., Schut, H., & Boerner, K. (2010). Continuing bonds in adaptation to bereavement: Toward theoretical integration. *Clinical Psychology Review, 30*(2), 259–268. doi:http://dx.doi.org/10.1016/j.cpr.2009.11.007

Stroebe, M. S., Schut, H., & Stroebe, W. (2005). Attachment in coping with bereavement. *Review of General Psychology, 9*, 48–66.

Uren, T. H., & Wastell, C. A. (2002). Attachment and meaning-making in perinatal bereavement. *Death Studies, 26*(4), 279–308.

Valentich, M. (2011). Feminist theory and social work practice. In F. J. Turner (Ed.), *Social work treatment: Interlocking theoretical approaches* (4th ed., pp. 282–318). New York, NY: Oxford University Press.

Wayment, H. A., & Vierthaler, J. (2002). Attachment style and bereavement reactions. *Journal of Loss & Trauma, 7*(2), 129–149. doi:10.1080/153250202753472291

Weissman, M., Markowitz, J., & Klerman, G. (2000). *Comprehensive guide to interpersonal psychotherapy.* New York, NY: Basic Books.

Wing, D. G., Clance, P. R., Burge-Callaway, K., & Armistead, L. (2001). Understanding gender differences in bereavement following the death of an infant. *Psychotherapy: Theory, Research, Practice, Training, 38*(1), 60–73. doi:10.1037/0033-3204.38.1.60

CHAPTER 3

Caregiving as a Theoretical Framework in Perinatal Palliative Care

Rana Limbo, Anthony Lathrop, and Jane Heustis

While I was pregnant, my biggest hope was that Eden would be born alive and that we would all get to hold her before she died. When that hope was realized, I think my hope was that we could keep her comfortable and that she wouldn't suffer. I hoped her life would have meaning. I hoped I would have courage and strength to watch my child die.

> (Maureen, mother of Eden, who lived at home with her family for 11 days after birth with a diagnosis of trisomy 18 and hypoplastic left heart)

*A*pproximately 5,600 babies die during the first year of life from birth defects. Most conditions are diagnosed during pregnancy through prenatal testing. Perinatal palliative care (PPC) has come to the forefront of bereavement care as increasing numbers of families continue a pregnancy after receiving a prenatal diagnosis of a life-threatening condition. PPC encompasses family-centered comfort care throughout the baby's life. Recent research highlights the critical role of caregiving in the parents' relationship with their child both before and after birth. Health care providers have the opportunity to assist with birth and advance care planning, guide families in communicating with others, and prepare for their child's living and dying.

The theory of attachment/caregiving (Bowlby, 1988; Pridham et al., 2012) frames PPC within the functions of protecting, nurturing, socializing (Bowlby, 1969; Bowlby, 1982; George & Solomon, 1999; Pridham et al., 2010; Ruddick, 1995), and final acts of caregiving (Limbo & Lathrop, 2014). Parents of babies diagnosed prenatally with a life-threatening condition often describe expectations of themselves in relation to their baby by talking about hopes (Gum & Snyder, 2002). Hope is central to PPC from the perspective of caregiving. Parents' hopes are embedded in all caregiving aspects (see Chapter 13). The power of parents' stories includes wanting to protect, nurture, socialize, and say their final good-byes. Maureen writes about all four in the previous brief description of her hopes for Eden and herself.

In her book, *Waiting With Gabriel: A Story of Cherishing a Baby's Brief Life* (2003), author and mother Amy Kuebelbeck described her family's experiences after learning during pregnancy that her unborn son Gabriel had a hypoplastic left heart. The diagnosis meant Gabriel would die shortly after birth. She poignantly wrote about caring for Gabriel during her pregnancy:

> Many times we spoke of doing something "with Gabriel."
> We took him fishing on a secluded lake near the North Shore
> of Lake Superior . . . I took Gabriel swinging on the girls'
> backyard swings. We took him to a Minnesota Twins game at
> the Metrodome (Mark's idea) and to a concert by the male vocal
> ensemble Chanticleer at Orchestra Hall (mine).

Kuebelbeck highlighted Gabriel's personhood and the hopes for him as a member of the family. Her words echoed the voices of many parents, providing a lens through which we can better understand what it means to have an unborn child with a life-threatening condition.

The purpose of this chapter is to establish caregiving as a "good fit" theoretical model for PPC. Specific aims are to (a) provide a brief historical overview of PPC, (b) summarize research findings, (c) relate the theory of caregiving, and (d) provide clinical practice guidelines.

BRIEF HISTORICAL OVERVIEW

Statistics

The rate of perinatal mortality (fetal losses and neonatal deaths combined) is 6.4 to 6.8 per 1,000 births (March of Dimes, 2014). Prematurity and the related entity of very low birth weight are the leading causes of perinatal mortality in the United States. Deaths associated with prematurity-related causes account for about 35% of all infant deaths (March of Dimes, 2014). Periviable births—those occurring at or near the early limits of preterm survivability—account for up to 1.9% of all births (Chauhan & Ananth, 2013).

Birth defects are another leading cause of fetal and infant losses. In 2010 in the United States, 5,107 infants died from congenital malformations, syndromes, and chromosomal abnormalities. These deaths accounted for 20.8% of U.S. infant deaths (Murphy, Xu, & Kochanek, 2013). According to the most recent statistics, approximately 25,000 fetal deaths occur annually in the United States, a number that has remained relatively stable since 2003 (Macdorman & Kirmeyer, 2009). About 35% of fetal losses are associated with birth defects such as malformations, dysplasias, or syndromes, with about 12% attributed to chromosomal abnormalities (Silver, 2007).

In addition to prematurity-related conditions, a wide variety of fetal conditions can lead families to perinatal hospice (PH) or PPC services. Combining data from two published PH series (N = 43), the most common diagnoses were anencephaly (n = 11), trisomy 18 (n = 11), other aneuploidies (n = 7), severe skeletal anomalies (n = 4), renal or urinary anomalies leading to anhydramnios and subsequent pulmonary hypoplasia (n = 4), and central nervous system anomalies (n = 3) (D'Almeida, Hume, Lathrop, Njoku, & Calhoun, 2006; Lathrop & VandeVusse, 2011a). The same two series showed 66% of infants born alive, when survival time ranged from 20 minutes to 17 months (D'Almeida et al., 2006; Lathrop & VandeVusse, 2011a). Nelson, Hexem, and Feudtner (2012) made a comprehensive study of data on children born with trisomy 13 or trisomy 18 that showed many lived beyond 1 year of age and required numerous hospitalizations. Formerly defined as "lethal" diagnoses, these two conditions may involve multiple hospitalizations and decision making about ongoing health care.

Evolution of Terminology and Care Terminology

In the past 15 to 20 years, concepts related to the care of infants and families affected by adverse conditions have evolved. In 1997, Calhoun, Hoeldtke, Hinson, and Judge used the term *perinatal hospice* to describe a model of supportive care for women and families who continue their pregnancies after prenatal diagnosis of severe fetal anomalies. The PH model offered a minimal intervention approach, physical and psychosocial support to newborns and their families, and avoidance of treatments that would hasten or delay the delivery of the pregnancy or the death of the newborn (Hoeldtke & Calhoun, 2001).

In a parallel development, authors involved in the care of neonates began using the term *perinatal palliative care* (Carter & Bhatia, 2001; Catlin & Carter, 2002). PPC is a more general term, encompassing both fetuses diagnosed with severe anomalies and those born prior to viability and/or overwhelming disease not responsive to treatment (Leuthner, 2004). Parents who wanted their voices to be heard, different and better care for their infants, and to be told the truth about infants' prognoses strongly influenced the development of this area of palliative care (Catlin, 2013).

As new models were evolving, parents and clinicians recognized that the terminology used to describe infants' conditions was at times inaccurate, confusing, and/or unnecessarily distressing to parents. Some authors and clinicians used the term *lethal anomalies* or *lethal diagnoses* (D'Almeida et al., 2006; Hoeldtke & Calhoun, 2001; Leuthner, 2004). Others used the phrase *incompatible with life* (Jenkins & Wapner, 2004; Ramer-Chrastek & Thygeson, 2005), despite the observed range of survival time for affected infants being 20 minutes to 256 days (D'Almeida et al., 2006). One mother reported experiencing additional distress when she heard care providers use the phrase *incompatible with life* because she and her husband thought this meant their fetus's condition was dangerous to her own life (Lathrop, 2010). For these reasons, some authors and care providers use the term *life threatening* to describe conditions associated with a radically shortened expected life span (Boss, Kavanaugh, & Kobler, 2010).

Care Models

The original PC model, primarily focused on the individual and pain relief, evolved to a broader notion of family-centered and comfort care. More recently, PH and PPC include bereavement care from the time of diagnosis as part of an integrative model (Balaguer, Martin-Ancel, Ortigoza-Escobar, Escribano, & Argemi, 2012; Milstein, 2015). This model (Figure 3.1) includes *hope* as central to decision making, treatment and palliative goals, and parental motivations (Kobler & Limbo, 2011; Pridham et al., 2012).

IDENTIFYING FAMILIES IN NEED OF SERVICES

Because of ways statisticians define and collect statistics of perinatal mortality, precise numbers of potential PH/PPC candidates cannot be identified. However, available statistics give some sense of the scope of the problem and the potential number of affected infants and families.

Professional caregivers can identify a fetus or newborn as a possible candidate for PH or PPC through a variety of pathways. These include (a) antenatal diagnosis of life-threatening conditions, (b) previable premature birth, and (c) infants whose diseases do not respond to current treatments. These diverse pathways provide parents with varying periods of time to consider options and plan for their baby's care.

Advances in technology have made it possible to diagnose fetal conditions at increasingly early gestations. Combined ultrasound and maternal serum screening methods can identify increased risk for some fetal anomalies as early as 11 to 14 weeks gestation (Nicolaides, 2004). Techniques for testing fetal free DNA in maternal serum are making noninvasive genetic

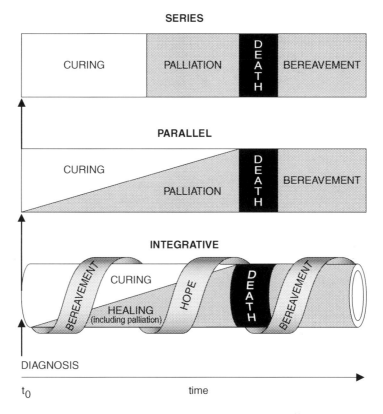

FIGURE 3.1 Integrative model of curing and healing.

Milstein (2005). Copyright 2005. Modified by Limbo and Kobler (2010).

screening possible at earlier gestational ages (i.e., as early as 10 weeks), with near-diagnostic certainty (Palomaki et al., 2011). Because development of maternal identity and maternal–fetal attachment are progressive processes throughout pregnancy (see Chapter 4) and because early detection technologies are new, researchers and health care providers are uncertain about how early diagnosis of adverse fetal conditions might affect mothers' decisions and experiences (Wool & Dudek, 2013).

LAYERED, PROGRESSIVE NEWS VERSUS SUDDEN, UNEXPECTED REALIZATION

Learning of life-threatening conditions can pose different time lines for families. For some, the process may involve gathering fragments of information that cause increasing concern. For example, one woman might learn at her first ultrasound appointment that she has a shortened cervical length, which increases her risk of an early preterm birth (Cahill et al., 2010; Crane &

Hutchens, 2008). Subsequent ultrasonography might show further shortening, dilation, or presentation of fetal parts, signifying an ever-increasing risk of imminent previable delivery. Another woman with no previously identified risk factors might experience an early labor and delivery of an equally threatened baby, all in a matter of a few hours. Although the outcomes may be similar, these mothers and families traveled very different paths.

Some women face difficult options of termination or continuation of pregnancy after learning of a life-threatening fetal condition. Those who choose to continue pregnancies may have weeks or months to prepare for their child's birth and make plans for how they want to socialize, nurture, and protect their child. Others may receive a less definitive diagnosis or defined newborn expectations, so they must anticipate and plan for a range of possible outcomes, including their baby's death prior to birth, early newborn death, or unexpected survival resulting in potential burden of care mingled with joy.

Decisions to continue or end a pregnancy are not dichotomous. Rather, decision making is on a continuum, with changing hopes and expectations influencing choices and options. Parents include caregiving expectations in how they protect, nurture, socialize, and prepare for the final good-bye. The dynamic nature of hope (Feudtner, 2009; Chapter 13, this text), and, therefore, of caregiving goals (Roscigno et al., 2012), plays a critical role in how professionals support PPC families throughout their child's life.

PPC RESEARCH

Wool (2011, 2013) systematically reviewed the existing literature on PPC. Parents described the experience of an adverse fetal diagnosis as a traumatic life event in which they were compelled to choose from among limited options (Wool, 2011). Intense emotions figured prominently in Fonseca, Nazare, and Canavarro's (2013) study of parents' initial reactions to adverse fetal diagnoses. Commonly experienced emotions included guilt, anger, anxiety, sadness, shock, despair, frustration, and hope (Fonseca et al., 2013). Parents experienced intense grief reactions regardless of their choice to continue or terminate affected pregnancies (Wool, 2011). Many parents attempted to find meaning in their experiences and, despite the intense grief and pain, reported experiences of personal growth (Wool, 2013).

Black and Sandelowski's (2010) qualitative study of women and their partners who experienced adverse fetal diagnoses focused on personal growth. Using directed content analysis guided by subscales of the Posttraumatic Growth Inventory (PTGI; Tedeschi & Calhoun, 1996), they found positive personal change in 18 of 25 participants. The PTGI subscale Relating to Others (Tedeschi & Calhoun, 1996) encompassed the most consistent and prolonged changes. The authors concluded it was important to recognize the potential for personal growth, even in the aftermath of a traumatic event, such as an adverse pregnancy outcome (Black & Sandelowski, 2010; Black & Wright, 2012).

Côté-Arsenault and Denney-Koelsch (2011) also conducted a qualitative study of parents' experiences after adverse fetal diagnoses. They found that parents grieved several losses, specifically, loss of a normal pregnancy, of a healthy baby, and of future parenting. The authors used the term *arrested parenting* to describe the sudden interruption in the process of becoming parents (2011). The key finding, *my baby is a person,* described parents' desire to honor and legitimize the humanity of their affected fetuses or newborns.

PH mothers in Lathrop and VandeVusse's (2011b) qualitative study emphasized the importance of affirmation. Participants identified themselves as mothers and their fetuses or newborns as babies, and they actively sought validation of their status from others. Validation described by the mothers came from their own caring behavior toward their babies, such as gestures of affection and closeness, and dressing, bathing, and swaddling their babies. Some mothers described intensely challenging caregiving needs for babies who survived longer than expected (Lathrop & VandeVusse, 2011b). One outcome of the caregiving relationship for mothers was an ongoing sense of love and connection after their babies' deaths (Lathrop & VandeVusse, 2011a). For some mothers, the ongoing connection was experienced as their babies' comforting, protective, or angelic presence in their lives. Many of the mothers visualized their babies' restoration to wholeness and well-being in an afterlife (Lathrop & VandeVusse, 2011a).

The importance of the caregiving relationship between mothers and babies is also reflected in an emerging body of scholarship on the care of critically ill infants in intensive care units. Models of developmental care (Montirosso et al., 2014; NIDCAP Federation, 2013) and family nurture interventions emphasize the importance of involving parents, particularly mothers, in the care of their critically ill newborns. Components of these models include: (1) encouraging skin-to-skin contact between mothers and infants, (2) enhancing mothers' competence and confidence in meeting their infants' specialized needs (Montirosso et al., 2014; NIDCAP Federation, 2013; Welch et al., 2013), and (3) enhancing affective communication and emotional connection between mothers and infants (Welch et al., 2013).

These studies represent an emerging body of scholarship relating to PH/PPC, parents' responses to adverse fetal diagnoses, and parents as caregivers to critically ill newborns. Adverse diagnoses or critical illness in the fetus or newborn affirm the intensity, complexity, and importance of the relationship between parents and their children.

THE IMPORTANCE OF CAREGIVING

The term *attachment* is often used broadly to describe a connection between persons, serving as shorthand for a connected and engaged relationship. Bowlby's (1969, 1982) theory of attachment is more precise, referring to what he terms a "behavioural system" (p. 95) that is hard-wired, species-specific, and includes goals related to a child's need for safety and security from his or her parent or primary caregiver. To accommodate the reciprocal nature of such a relationship, Bowlby developed the theory of caregiving, advancing the idea that caregiving goals are initiated by the parent and designed to nurture, protect, and socialize the child as he or she grows and develops. Researchers studying PH mothers' narratives (Limbo & Lathrop, 2014) identified a fourth caregiving goal when a baby died or was dying: caregiving acts related to the final good-bye.

George and Solomon's (1999) work is pivotal in helping understand the principles of attachment and caregiving theories. They emphasized the reciprocal nature of the parental caregiving goal of *providing* protection to a child (caregiving theory) and a child *seeking* protection from the parent (attachment theory). They described caregiving theory as a way of organizing a parent's internal experience with child outcomes. With this understanding of attachment and caregiving as separate, distinct, yet reciprocal, behavioral systems with different goals, attachment and caregiving researchers helped explain and describe relationships (Bowlby, 1988; Limbo & Pridham, 2007; Main, Kaplan, & Cassidy, 1985; Pridham et al., 2012). In essence, George and Solomon (1999) identified caregiving goals and helped scientists and clinicians move from a static model of reciprocal behaviors to a dynamic model of *being in relationship*.

THE INTERNAL WORKING MODEL OF CAREGIVING

Bowlby (1969, 1982) hypothesized the caregiving behavioral system functioned through internal working models (IWMs). An IWM is a metaphor for self, other, and the relationship, dynamically driven (hence the term *working*), remembered, and held in mind across time (Bowlby, 1988; Pridham et al., 2012). The IWM includes expectations, intentions, motivations, and feelings; affects and is affected by meaning and representation; and is influenced by past experience and what one anticipates in the future (Pridham, 1993). IWMs can be deconstructed and reconstructed by processing information in new and different ways (Bretherton, 1985). For example, a psychotherapist may help a couple reconstruct their shared IWM of their marriage, leading to a healthier, happier relationship.

The literature provides numerous examples of IWMs of caregiving in those interacting with children. Pridham and colleagues (2012) described a unique definition and description of parenting transitions within the framework of feeding. They identified the dynamic nature of transitions as the primary caregiver adapted feeding goals and motivations based on two major conditions: the infant's growth and development and the parent's *anticipation* of how the infant's development would change. In another study, findings showed support for caregiving responses, based on knowing what to expect or anticipate, characterized mothers who were more highly attuned to their infants overall (Limbo & Pridham, 2007).

Langer and colleagues (2013) studied German and Turkish mothers' reactions to their child developing a fever. Mothers interpreted fever as a potential serious threat to their child's well-being. This interpretation led the mothers to rapidly intervene to protect their child (protective caregiving). Researchers identified the mothers' instant emotional response and a need to do something to understand the cause and treat the fever. A child's fever led to activation of the caregiving system because the parent and child are in relationship with each other. All 20 mothers who were interviewed described a "deeply rooted urge to protect" (p. 1). The authors noted that "By applying the caregiving system model . . . maternal actions can be understood as an understandable attempt to protect the child from harm" (p. 1). They concluded that attachment/caregiving theory offers a "promising theoretical approach" (p. 8) for understanding the responses and goals of parents whose children are ill. Finally, they established a link to caregiving in bereaved parents by concluding that "the goal to protect the child and maintain its life was a powerful motivation . . . and represents a central element in the caregiving system model" (p. 7).

CAREGIVING IN BEREAVED PARENTS

Elements of what is often called *parenting* appear in the literature about perinatally bereaved parents (Limbo & Wheeler, 1986, 1998, 2003; see Chapter 11, this text) and bereaved parents of older children. For example, researchers based in the pediatric intensive care unit identified three overall themes of parent responses to their child's dying: "Parenting in the pediatric intensive care unit" (McGraw et al., 2012) included providing love, comfort, and care; creating security and privacy; and exercising responsibility.

Parent stories about their baby's death often demonstrate the importance of spending time with their child (Gold, 2007). The time spent may include performing tasks like bathing, encouraging siblings and other family members to have contact with the baby, and creating lasting memories through rituals, photography, and keepsakes (Limbo & Kobler, 2010). Limbo and Lathrop (2014) applied caregiving theory (Bowlby, 1988) to the analysis of PH mothers' narratives as they described being in relationship with their babies (before and after birth and before and after death). The research findings described the hard-wired caregiving system—organized around the IWM—triggered by the innate goals of caring for a child, living or dead. Such an understanding—when used as a framework for clinical care of bereaved parents—focuses on their role as parent, not on whether their child is physically alive or not. The following section summarizes the essential caregiving goals: protecting, nurturing, socializing, and final acts of caregiving. Each is part of a framework for evidence-based clinical care.

Protecting

Those who listen to bereaved parents often hear them refer to their grief over not being able to protect their baby from death.

> I was journaling a lot so I would write in the journal like, "I'm sorry [baby's name] that I can't give you more time" because I knew that when we induced, you know, she was going to die sooner than she would have if I had given her more time. (Lathrop, 2010)

> I mean really when I, when I was still carrying her, I think that's when I felt like I was really able to mother her, you know, like I knew she was safe; we knew, we knew that as long as she was in my womb, she was safe, you know, and that nothing could happen to her. (Lathrop, 2010)

Photographs of the baby can serve as a way of helping loved ones who may not have seen the baby alive establish a connection with the baby. One mother whose baby had an obvious anomaly protected her baby by carefully selecting the people with whom she shared the images (Limbo & Lathrop, 2014).

Nurturing

Pridham et al. (2012) identified nurturing as a type of caregiving motivation in mothers of babies born prematurely. Mothers nurtured their babies by learning about and providing proper nutrition (amount and type), monitoring that their growth was appropriate for their age, and enhancing their skill level (e.g., feeding competency, motor development).

PH mothers (Limbo & Lathrop, 2014) also spoke of nurturing in terms of feeding. Several mothers described expressing a few drops of breast milk and placing them on the lips of their babies. Nurturing may include keeping the baby in a skin-to-skin position until the baby is handed to a funeral director or another person responsible for final disposition. Cleaning the baby's skin (i.e., bathing), shampooing the hair, removing dried blood, and placing a clean and dry blanket around the baby could represent nurturing for a parent.

Socializing

It may be difficult to imagine that parents think about their baby's relationship with others, even after the baby has died. Yet such is true. A mother may comment on how a nurse held the baby close to her, patting the baby's buttocks as she swayed from side to side. Photographs are important tools for introducing the baby to others. A mother may use a photograph generated from an ultrasonogram to proudly show others special features of her precious child. This mother noted, "It helped so much to know that yeah, that . . . other people were sort of sharing in the joy that we had for her . . . We wanted them to be able to share in the joy of her life" (Lathrop, 2010). A baby's connection with others may be established or strengthened through seeing and holding, participating in a formal (blessing) or informal (reading to the baby) ritual, and using the baby's name in conversation.

Final Acts of Caregiving

Health care providers may have overlooked the importance of the last moments parents have with their baby's physical body. Researchers identified the profound impact these final acts of caring for their baby's body had on parents (Limbo & Lathrop, 2014). The critical element of the final acts of caregiving involved the parent or parents choosing how they wished these last moments to play out. A mother might feel overwhelmed by having to turn her baby's body over to someone else and choose not to participate. Another mother may wish to be the person placing her baby's body in the crematory. Often parents ask to place their baby's body in the casket as their final act of caregiving. Again, understanding that these expectations, intentions, and motivations are hard-wired helps clinicians let the parent take the lead.

CLINICAL GUIDELINES: CAREGIVING IN PERINATAL PALLIATIVE CARE

Research and clinical guidelines provide support for offering perinatal palliative services using a caregiving theoretical framework. Limbo and

Lathrop (2014) provided examples of PH mothers' narratives that included nurturing, protecting, socializing, and final acts of caregiving. The mothers reported experiences that occurred up to 10 years previously, indicating that caregiving is memorable and meaningful. PPC can offer the family vital support in continuing to protect, nurture, and socialize their unborn baby in a safe and respectful venue, providing a sense of normalcy during the baby's life. Professionals offering PPC services assist family and staff in cocreating a plan that incorporates acts of protecting, nurturing, socializing, and creating or deciding on the final acts of caregiving. Support staff can carefully guide families in available options and assist them in beginning to tell the story of their precious baby. PPC can also prepare those directly caring for mothers and their families so that they are ready to offer the best and right supportive care. Bedside staff will participate in acts of protecting, nurturing, socializing, and final acts of caregiving involving the baby, parents, and their extended family.

BIRTH AND ADVANCE CARE PLANNING

Caring for families whose baby has a life-threatening condition requires thinking beyond the moment. Anticipating questions and comments of parents, communicating with the total care team, or documenting the plan that is accessible to all team members (such as an electronic health record) are examples of conditions to be considered in establishing a seamless process for families.

The structure of PPC services can be offered within a traditional hospice agency, stand-alone PH programs, or an existing perinatal bereavement or palliative care program (Kobler & Limbo, 2011). The website perinatalhospice.org provides a list of programs worldwide that reflect different models of implementation, yet share values and goals that support quality of life for babies and their families. PPC programs can also provide a framework that supports caregivers using comprehensive services; nonjudgmental values; and individualized, family-centered models of care.

BEGINNING THE JOURNEY WITH THE FAMILY

Early initiation of an interprofessional and integrative care process is essential for optimum outcomes in PPC. However, the process of prenatal testing and subsequent diagnosis of a life-threatening fetal condition is a time of great shock and confusion for parents. They frequently feel unprepared to fully grasp its intensity, let alone make important decisions about the life and death of their yet-to-be-born baby. The family may need time to digest all that has happened, reconstruct their hopes regarding the pregnancy, and consider alternatives before moving forward with a plan. Beginning the palliative care process must take into consideration the concept of time, moving at the pace that best fits the needs and desires of the family. For some families, beginning conversations can take place at diagnosis; for others, conversations about planning for the baby could take place days, weeks, or even months postdiagnosis. The key is to initiate a connection soon after diagnosis to ensure family members are aware of services, even if they elect to postpone planning.

The essence of family-supportive PPC is based on the relationship between family and caregivers. Families appreciate having one person, a liaison, who acts as their primary contact and assists them in connections to all services (Leuthner & Jones, 2007; Limbo, Toce, & Peck, 2008). The PPC liaison can be vital in bridging the gap from the outpatient arena to the inpatient unit to home care services, if needed. The PPC liaison:

- Participates in the diagnostic process and connects with the family soon after diagnosis
- Enters into relationship with the family and explores their expectations, intentions, motivations, hopes, beliefs, and spiritual practice needs
- Mobilizes the support team for family
- Assures family that their wishes and desires are communicated through the multisystem team

The first conversation is often the most critical when initiating a PPC relationship. Parents and family may still have many questions about the future of their unborn baby. They may also still be centered on hope of recovery. The PPC liaison can carefully establish a family's current needs by asking open-ended questions, such as, *What is important to you? What is the hardest part? What are you most concerned about? What could be helpful to you and your family right now?* Initial conversations often center on the act of protecting—assuring family that nothing will be done without their permission, affirming respect for this chaotic time, as well as simple explanations of what PPC can offer in the next weeks and months.

THE ROLE OF THE PPC TEAM

An interprofessional team provides comprehensive support to families. Team members create a safe place for the family to explore options of care and cope with this new experience. The PPC team consists of multiple disciplines: medicine, genetic counseling, nursing, chaplaincy, social work, and child life, among others. In addition, the support includes multiple care teams: maternity, maternal fetal medicine, neonatal intensive care, hospice, home health, and others. PPC teams may also include out-of-facility support, such as childbirth education (Kobler, Limbo, & Oakdale, 2012), organ procurement, home health, and milk bank (Moore & Catlin, 2003).

Lay support may include volunteer photographers (e.g., those in a program such as Now I Lay Me Down To Sleep) and other bereaved parents (through support groups, in-person, and online connections) (Carlson, Lammert, & O'Leary, 2012). Together, they provide an integrative, seamless level of care coordinated by the PPC liaison. From the physician's office, to the inpatient unit, to postdischarge care, the key for a well-coordinated team is communication: All team members must be up to date on family needs and know what services are being provided. The PPC care team ensures essential elements and creates a framework for future families that include:

- Protocols and care maps that outline palliative care
- Processes for adjusting or altering standard operating procedures to anticipate family needs. These processes presume positive answers to questions such as *Are photographers allowed in the delivery room? Can family members have a blessing service in the hospital chapel? Can the baby stay in the labor and delivery area rather than be admitted to the neonatal intensive care unit?*
- Tools for seamless communication throughout the care team, such as electronic health record documentation and checklists
- Guidance and mentoring for bedside staff throughout the family's hospital stay

SUPPORT DURING THE PREGNANCY

Once a connection has been made between the family and a health care provider liaison, PPC planning becomes fluid, depending on the needs and desires of family members. Some families are eager to plan from the initial diagnosis, while others need more time.

The authors provide examples of four families who receive similar life-threatening diagnoses about their unborn baby, yet each family has different expectations, hopes, and values: They describe varied responses, using pseudonyms, but real-life decisions. Family 1: After the diagnosis of trisomy 18, Samantha and David called the palliative care team immediately, wanting everything to be "perfect for our perfect daughter." Family 2: When the PPC liaison approached Brittany, she responded she did not "want anything to do with all that." However, her mother wanted to explore options. Family 3: Misty declined PPC support at the time of diagnosis but called the PPC liaison on the day prior to her scheduled induction, ready to consider options of care for her baby. Family 4: The Lombardo family elected to not preplan their baby's special day. Consequently, they spent approximately the first 2 hours of their admission creating an impromptu plan. Whether contacts were made at prenatal appointments, during telephone conversations, or at the bedside, all families reported that connections to caregivers prior to delivery made the difference in how they coped with their baby's illness and death. These families' experiences provide evidence that relationship-based care is the critical link to effective PPC.

During the pregnancy, families most appreciate information and support regarding these five domains: (a) their baby's diagnosis, (b) affirmation of the pregnancy, (c) facilitating information from outside sources, (d) connections to people who understand, and (e) cocreating a birth plan.

Their Baby's Diagnosis

Families have continued questions about causes and treatment plans. On Latasha's fourth visit after diagnosis of renal agenesis, she quietly asked the PPC liaison if a kidney transplant were possible for her baby. Families often need continued information about what is happening with their baby and what will happen after birth. First-time parents may also need childbirth education, typically in individual sessions.

Affirmation of the Pregnancy

After a life-threatening diagnosis, families often are uncomfortable talking about their baby to family and friends. Families can be guided to discuss what has happened and ways to continue honoring their baby through journaling, art, and Internet sharing (e.g., blogs and other social media options).

Facilitating Information From Outside Sources

Families often need guidance in evaluating information from Internet sites, books, magazines, and stories from family members and friends. Juan and Isabella wanted to change their birth plan after hearing about a child with trisomy 13 who lived into her teenage years. After the PPC coordinator connected them with cardiology, pediatric surgery, neonatology, and medical genetics specialists, and other bereaved parents, they were able to reformulate their hopes and expectations for their baby. In the end, they elected palliative care. Some families also need assistance in how to tell others about what is going to happen. Christine struggled with how to tell her four children. Child life specialists assisted her in child-appropriate explanations and ways to involve the children in the birth plan.

Connections to People Who Understand

During a prenatal appointment, Vanessa admitted she had no one to talk to. "I love my sister. She is my best friend, but she doesn't understand what I'm going through and, frankly, I feel pretty lonely." Frequent connections to the PPC team chaplain and to the local parents' group gave Vanessa alternative support.

Parents and family members often make assumptions about what is possible or not possible. For example, Tasha, a mother of four children, expressed surprise when the PPC coordinator offered traditional options: "He can still cut the cord? I can still put my baby to my breast right after delivery? I figured those things were *out* considering the circumstances." Stephanie's greatest hope was that her baby would be born alive. When the ultrasonographer did not find her baby's heart beat at her 34-week appointment, she was devastated. Her PPC liaison was able to help her reconstruct her hopes and offer additional alternatives prior to delivery. When PPC caregivers draw a virtual picture of possibilities, family members can begin framing what is important to them.

Cocreating a Birth Plan

A birth plan is a communication tool, a relatively simple way for the mother and family to communicate hopes, wishes, and expectations to their caregivers during labor and delivery. A birth plan creates a framework for conversation about the future for the baby and the baby's family. The PPC birth plan is a working document, changing as family's hopes and wishes evolve as delivery approaches. Bailey and her partner Dustin were adamant in the weeks before their baby's delivery that extended family members (e.g., the baby's grandparents) would not participate in their baby's birth. The PPC team prepared a special space and designated staff to support the parents' plans. Bailey changed her mind and asked for both grandmothers to be part of the experience. Family-centered, relationship-based birth plans always include contingency plans.

The PPC birth plan should include (a) admission to the hospital, (b) early and active labor, (c) delivery, (d) mother/baby care, and (e) neonatal care. When helping families evaluate their options, it may be helpful to start with more concrete ideas of protecting, nurturing, and socializing, and then slowly introduce concepts related to final acts of caregiving. Asking questions such as, "Tell me what you have been thinking about," "What are you hoping for?" and "What might make your baby's birth the special day you want it to be?" will help the family clarify what is important to them.

Elements of the PPC birth plans may include processes that can be initiated prenatally, such as connections to organ donation procurement and support, volunteer photographers, and lactation support and/or breast milk donation.

DOCUMENTATION

The PPC journey is a story worth telling. Complete and thorough documentation creates an impression of the baby's family legacy. Detailed and accessible documentation benefits both the family and staff who provide the care. It enhances the family experience: Parents do not have to tell their story in multiple venues and state their wishes repeatedly. Knowing the parents' story creates an atmosphere of respect and caring.

Reliable documentation also enhances staff satisfaction. Bedside caregivers want to be part of the family's experience and want to prepare for supporting the parents in protecting, nurturing, socializing, and designing the final acts of caregiving for their baby. Knowing the story before their patient arrives helps bedside staff enter into relationship with the family and feel part of the team.

Each facility has its own policies and procedures for documentation. Whether done electronically or by paper, it is important to document each step of outpatient, inpatient, and postdischarge care. For example, Tamika arrived at the hospital on a Saturday evening at 33 weeks gestation, fully dilated and ready to deliver. The staff read her chart upon her arrival, quickly reviewed her birth plan, and moved her to the delivery area. Complete documentation enabled staff to provide the experience Tamika and her family planned, even when time did not allow for detailed conversation.

Documentation should include the following:

- Names and contact information of PPC team members working with the family
- Current list of family's expectations
- Explanations of baby's diagnosis and diagnostic processes
- Initial discussions with the family regarding diagnosis and options offered
- Ethics consultation, if applicable
- Discussions about birth planning
- Interprofessional notes and/or consults

CONCLUSION

Sensitive, empathic guidance and cocreation of a plan of care serve as foundations of a relationship between families and those caring for them.

Relationships provide hope in the midst of intense human suffering. Nurturing, protecting, socializing, and creating final acts of caregiving frame the life-changing moments families have with their baby whose life ended or will end far too soon.

CASE STUDY

Kira is a 31-year-old patient who is in the third trimester of her second pregnancy. She and her husband, Tom, were told of a severe fetal anomaly early in the pregnancy. They chose to continue the pregnancy and were offered PPC. They named the baby Erin and have encouraged their 3-year-old son, Aiden, to talk with Erin and plan rituals after her death. Kira's mother was not in favor of their decision to continue the pregnancy, and feels that Aiden should not be involved. But Tom's family feels that the decision to continue the pregnancy to its natural end is congruent with their religious views and they wholeheartedly support their choice. Kira is now seeking care for signs of labor and is admitted to the labor and delivery unit.

FOCUS QUESTIONS

1. How could the theory of caregiving be used to guide Kira and Tom's care?
2. How do the perspectives of Kira's mother and Tom's parents impact the care that should be planned for this family?
3. In terms of family support:
   a. What type of support should be offered to Kira and Tom?
   b. How should Aiden be incorporated into the plan of care?
   c. How does Kira's mother's perspective affect the plan of care?
4. What types of supportive care should be offered to Kira and Tom after Erin's birth?

REFERENCES

Balaguer, A., Martin-Ancel, A., Ortigoza-Escobar, D., Escribano, J., & Argemi, J. (2012). The model of palliative care in the perinatal setting: A review of the literature. *BMC Pediatrics, 12*, 25. doi:10.1186/1471-2431-12-25

Black, B., & Sandelowski, M. (2010). Personal growth after severe fetal diagnosis. *Western Journal of Nursing Research, 32*(8), 1011–1030. doi:10.1177/0193945910371215

Black, B., & Wright, P. M. (2012). Posttraumatic growth and transformation as outcomes of perinatal loss. *Illness, Crisis, & Loss, 20*(3), 225–237. doi:10.2190/IL.20.3.b

Boss, R., Kavanaugh, K., & Kobler, K. (2010). Prenatal and neonatal palliative care. In J. Wolfe, P. Hinds, & B. Sourkes (Eds.), *Textbook of interdisciplinary pediatric palliative care* (pp. 387–401). Philadelphia, PA: Saunders.

Bowlby, J. (1969). *Attachment and loss.* New York, NY: Basic Books.

Bowlby, J. (1982). *Attachment.* New York, NY: Basic Books.

Bowlby, J. (1988). *A secure base: Parent-child attachment and healthy human development.* New York, NY: Basic Books.

Bretherton, I. (1985). Attachment theory: Retrospect and prospect. In I. Bretherton & E. Waters (Eds.), *Monographs of the Society for Research in Child Development, growing points of attachment: Theory and research* (Vol. 50(1–2), Serial No. 209, pp. 3–35). Chicago, IL: University of Chicago Press.

Cahill, A. G., Odibo, A. O., Caughey, A. B., Stamilio, D. M., Hassan, S. S., Macones, G. A., & Romero, R. (2010). Universal cervical length screening and treatment with vaginal progesterone to prevent preterm birth: A decision and economic analysis. *American Journal of Obstetrics and Gynecology, 202*(6), 548.e1–548.e8. doi:10.1016/j.ajog.2009.12.005

Calhoun, B. C., Hoeldtke, N. J., Hinson, R. M., & Judge, K. M. (1997). Perinatal hospice: Should all centers have this service? *Neonatal Network: NN, 16*(6), 101–102.

Carlson, R.; Lammert, C., & O'Leary, J. M. (2012). The evolution of group and online support for families who have experienced perinatal or neonatal loss. *Illness, Crisis & Loss, 20*(3), 275–293.

Carter, B. S., & Bhatia, J. (2001). Comfort/palliative care guidelines for neonatal practice: Development and implementation in an academic medical center. *Journal of Perinatology: Official Journal of the California Perinatal Association, 21*(5), 279–283. doi:10.1038/sj.jp.7210582

Catlin, A. (2013). Perinatal hospice care during the antepartum period. *Journal of Obstetric, Gynecologic, and Neonatal Nursing: JOGNN/NAACOG, 42*(3), 369–371. doi:10.1111/1552-6909.12029

Catlin, A., & Carter, B. (2002). Creation of a neonatal end-of-life palliative care protocol. *Journal of Perinatology: Official Journal of the California Perinatal Association, 22*(3), 184–195. doi:10.1038/sj.jp.7210687

Chauhan, S. P., & Ananth, C. V. (2013). Periviable births: Epidemiology and obstetrical antecedents. *Seminars in Perinatology, 37*(6), 382–388. doi:10.1053/j.semperi.2013.06.020

Côté-Arsenault, D., & Denney-Koelsch, E. (2011). "My baby is a person": Parents' experiences with life-threatening fetal diagnosis. *Journal of Palliative Medicine, 14*(12), 1302–1308.

Crane, J. M., & Hutchens, D. (2008). Transvaginal sonographic measurement of cervical length to predict preterm birth in asymptomatic women at increased risk: A systematic review. *Ultrasound in Obstetrics & Gynecology: The Official Journal of the International Society of Ultrasound in Obstetrics and Gynecology, 31*(5), 579–587. doi:10.1002/uog.5323

D'Almeida, M., Hume, R. F., Lathrop, A., Njoku, A., & Calhoun, B. C. (2006). Perinatal hospice: Family-centered care of the fetus with a lethal condition. *Journal of American Physicians and Surgeons, 11*(2), 52–55.

Feudtner, C. (2009). The breadth of hopes. *The New England Journal of Medicine, 361*(24), 2306–2307.

Fonseca, A., Nazare, B., & Canavarro, M. C. (2013). Clinical determinants of parents' emotional reactions to the disclosure of a diagnosis of congenital anomaly. *Journal of Obstetric, Gynecologic, and Neonatal Nursing: JOGNN / NAACOG, 42*(2), 178–190. doi:10.1111/1552-6909.12010

George, C., & Solomon, J. (1999). Attachment and caregiving: The caregiving behavioral system. In J. Cassidy & P. R. Shaver (Eds.), *Handbook of attachment: Theory, research, and clinical applications* (pp. 649–670). New York, NY: Guilford Press.

Gold, K. J. (2007). Navigating care after a baby dies: A systematic review of parent experiences with health providers. *Journal of Perinatology: Official Journal of the California Perinatal Association, 27*(4), 230–237. doi:10.1038/sj.jp.7211676

Gum, A., & Snyder, C. R. (2002). Coping with terminal illness: The role of hopeful thinking. *Journal of Palliative Medicine, 5*(6), 883–894. doi:10.1089/10966210260499078

Hoeldtke, N. J., & Calhoun, B. C. (2001). Perinatal hospice. *American Journal of Obstetrics and Gynecology, 185*(3), 525–529. doi:S0002-9378(01)87556-6

Jenkins, T. M., & Wapner, R. J. (2004). Prenatal diagnosis of congenital disorders. In R. K. Creasy, R. Resnik & J. D. Iams (Eds.), *Maternal-fetal medicine: Principles and practice* (5th ed., pp. 235–280). Philadelphia, PA: WB Saunders.

Kobler, K., & Limbo, R. (2011). Making a case: Creating a perinatal palliative care service using a perinatal bereavement program model. *The Journal of Perinatal & Neonatal Nursing, 25*(1), 32–41; quiz 42-43. doi:10.1097/JPN.0b013e3181fb592e

Kobler, K., Limbo, R., & Oakdale, C. (2012). Childbirth education for parents receiving perinatal palliative care. *International Childbirth Education Association Journal, 27*(2), 26–32.

Kuebelbeck, A. (2003). *Waiting with Gabriel: A story of cherishing a baby's brief life.* Chicago, IL: Loyola Press.

Langer, T., Pfeifer, M., Soenmez, A., Kalitzkus, V., Wilm, S., & Schnepp, W. (2013). Activation of the maternal caregiving system by childhood fever—a qualitative study of the experiences made by mothers with a German or a Turkish background in the care of their children. *BMC Family Practice, 14*, 35. doi:10.1186/1471-2296-14-35

Lathrop, A. (2010). *A narrative analysis of perinatal hospice stories.* (Doctoral dissertation). Retrieved from ProQuest Dissertations and Theses database. (UMI No. 3398940)

Lathrop, A., & VandeVusse, L. (2011a). Affirming motherhood: Validation and invalidation in women's perinatal hospice narratives. *Birth. 38*(3), 256–265. doi:10.1111/j.1523-536X.2011.00478.x

Lathrop, A., & VandeVusse, L. (2011b). Continuity and change in mothers' narratives of perinatal hospice. *The Journal of Perinatal & Neonatal Nursing, 25*(1), 21–31. doi:10.1097/JPN.0b013e3181fa9c60

Leuthner, S., & Jones, E. L. (2007). Fetal concerns program: A model for perinatal palliative care. *MCN, The American Journal of Maternal Child Nursing, 32*(5), 272–278. doi:10.1097/01.NMC.0000287996.90307.c6

Leuthner, S. R. (2004). Fetal palliative care. *Clinics in Perinatology, 31*(3), 649–665. doi:10.1016/j.clp.2004.04.018

Limbo, R., & Kobler, K. (2010). The tie that binds: Relationships in perinatal bereavement. *MCN, The American Journal of Maternal Child Nursing, 35*(6), 316–321; quiz 321–323. doi:10.1097/NMC.0b013e3181f0eef8

Limbo, R., & Lathrop, A. (2014). Caregiving in mothers' narratives of perinatal hospice. *Illness, Crisis, & Loss, 22*(3), 43–65.

Limbo, R., & Pridham, K. (2007). Mothers' understanding of their infants in the context of an internal working model of caregiving. *ANS. Advances in Nursing Science, 30*(2), 139–150. doi:10.1097/01.ANS.0000271104.34420.b6

Limbo, R., Toce, S. & Peck, T. (2008). *Resolve through sharing (RTS) position paper on perinatal palliative care*. La Crosse, WI: Gundersen Lutheran Medical Foundation, INC. Retrieved from http://www.bereavementservices.org/documents/FINAL9.11.08 .pdf

Limbo, R., & Wheeler, S. R. (1986, 1998, 2003). *When a baby dies: A handbook for healing and helping*. La Crosse, WI: Bereavement Services.

Macdorman, M. F., & Kirmeyer, S. (2009). The challenge of fetal mortality. *NCHS Data Brief, (16)*, 1–8.

Main, M., Kaplan, N., & Cassidy, J. (1985). Security in infancy, childhood, and adulthood: A move to the level of representation. *Monographs of the Society for Research in Child Development, 50*(1/2), 66–104.

March of Dimes. (2014). Peristats: Updated fetal and infant mortality data. Retrieved from www.marchofdimes/peristats

McGraw, S. A., Truog, R. D., Solomon, M. Z., Cohen-Bearak, A., Sellers, D. E., & Meyer, E. C. (2012). "I was able to still be her mom"—parenting at end of life in the pediatric intensive care unit. *Pediatric Critical Care Medicine, 13*(6), e350–e356. doi:10.1097/ PCC.0b013e31825b5607

Milstein, J. (2005). A paradigm of integrated care: Healing with curing throughout life, 'being with' and 'doing to'. *Journal of Perinatology, 25*, 563–568.

Milstein, J. M. (2015). Our moral imperative: Finding a path to wholeness. *Clinical Pediatrics, 54*(3), 205–207.

Montirosso, R., Fedeli, C., Del Prete, A., Calciolari, G., Borgatti, R., & NEO-ACQUA Study Group. (2014). Maternal stress and depressive symptoms associated with quality of developmental care in 25 Italian neonatal intensive care units: A cross sectional observational study. *International Journal of Nursing Studies, 51*(7), 994–1002. doi:10.1016/j.ijnurstu.2013.11.001

Moore, D. B., & Catlin, A. (2003). Lactation suppression: Forgotten aspect of care for the mother of a dying child. *Pediatric Nursing, 29*(5), 383–384.

Murphy, S. L., Xu, J., & Kochanek, K. D. (2013). Deaths: Final data for 2010. *National Vital Statistics Reports, 61*(4), 1–117.

Nelson, K. E., Hexem, K. R., & Feudtner, C. (2012). Inpatient hospital care of children with trisomy 13 and trisomy 18 in the United States. *Pediatrics, 129*(5), 869–876. doi:10.1542/peds.2011-2139

Nicolaides, K. H. (2004). *The 11 to 13+6 weeks scan*. London, UK: Fetal Medicine Foundation.

NIDCAP Federation. (2013). *Newborn individualized development care and assessment program: An education and training program for health care professionals*. Boston, MA: NIDCAP Federation International.

Palomaki, G. E., Kloza, E. M., Lambert-Messerlian, G. M., Haddow, J. E., Neveux, L. M., Ehrich, M., . . . Canick, J. A. (2011). DNA sequencing of maternal plasma to detect Down syndrome: An international clinical validation study. *Genetics in Medicine, 13*(11), 913–920. doi:10.1097/GIM.0b013e3182368a0e

Pridham, K., Harrison, T., Brown, R., Krolikowski, M., Limbo, R., & Schroeder, M. (2012). Caregiving motivations and developmentally prompted transition for mothers of prematurely born infants. *ANS. Advances in Nursing Science, 35*(3), E23–E41. doi:10.1097/ANS.0b013e3182626115

Pridham, K., Harrison, T., Krolikowski, M., Bathum, M. E., Ayres, L., & Winters, J. (2010). Internal working models of parenting: Motivations of parents of infants with a congenital heart defect. *ANS. Advances in Nursing Science, 33*(4), E1–E16. doi:10.1097/ ANS.0b013e3181fc016e

Pridham, K. F. (1993). Anticipatory guidance of parents of new infants: Potential contribution of the internal working model construct. *Image—the Journal of Nursing Scholarship, 25*(1), 49–56.

Ramer-Chrastek, J., & Thygeson, M. V. (2005). A perinatal hospice for an unborn child with a life-limiting condition. *International Journal of Palliative Nursing, 11*(6), 274–276.

Roscigno, C. I., Savage, T. A., Kavanaugh, K., Moro, T. T., Kilpatrick, S. J., Strassner, H. T., . . . Kimura, R. E. (2012). Divergent views of hope influencing communications between parents and hospital providers. *Qualitative Health Research, 22*(9), 1232–1246. doi:10.1177/1049732312449210

Ruddick, S. (1995). *Maternal thinking: Toward a politics of peace; with a new preface.* Boston, MA: Beacon Press.

Silver, R. M. (2007). Fetal death. *Obstetrics and Gynecology, 109*(1), 153–167. doi:109/1/153

Tedeschi, R. G., & Calhoun, L. G. (1996). The posttraumatic growth inventory: Measuring the positive legacy of trauma. *Journal of Traumatic Stress, 9*(3), 455–471.

Welch, M. G., Hofer, M. A., Stark, R. I., Andrews, H. F., Austin, J., Glickstein, S. B., . . . FNI Trial Group. (2013). Randomized controlled trial of family nurture intervention in the NICU: Assessments of length of stay, feasibility and safety. *BMC Pediatrics, 13,* 148–158. doi:10.1186/1471-2431-13-148

Wool, C. (2011). Systematic review of the literature: Parental outcomes after diagnosis of fetal anomaly. *Advances in Neonatal Care, 11*(3), 182–192. doi:10.1097/ANC.0b013e31821bd92d

Wool, C. (2013). State of the science on perinatal palliative care. *Journal of Obstetric, Gynecologic, and Neonatal Nursing, 42*(3), 372–382; quiz E54–E55. doi:10.1111/1552-6909.12034

RESOURCES

- perinatalhospice.org
- Position Paper on Perinatal Palliative Care, downloadable from www.bereveamentservices.org
- *Waiting for Birth and Death* available from bereavementservices.org/catalog

CHAPTER 4

When an Expected Baby Dies: Maternal–Fetal Attachment in Context of Loss

Beth Perry Black

Grief is "the intense and painful pining for and preoccupation with some-body or something, now lost, to whom or to which one was attached" (Parkes, 2006, p. 23). More poetically, perhaps, Parkes (2015) described the pain of grief as "just as much a part of life as the joy of love, the price we pay for love, the cost of commitment" (Part 1: Love and Grief). These simple and poignant words are particularly apt in describing the sadness and yearning experienced by pregnant women, their partners, and families when their expected child dies before birth or soon thereafter. Pregnancy and birth are not simply biological events; they have deep social meanings. Nurse Reva Rubin (1975), in her groundbreaking work on maternal role attainment, described a pregnant woman's growing awareness of "the child within her and attaches so much value to him that she possesses something very dear, very important to her" by the end of the second trimester (p. 145). Sociologist Barbara Katz Rothman noted, "Birth is not only about making babies. Birth is about making mothers. . ." (Rothman, n.d.). A perinatal loss is a complex event because it means that a woman has lost not only her expected child but she has lost her opportunity to become the mother to this baby—even if she already has other children.

The maternal–infant relationship has been the focus of attention of researchers across a variety of disciplines in the past few decades. In the 1970s, "bonding" as a mechanism by which the early maternal–infant relationship was forged changed childbirth practices in the United States. Within a decade, technological advances in fetal screening including electronic fetal monitoring and ultrasonography gave rise to increased knowledge about the developing fetus and moved the discourse around the maternal–infant relationship into the prenatal period. Known as *maternal–fetal attachment* (MFA), researchers and clinicians became interested in this phenomenon, which some think may predict the quality of the eventual maternal–infant relationship. Alternately, this phenomenon may be known as *prenatal* or *antenatal attachment* when referring to male partners' experiences vis-à-vis the fetus.

In this chapter, the historical and cultural roots of attachment are explored, as used in childbirth settings in the United States over the past 40 years. First, the concept of bonding is discussed, as it was used in the 1970s to promote the development of a strong maternal–infant relationship immediately after birth. Then, the development and widespread use of prenatal technologies are shown. Specifically, ultrasonography in the 1980s began to move the bonding/attachment discourse into pregnancy, at which point the construct of MFA was developed, defined, and (presumably) measured. The various definitions of MFA and criticisms of the construct and how ultrasonography has affected both the attachment and grief discourse surrounding pregnancy are discussed. Finally, using data from two ethnographic studies of women and families with a prenatal diagnosis of a severe (life-limiting or lethal) fetal defect, ways in which expectant parents acknowledged that their baby was likely to die, expressed their commitment to the well-being of their baby, simultaneously prepared for his or her death, and grieved the multiple losses that accompany death in the context of birth are demonstrated.

THEORETICAL ROOTS OF ATTACHMENT AND BONDING

The work of John Bowlby is usually cited as central in the development of attachment theory; however, his 40-year collaboration with Mary Ainsworth is often overlooked in discussions of attachment theory. In the context of robust, intense longitudinal research, Ainsworth and Bowlby developed and continued to refine their understanding of the nature of human attachments. To cite Ainsworth and Bowlby at any one point is to capture only a cross-section of their decades-long work on how human attachments are developed. In fact, in her published address upon receipt of the 1989 American Psychological Association Award, Ainsworth detailed the long history of the development of the theory, its eclectic roots stretching across a number of disciplines (e.g., developmental, social, cognitive, and personality psychology; systems theory; biological sciences; Ainsworth & Bowlby, 1991). Attachment theory, as per Ainsworth, is primarily "an ethological approach to personality development" (p. 333). Ethology is the study of animal behavior occurring in its natural setting. Acknowledging the ethological foundation of attachment theory provides an interesting point of departure for the discussion of the concept of bonding as developed and implemented in the 1970s in childbirth settings.

Bonding: Fact and Fiction

The science of the formation of human relationships is complex. Humans as the biological species *Homo sapiens* (Latin: "wise man") are altricial, meaning that human offspring are very immature at birth and require years of physical, cognitive, and social development before becoming fully mature and able to survive independently. Other species are precocial, meaning that mobility occurs early after birth, raising the possibility that a newborn animal could wander from the safety of its mother (the main source of nutrition) and of the herd or flock. Among precocial animals, newly born or hatched offspring "imprint" during a critical period soon after birth, a behavioral response to a biological innate drive to form a bond of attachment to its mother. As a matter of survival, precocial animals must attach quickly to their mothers.

Childbirth practices in the 1970s were shaped by the work of pediatricians Kennell and Klaus (1976), who in their book *Maternal–Infant Bonding: The Impact of Early Separation or Loss on Family Development* described a theoretical critical period in which human infants and mothers form bonds of attachment ("bonding") in the early moments and hours following birth, drawing on animal models of imprinting. Their work was highly influential in shaping childbirth practices to include rooming-in of the newborn with the mother, early initiation of breastfeeding, skin-to-skin contact immediately after birth, and other acts intended to promote bonding during the putative critical period after birth. These practices were widely accepted and institutionalized, although by the early 1980s, researchers and social critics judged the scientific basis for these practices as being methodologically and epistemologically weak (Eyer, 1992).

Critics of institutionalized bonding practices expressed concern that these measures reduced women to simple enactors of an instinct to mother. Moreover, premature birth, neonatal or maternal illness, adoption, or other contingencies may delay early interaction of a mother with her infant. As a consequence, the mother would presumably miss the opportunity to "bond with" her baby. These rather common contingencies of early parenting left women and their partners unnecessarily guilt-ridden and fearful that the lack of early contact might have long-term negative consequences on their relationship with their child. The presumably well-meaning institutionalization of practices to promote bonding in perinatal settings was met with substantial criticism regarding the unintentional consequences of a narrow, simplistic view of the development of the highly complex relationship between mothers (and fathers) and their infants, a view that Eyer referred to as "a scientific fiction" (1992).

Prenatal Technology: Extending Attachment Into Pregnancy

Interest that arose in the 1960s to 1970s with regard to the maternal–infant relationship immediately postbirth soon extended to the possibility of a relationship between the pregnant woman and her developing fetus prior to birth (DiPietro, 2010). The development of fetal monitoring technologies, especially ultrasonography in the late 1970s and 1980s, proved to be a powerful agent in shaping pregnancy experiences in the United States. This visual technology gave women and partners previously unavailable information about the developing fetus, and being able to "see" images of the developing fetus changed the work of expectant parenthood and raised questions about the issue of parental–fetal attachment, specifically with regard to what is known about the developing fetus and when it is known (Sandelowski & Black, 1992).

Currently, the American College of Obstetricians and Gynecologists recommends a mid-pregnancy ultrasound scan to survey the developing fetal anatomy (ACOG, 2009), and although the background risk for a fetal defect of any severity is 3%, prenatal ultrasonography is widespread in the United States (MacDorman, Munson, & Kirmeyer, 2007). Research has yet to demonstrate long-lasting effects on attachment of the expectant woman to the developing fetus after an ultrasound scan, nor is there long-lasting effect on health behaviors initiated after seeing images of the fetus. Baille, Mason, and Hewison (1997) cautioned practitioners against overinterpreting a woman's enjoyment of a scan as evidence that the scan has in fact been therapeutic or has precipitated an increase in maternal attachment to the fetus. The enjoyment of seeing images of the fetus during the second trimester anatomical exam often obscures its purpose—scanning for fetal defects—and leaves pregnant women and their families unprepared for adverse findings (Garcia et al., 2002; Lalor & Begley, 2006).

Furthermore, critics of pregnancy and childbirth technologies have described their use as fetocentric and medicalized, leaving women's experiences of pregnancy secondary to protection of the fetus from the (unlikely) threat of harm (Parry, 2006). Katz (1993) reflected enthusiastically on the modification of "bonding patterns developed over thousands of years" that occurred "within a span of a single generation" (p. 53) as a result of ultrasonography; he furthermore described new, greater emphasis on "two patients, rather than on the mother alone" (p. 54). Maher (2002) noted that visual technologies of pregnancy have served to disconnect pregnant women from their developing fetuses, and have thus "cast women as the objects rather than the subjects of their pregnancies" (Palmer, 2009, p. 67). Taken to its extreme, some states have enacted legislation (e.g., North Carolina General Statutes Women's Right to Know Act, 2011) requiring women seeking a legal abortion to have an obstetric-quality ultrasound exam at least 4 hours prior to a scheduled abortion, during which the person performing the exam is required to explain what the display is depicting and to give the woman the opportunity to hear the fetal heart tones. Legislation of this type is predicated on the assumption that the visual image of the fetus, combined with the state-mandated narration of the exam by the technologist, will invoke a response in women that will outweigh other factors that have led them to seek an abortion.

DESCRIBING AND DEFINING WOMEN'S RELATIONSHIP TO THE DEVELOPING FETUS

The construct of MFA grew out of early work by Rubin (1967a, 1967b) exploring attainment of the maternal role. In the early 1960s, Rubin took what was fundamentally an ethological approach to her research of childbearing women, identifying in both primigravidas and multiparas operations associated with assuming the maternal role: taking in; taking on; letting go; and maternal identity. Taking in and taking on both occur during pregnancy as the expectant woman's thinking about herself as a mother evolves. She mimics behaviors of other mothers and fantasizes about her expected baby and how she herself will behave as a mother. Interestingly, Rubin noted that in becoming mothers, women had to let go of previous conceptualizations of themselves, a process that required grief work to fully relinquish previous roles in order to become mothers. The development of this new self-system began during pregnancy, according to Rubin (Mercer, 1986).

Rubin's early work in describing pregnant women's psychological and emotional adjustments to expectant motherhood served as a springboard for further research on maternal adaptation processes during pregnancy. In the late 1970s and 1980s, researchers reported on the development of maternal attachment to the fetus and the kinesthetic experiences of pregnancy through which women came to know their expected infants, such as their sleep–wake cycles and personalities (Carter-Jessop, 1981; Cranley, 1981a; Cranley, 1981b; Josten, 1981; Leifer, 1977; Lumley, 1982). According to Shereshefsky and Yarrow (1973) and Leifer (1977), women's adjustment to pregnancy and the extent of their interactions and attachment to the fetus seemed to contribute to how they adapted to motherhood during the postpartum period.

Lumley (1972) described pregnant women's imagined representations of the fetus, which became increasingly "human" over the course of the pregnancy, and later described attachment as the development of a relationship with the fetus in the imagination, occurring at the point where women thought of the fetus as a person separate from themselves.

Lumley (1980) later described women's differentiation of the fetus as a "little person" after seeing the fetus via an ultrasonography. Women's conceptualization of the fetus as real grew over the course of the pregnancy, ranging from 30% experiencing this in the first trimester to 92% by the third trimester (Lumley, 1982). For families for whom pregnancy will end in loss, some appreciate the opportunity for continuing ultrasounds throughout the pregnancy; however, for other families, choosing "fetal anonymity" may be a strategy to protect and preserve oneself against the prospect of another devastating loss (Sandelowski & Black, 1992); Sandelowski and Black noted, "Resisting fetal knowledge is not the same as resisting a baby" (p. 611).

Defining Maternal–Fetal Attachment

Descriptions of maternal emotional development in relation to the fetus led to a body of work in which the concept of maternal attachment to the fetus was defined and measured. Variously known as maternal–fetal attachment, antenatal attachment, or prenatal attachment, researchers across a number of disciplines hypothesized that high levels of emotional investment in the fetus could or would positively influence the maternal–child relationship. Furthermore, antenatal emotional attachment could—theoretically—explain maternal health behaviors while pregnant; assist in understanding grief subsequent to pregnancy loss (O'Leary, 2004); and explain maternal responses during pregnancy to events such as amniocentesis, ultrasonography, and other antenatal testing (Van den Bergh & Simons, 2009).

The earliest research on the construct of MFA was by nurse Mecca Cranley (1981a), who defined MFA as "the extent to which women engage in behaviors that represent an affiliation and interaction with their unborn child" (p. 282). Cranley developed an instrument to measure MFA as a central part of her doctoral dissertation. In her definition, she assumed that the presence (and by default, absence) of specific behaviors was reflective of the extent of pregnant women's "attachment" to their fetus. The Maternal Fetal Attachment Scale (MFAS) is a 24-item (originally 37) Likert scale that has been widely used in perinatal research and has been refined over time for use at various times during pregnancy. The five original dimensions of the MFA were derived theoretically; Cranley's small sample precluded adequate factor analysis, although subsequent work by others (i.e., Müller & Ferketich, 1993; Van den Bergh & Simons, 2009) in larger samples has determined there are valid subscales. The findings of research using the MFAS were often inconclusive and sometimes contradictory (Brandon, Pitts, Denton, Stringer, & Evans, 2009), which led other researchers to redefine MFA or otherwise expand on Cranley's initial definition.

Müller found the focus of Cranley's definition of MFA on maternal behaviors to be limiting, believing instead that women's thoughts and fantasies about the developing fetus signaled a growing relationship between the woman and her expected child. In 1993, Müller published her definition of prenatal attachment as "the unique relationship that develops between a woman and her fetus. These feelings are not dependent on the feelings the woman has about herself as a pregnant person or her perception of herself as a mother" (p. 11). Müller's definition of prenatal attachment was shaped by her secondary analysis of interview data collected by Mercer et al. (1988), which she noted included nonbehavior words such as *wish*, *hope*, and *imagine* (Brandon et al., 2009). Müller subsequently developed the Prenatal Attachment Inventory (PAI) of 29 items designed to measure "affectionate attachment" (Brandon et al., 2009).

In 1993, Condon published his version of a scale to measure MFA. The 19-item Maternal Antenatal Attachment Scale (MAAS) was designed to focus entirely on women's thoughts and feelings about the developing fetus, and not on their attitudes or feelings toward the pregnancy experience or maternal role, which he thought were shortcomings of the MFAS and PAI. The MAAS had two factors—quality and intensity—that Condon conceptualized as perpendicular constructs, the intersection of which formed four quadrants: strong or healthy attachment; positive attachment/low preoccupation; uninvolved or ambivalent with low preoccupation; and preoccupation characterized by anxiety, ambivalence, or lack of affect (Brandon et al., 2009).

Despite shortcomings in the conceptual underpinnings of MFA, researchers and clinicians remain interested in the idea that attachments are created during pregnancy and that they can be measured and possibly influenced. Alhusen and colleagues at Johns Hopkins University have used the MFAS in recent research on maternal attachment and infant developmental outcomes in low-income urban women (Alhusen, Gross, Hayat, Rose, & Sharps, 2012; Alhusen, Gross, Hayat, Woods, & Sharps, 2012; Alhusen, Hayat, & Gross, 2013). Importantly, however, Van den Bergh and Simons (2009), in their review of measures of attachment in the prenatal period, suggested that because of the lack of reciprocity between the pregnant woman and fetus, the concept of attachment in this context is an incorrect use of Bowlby's and Ainsworth's definition of attachment. Furthermore, the various measures of the maternal–fetal/antenatal/prenatal attachment construct are inadequate to explore representations of attachment that are less tangible than overt behaviors (Van den Bergh & Simons, 2009).

Questions of Attachment After a Severe Fetal Diagnosis

The diagnosis of a severe (life-limiting or clearly lethal) fetal defect poses challenges to expectant parents, whose hopes, dreams, and plans for their expected baby are challenged by the threat of severe disability and death. The question of prenatal attachment, one that is difficult to answer even when the fetus is deemed healthy, becomes especially problematic when pregnancy is likely to end in stillbirth or death soon after birth. McKechnie, Pridham, and Tluczek (2014) described three distinct parental trajectories of relating to the impaired fetus: (a) claiming the child as one's own; (b) delaying connection to the fetus; and (c) doing the routine of pregnancy. The underlying assumption of this work was that the transition to parenthood and the formation of the parent–child relationship begin during pregnancy, and that a severe fetal diagnosis "poses threats to a psychologically healthy transition to parenthood and to the parent-child relationship that begins before birth" (p. 1). Claiming the child as one's own paralleled for some parents Rubin's "binding-in" stage, when an expectant mother formed an emotional tie with the developing fetus. McKechnie, Pridham, and Tluczek (2014) argued that some expectant parents demonstrated "prenatal commitment and attachment" to their expected child with congenital defects, which may in turn "promote higher-quality, adaptive parenting for a child requiring special care" (p. 13). Expectant parents who delayed forming attachments to their severely impaired fetus "derailed many aspects of the initial stage of becoming a parent and could be considered counter to the development of parental caregiving" (p. 13), which could in turn lead to less sensitive parenting of an infant with congenital anomalies (McKechnie, Pridham, & Tluczek, 2014).

An alternative explanation for delaying attachment may arise from grief theory. From a grief perspective, becoming a parent as a task of pregnancy may be overridden by the "inherently disorganizing/disorienting" nature of grief (Thomson, 2010) when an expected child is diagnosed with a severe defect. Neimeyer, Holland, Currier, and Mehta (2008) described grief as "a struggle to reaffirm or reconstruct a world of meaning that has been challenged by loss" (p. 270). Pregnancy itself is a development stage and life event characterized by its own reorganizing features, and includes profound shifts in identity, roles, and behaviors. Notably, Rubin (1967a) described grief work as fundamental to childbearing, even if the baby is healthy. Drawing from Lindemann's definition of "grief work," Rubin described the grief work associated with childbearing as the review "in memory, of the attachments and associated events of a former self" (p. 243) as a function of what she referred to as the "taking in" of the role of mother for the first time or for subsequent children.

NARRATIVES FROM THREE EXPECTANT FAMILIES WITH A SEVERE FETAL DIAGNOSIS

The complexities of the human experience are especially profound when childbearing is complicated by grief. Health care providers in perinatal settings must avoid overly simplistic explanations for responses and behaviors of expectant parents when their hopes and dreams of a healthy infant vanish in the wake of a diagnosis of a severe fetal defect. From two ethnographic studies[1] with the families under these circumstances, wide variation was found in responses across families and even between partners as they worked to make sense of the diagnosis and the impending death of their expected infant and to live into a future deeply changed by their experience of perinatal loss. Here are three examples of families whose similarities stop at the diagnosis of a severe fetal defect; it is difficult to argue, however, that any one of these responses is more or less adaptive or healthy. Although identifying details including names have been altered, the meanings of these families' stories remain intact.

Juanita and Julio

Juanita (20) and Julio (28) were a married Latino couple with a healthy 2-year-old daughter Carla. Juanita stayed at home to care for Carla; Julio worked as a brick mason during the week and as a pastor at a small local church on the weekends. Their income was less than $15,000 per year. Juanita had the equivalent of a sixth-grade education, while Julio was a high school graduate. During Juanita's 20-week ultrasound scan of fetal anatomy, her obstetrician discovered that the male fetus had anencephaly. For Juanita and Julio, the prospect of limited time with their baby intensified their attachment to him. They responded in terms of being both denied their baby and holding on to him. Juanita described her initial response:

> Sentía como que, al instante cuando me dijeron que. . . más cuando me dijeron que mi bebé no iba a sobrevivir desde ahí me lo estaban quitando. [*I felt like, at the moment when they told me that. . .when they told me that my baby wasn't going to survive, from that moment they were taking him away from me.*]

After deciding to continue her pregnancy despite the dire diagnosis, she noted:

> Pues, uh, ¿cómo le puedo decir? En estos momentos pues no sé qué, siento algo bonito verdá' que tengo a mi bebé, pero también tengo en mente que no va a durar mucho conmigo y trato de disfrutar más de este momento. [*I really feel, well, how do I tell you this? I guess it's just, I feel like I know that uh, I, there's something very beautiful about having my child with me right now and I know it is not going to last very long . . . so I just try to, to enjoy it as much as I can now.*]

Julio compared their feelings toward their expected baby with what they felt during their first pregnancy when the fetus was normal:

> Pues un poco, por causa de que sabíamos de que lo que iba a pasar, aunque tratábamos de tenerlo con más, con más este, con más amor, tratábamos de. . ." [*Well, this time knowing what we did know about was going to happen, I think this time we tried to have a little bit of more love for [the baby]. . .*]

When their hope for a healthy baby was denied to them, this couple responded by cherishing what time they had with their expected son, and being purposeful in loving him. Similarly, Juanita described the intentionality of caring more for her daughter as a result of the death of their son:

> Pues la verdad sí, este, yo me siento de todo lo que pasó y todo esto me, me ayudó mucho también. . . saber, o sea, más de la vida, más como poder cuidar a los hijos que Dios nos da, como Carla que ya está conmigo que debo cuidarla más. [*Well, the truth is, yes uh, I do feel everything that happened and all this has, has helped me a great deal too. . . to know, I mean, more about life, more about how to take care of the children that God gives us, like Carla, who is already with me, that I must take care of her more.*]

Juanita and Julio described much of their experience in terms of feelings about their baby, who had an unequivocally lethal condition, and their healthy toddler. This is in contrast to the following couple, who described their experience in terms of behaviors.

Michelle and William

Michelle (24) and William (26), a White married couple expecting their first child, described being intentional in creating their family prior to the birth of their son, who, like Juanita and Julio's son, was diagnosed mid-pregnancy with anencephaly. Michelle had a 2-year associate degree and William was in graduate school to become a counselor. They lived in student housing and had an annual income of $24,000. William described their activities as more purposeful than had their son Justin been healthy:

> We're going to concerts and taking pictures and making as many memories as possible. You know, treating it even more so than we might have, you know, if we were just waiting for him to come. Just thinking of like family events that we can do 'cause she's a mom and I'm a dad even though baby Justin is not doing so well.

After their son's birth, Michelle described what the remainder of her pregnancy was like:

> Well, throughout the pregnancy, we did special things, as if he were like any other baby, and, you know, we raised him. So we did things like, we went apple picking in the mountains, which our family does every year, and we want to make that our family tradition as well. So, um, we just got the idea from a friend to just do things you would normally do. . . .Just to think of, like, you know, enjoying him while he's here instead of, you know, focusing so much on, like, what's to come.

Michelle and William focused on an "as if" quality to the pregnancy but with more intensity than they thought they would have had without getting the lethal diagnosis. Their pregnancy and grief discourse was characterized by detailed descriptions of activities that they did, rather than how they felt, in living out what they understood was to be a "short life" for their son Justin, who was stillborn at term. Michelle created an elaborate digital scrapbook detailing the pregnancy, birth, and memorial service; Michelle and William planned to share this scrapbook with their next child, so he or she would "know their older brother."

Susan

Susan was a 41-year-old White single woman who entered the study after terminating her first pregnancy at 19 weeks when the physical condition of the male fetus diagnosed with trisomy 21 and severe hydrops deteriorated precipitously. Susan had a graduate degree, was employed full time in a tech industry, and had an annual income of $140,000. She was engaged to her long-term partner Dennis, who, because of his frequent work-related travel, did not participate in the study. Within 6 months of the pregnancy termination, she unexpectedly became pregnant with identical female twins. During the second pregnancy, she described her efforts to take care of herself for the sake of the developing twins, and also explained her guarded emotional response with regard to the pregnancy:

> Here's how I have dealt with things, sometimes I can just shut it down. Like, try to, and I don't know if it's really good or not, it's called stuffing, I guess, so you just push it down, you just don't even think about it, like just don't think about it, so you know, with the babies, I am just trying to think about right now so I eat what I can, I can sleep, I can go to the doctor, and I've got the best care right now.

When Susan was asked specifically about her feelings toward the developing twins, she responded:

> I don't know when the bonding starts. I think the bonding may start, I mean to me it seems like it's logical that the bonding would start after they're born and, not that I'm not bonding with them, I mean I'm carrying them, but it's just not the same, like I'm not interacting with them directly. Right now I can't really see their faces and I can't see their personalities because I know that's going to be a lot of their essence and who they are and what they do, and how they respond, and how they act, and just that whole, um, that whole process.

Interestingly, she described her tempered excitement as being a response to the sex of the twins:

> I don't want to be too excited about the girls because that feels disrespectful to that first baby because it was a boy. . .in a way I feel guilty for saying that because I feel like that was disrespectful of the other child. Because it was a boy and you know, it didn't happen.

Susan had frequent ultrasounds because of the concern of twin-to-twin transfusion. Although this did not occur, she found herself "overly concerned with a millimeter and a half"—the difference in head circumferences between the developing twins. Susan recognized that her concern was magnified by her age, the previous fetal diagnosis and loss, and "the sheer miracle of identical twins." In her effort to protect the twins, she asked to forego the final interview of the study because, "I only think of him [the previous baby] when you are here, and I don't want to feel sadness unnecessarily because it may not be good for the girls." She worked to both "stuff" her concern over the current pregnancy and to avoid negative thoughts and sadness associated with the first pregnancy that may impinge on the well-being of the twins she was expecting.

Best Intentions and Deep Commitment

Parents narratives were characterized by their intentional efforts in addressing the likely death of their expected baby. Despite their divergent stories and life circumstances, they each made conscious decisions in terms of how they related to their expected infants: by increasing their love for the baby; by participating in planned family activities prior to the birth; and by taking care of oneself while holding back full emotional investment until after birth. There is little doubt that each of these persons was deeply committed to their expected child/children; however, it is unlikely that the depth of their various forms of commitment could be described and measured through the definitions and tools described in this chapter. Idiosyncratic and intimate, these families' responses were contextually and culturally located in ways that make simple measurement of the elusive construct of prenatal attachment impossible. At worst, researchers and clinicians alike risk reducing the exceptional complexity of grief in the context of childbirth to a measurable, singular construct.

CONCLUSION

Examining questions of grief and bereavement always involves gaining access to the inner lives of persons when they are most vulnerable. When grief and bereavement result from pregnancy loss, the expectant woman, her partner, and family are at an especially sensitive and vulnerable place in their lives. For many couples, future childbearing becomes uncertain and the size and constitution of their planned family may no longer be possible. How they interact with their current and future children may be affected by the loss; however, for other families, the loss may be intense at the moment but the long-term effects of the loss may be minimal.

Maternal–fetal/prenatal attachment as a construct and a measure offers only limited understanding of the complicated dimensions of women and their partners as they begin to form their relationship during pregnancy with their expected child. There is little doubt that in most cases expectant parents form some element of commitment to the expected child, and the death of the expected child leaves the parents bereft and grieving, experiencing what Parkes called "the price we pay for love."

The narratives of parents provide some of the clearest insights into the meanings of birth accompanied by death that no measure can aspire to capture. In *An Exact Replica of a Figment of My Imagination*, author Elizabeth McCracken (2008) created the memoir of her son Pudding's stillbirth and her subsequent pregnancy within a year that resulted in the birth of her second son Gus. McCracken ends her account: "It's a happy life, but someone is missing. It's a happy life, *and* someone is missing. It's a happy life" (p. 184).

NOTE

1. The author acknowledges these funding sources: National Institute of Nursing Research, NIH; Grant No. 1R21NR011487-01A1. End-of-Life Care After Severe Fetal Diagnosis. Building Interdisciplinary Research Careers in Women's Health (BIRCWH); NICHD-NIH; Grant No. K12

HD01441. Mentored Clinical Scholars grant: Perinatal Care Options Study; M. Sandelowski, PhD, RN, FAAN, mentor. Perinatal Care Options Study—Spanish version. University of North Carolina at Chapel Hill Junior Faculty Development Award, IBM Fund.

CASE STUDY

Maria is a 40-year-old single woman with a career in advertising who became pregnant unexpectedly. She attended all of the scheduled prenatal visits but refused ultrasound exams until near term, when her midwife became concerned about the lack of fetal growth between visits. The ultrasound revealed that the fetus was not moving much, the placenta was calcified, and the amniotic fluid was decreased. Maria was counseled to have a cesarean section right away, but she refused. Two days later, she noticed that she had not felt fetal movement for several hours. She called her midwife and then went to the local hospital, where no fetal heart tones were heard. Fetal death was confirmed by ultrasound.

FOCUS QUESTIONS

1. Do you think that Maria's actions early in the pregnancy should concern a health care provider? Why or why not?
2. Describe what you think her actions mean in terms of maternal–fetal attachment.
3. What questions should Maria's providers ask of her regarding her response to the fetal death?

REFERENCES

ACOG Committee on Practice. (2009). Ultrasonography in pregnancy. *Obstetrics and Gynecology, 113,* 451–461.

Ainsworth, M. D. S., & Bowlby, J. (1991). An ethological approach to personality development. *American Psychologist, 46,* 333–341.

Alhusen, J. L., Gross, D., Hayat, M. J., Rose, L., & Sharps, P. (2012). The role of mental health on maternal-fetal attachment in low-income women. *JOGNN: Journal of Obstetric, Gynecologic and Neonatal Nursing, 41,* E71–E81.

Alhusen, J. L., Gross, D., Hayat, M. J., Woods, A. B., & Sharps, P. W. (2012). The influence of maternal-fetal attachment and health practices on neonatal outcomes in low-income, urban women. *Research in Nursing & Health, 35,* 112–120.

Alhusen, J. L., Hayat, M. J., & Gross, D. (2013). A longitudinal study of maternal attachment and infant development outcomes. *Archives of Women's Mental Health, 26,* 521–529.

Baille, C., Mason, G. & Hewison, J. (1997). Scanning for pleasure. *British Journal of Obstetrics and Gynaecology, 104,* 1223–1224.

Brandon, A. R., Pitts, S., Denton, W. H., Stringer, C. A., & Evans, H. M. (2009). A history of the theory of prenatal attachment. *Journal of Prenatal and Perinatal Psychology and Health, 23*(4), 201–222.

Carter-Jessop, L. (1981). Promoting maternal attachment through prenatal intervention. *MCN, The American Journal of Maternal Child Nursing, 6,* 107–112.

Condon, J. T. (1993). The assessment of antenatal emotional attachment: Development of a questionnaire instrument. *British Journal of Medical Psychology, 66,* 167–183.

Cranley, M. S. (1981a). Development of a tool for the measurement of maternal attachment during pregnancy. *Nursing Research, 30,* 281–284.

Cranley, M. S. (1981b). Roots of attachment: The relationship of parents with their unborn. *Birth Defects: Original Article Series, 17*(6), 59–83.

DiPietro, J. A. (2010). Psychological and psychophysiological considerations regarding the maternal-fetal relationship. *Infant and Child Development, 19,* 27–38.

Eyer, D. E. (1992). *Maternal-infant bonding: A scientific fiction.* New Haven, CT: Yale University Press.

Garcia, J., Bricker, L., Henderson, J., Martin, M-A., Mugford, M., Nielson, J., & Roberts, T. (2002). Women's views of pregnancy ultrasound: A systematic review. *Birth, 29*(4), 225–250.

Josten, L. (1981). Prenatal assessment guide for illuminating possible problems with parenting. *MCN, The American Journal of Maternal Child Nursing, 6,* 113–117.

Katz, V. (1993). Obstetric ultrasound: An overview. In J. W. Sparling (Ed.), *Concepts in fetal movement research* (pp. 53–76) [Kindle version]. Binghamton, NY: Haworth Press. Retrieved from Amazon.com

Kennell, M. H., & Klaus, J. H. (1976). *Maternal-infant bonding: The impact of early separation or loss on family development.* St. Louis, MO: Mosby.

Lalor, J., & Begley, C. (2006). Fetal anomaly screening: What do women *want* to know? *Journal of Advanced Nursing, 55*(11), 11–19.

Leifer, M. (1977). Psychological changes accompanying pregnancy and motherhood. *Genetic Psychology Monographs, 95,* 55–96.

Lumley, J. M. (1972). The development of maternal–fetal bonding in first pregnancy. Third International Congress, Psychosomatic Medicine in Obstetrics and Gynaecology. Conference proceedings, London, UK.

Lumley, J. M. (1980). Through a glass darkly: Ultrasound and prenatal bonding. *Birth, 17,* 214–217.

Lumley, J. M. (1982). Attitudes to the fetus among primigravidae. *Australian Paediatric Journal, 18,* 106–109.

MacDorman, M. F., Munson, M. L., & Kirmeyer, S. (2007). Fetal and perinatal mortality, United States, 2004. *CDC National Vital Statistics Reports, 56*(3), 1–19.

Maher, J. (2002). Visibly pregnant: Toward a placental body. *Feminist Review, 72,* 95–107.

McCracken, E. (2008). *An exact replica of a figment of my imagination: A memoir.* New York, NY: Little, Brown and Company.

McKechnie, A. C., Pridham, K., & Tluczek, A. (2014). Preparing heart and mind for becoming a parent following a diagnosis of fetal anomaly. *Qualitative Health Research,* 1–17. doi: 10.1177/1049732314553852

Mercer, R. (1986). *First-time motherhood: Experiences from teens to forties.* New York, NY: Springer Publishing Co.

Mercer, R. T., Ferketich, S., DeJoseph, J., May, K., & Sollid, D. (1988). Further exploration of maternal and paternal fetal attachment. *Research in Nursing & Health, 11*(4), 269–278.

Müller, M. E., & Ferketich, S. (1993). Factor analysis of the Maternal Fetal Attachment Scale. *Nursing Research, 42*(3), 144–147.

Neimeyer, R. A., Holland, J. M., Currier, J. M., & Mehta, T. (2008). Meaning reconstruction in later life: Toward a cognitive-constructivist approach to grief therapy. In A. Steffan, L. Thompson, & D. Gallagher-Thompson (Eds.), *Handbook of behavioral and cognitive therapies with older adults* (pp. 264–277). New York, NY: Springer.

North Carolina General Statutes House Bill 854/S.L.2011-405 (=S769). (2011). Women's Right to Know Act. Retrieved from ncleg.net

O'Leary, J. (2004). Grief and its impact on prenatal attachment in the subsequent pregnancy. *Archives of Women's Mental Health, 7,* 7–18.

Palmer, J. (2009). The placental body in 4D: Everyday practices of non-diagnostic sonography. *Feminist Review, 93,* 64–80.

Parkes, C. T. (2006). Dangerous words. *Bereavement Care, 26*(2), 23–25.

Parkes, C. T. (2015). *The price of love: The selected works of Colin Murray Parkes (World Library of Mental Health)* [Kindle version]. London, UK: Routledge. Retrieved from Amazon.com

Parry, D. C. (2006). Women's lived experiences with pregnancy and midwifery in a medicalized and fetocentric context: Six short stories. *Qualitative Inquiry, 12,* 459–471.

Rothman, B. K. (n.d.). Retrieved from www.barbarakatzrothman.com

Rubin, R. (1967a). Attainment of the maternal role: Part I. Processes. *Nursing Research, 16*(3), 237–245.

Rubin, R. (1967b). Attainment of the maternal role: Part II. Models and referents. *Nursing Research, 16*(4), 342–346.

Rubin, R. (1975). Maternal tasks in pregnancy. *MCN, The American Journal of Maternal Child Nursing, 4,* 143–153.

Sandelowski, M., & Black, B. P. (1992). The epistemology of expectant parenthood. *Western Journal of Nursing Research, 16,* 601–622. doi:10.1177/019394599401600602.

Shereshefsky, P. M., & Yarrow, L. J. (1973). *Psychological aspects of a first pregnancy and early postnatal adaptation.* New York, NY: Raven Press.

Thomson, P. (2010). Loss and disorganization from an attachment perspective. *Death Studies, 34,* 893–914.

Van den Bergh, B., & Simons, A. (2009). A review of scales to measure the mother–fetus relationship. *Journal of Reproductive and Infant Psychology, 27*(2), 114–126.

CHAPTER 5

The Pushing On Theory of Maternal Perinatal Bereavement

Patricia Moyle Wright

In this chapter, the Pushing On theory (POT) of maternal perinatal bereavement is presented within the context of the extant literature on women's experiences of pregnancy loss. The POT is a substantive theory developed through grounded theory research. The core category, pushing on, describes how perinatally bereaved women move beyond their grief and ultimately integrate pregnancy loss into their lives. The other six categories of experiencing the pregnancy, losing the baby, bearing the burden, working it through, coming to terms, and living a changed life describe various dimensions of the process of perinatal bereavement. It should be noted that the author has changed some of the wording from the original study to clarify concepts and to reflect her more recent thinking as the field of perinatal bereavement and her understanding of the process have evolved.

Pregnancy loss is a deeply personal experience that has not been recognized historically as a life-changing event. However, with the dawning of the women's movement, the deafening silence about pregnancy loss was broken as women began to feel more empowered to talk about their own life experiences, particularly those that were uniquely female experiences. They found that sharing their stories of loss with others created an environment of support and understanding, particularly among other women who shared the same history. Such close personal networks later evolved into formal groups in which women could support other women through their grief (Carlson, Lammert, & O'Leary, 2011). In this way, pregnancy loss came to be viewed as a unique experience that could be understood best by other bereaved women. To some extent, this viewpoint still permeates the literature on maternal perinatal bereavement.

The value of this point of view is that women's voices have not been usurped; instead, the scientific inquiry around this human experience has steadily increased. Indeed, most of the foundational research in this area has been qualitative, and has honored the unique perspectives of bereaved women. The work of pioneers such as Hutti (1986), Limbo and Vinge (1990), Swanson-Kauffman (1986), and Toedter, Lasker, and Alhadeff (1988) validated perinatal loss as a legitimate branch of mainstream grief studies. Their work and that of many others helped propel the field from clusters of personal stories with common themes to an evidence-based body of literature that informs our understanding of what this type of grief is like and how grieving women can be best supported.

Research conducted over the past three decades has broken new ground to elucidate various dimensions of the multifaceted and extremely complicated process of this form of human grief. For example, the association between pregnancy loss and negative psychoemotional variables indicates women often experience depression (Toffol, Koponen, & Partonen, 2013; van den Akker, 2011), anxiety (Murphy, Shevlin, & Elklit, 2014), altered family and social relationships (Kagami et al., 2012; Sutan & Miskam, 2012; van den Akker, 2011), and emotional and physical symptoms of grief (Barr & Cacciatore, 2008; Fenstermacher, 2014; St. John, Cooke, & Goopy, 2006) after pregnancy loss. Mediating factors include religiosity (Cowchock, Lasker, Toedter, Skumanich, & Koenig, 2010; Mann, Mannan, Quiñones, Palmer, & Torres, 2010), a strong spousal or partner relationship (Mann et al., 2010), social support (Cacciatore, Schnebly, & Froen, 2009), and time (Bennett, Litz, Maguen, & Ehrenreich, 2008). There is conflicting evidence on the influence of gestational age, previous live birth, and the length of time women are affected by the loss (Wright, 2011). Knowledge of the factors that influence women's responses to pregnancy loss has helped to enlighten scholars regarding what grieving women feel and the emotional struggles they face.

Several theories have been used to help explain maternal perinatal bereavement. For example, Swanson's (1991) theory of caring, Lazarus and Folkman's (1984) theory of stress, and Hogan's grief to personal growth theory (Hogan & Schmidt, 2002) have all been empirically tested for fit with good results (Jansson & Adolfsson, 2011; Sansoni & Giaquinto, 2001; Swanson, 2000). The natural progression of the excellent empirical and theoretical work that has been done in the field of perinatal bereavement should lead to the development of theories specifically designed to provide a comprehensive understanding of the entire process of maternal perinatal bereavement. Such theories can provide a roadmap of sorts, explaining what is involved in perinatal loss, how women and their loved ones might react, how relationships might change, and what outcomes can be expected. Such knowledge should be clinically useful in developing support interventions and services and in determining when women have turned a corner from a typical grief trajectory to a crisis.

Sometimes, theories can be constructed using the extant literature. However, the state of the science in the field of perinatal bereavement has not been conducive to this approach due to wide variations in the types of research conducted, instruments used, recruitment parameters, and inconsistent use of terms to define pregnancy or perinatal loss (Wright, 2011). In such instances, the grounded theory method can provide a means to develop theories that are rooted in the words of those who have lived the experience. The grounded theory method, when applied to specific life circumstances, can lead to the discovery of a substantive theory (Glaser & Strauss, 1967). A substantive theory is a midrange theory that is expected to be a good fit for clinical practice because it is grounded in the words of those who have lived the experience (Benoliel, 2001; Glaser, 1992).

One such theory, the POT was developed through grounded theory research with 19 perinatally bereaved women (Wright, 2010). It provides a comprehensive understanding of women's experiences of pregnancy loss. The six categories discovered through grounded theory inquiry describe how women navigate the processes of experiencing the pregnancy, losing the baby, bearing the burden, working it through, coming to terms, and living a changed life. The overarching experience, or the core category, as it is called in grounded theory language, was named "pushing on" because it describes the main action in the theory (Glaser, 1998). Pushing on captures women's struggle to move beyond the shock and grief inherent in their loss. This chapter is structured according to the categories of the POT. Current literature related to each category is incorporated and clinical implications are discussed. The chapter also offers a comparison of the POT with two other models of perinatal grief. The chapter concludes with a discussion of the POT and implications for further research.

PUSHING ON

The process of pushing on—that is, women's determination to continue on despite their pain—inherently involves work and conscious effort (Wright, 2010). This overarching core category indicates that women have to actively push themselves through the pain of loss and to re-engage in life, a finding consistent with other research indicating recovery from bereavement is an active process that involves engagement and effort (Freud, 1917/1957; Hogan, Morse, & Tasón, 1996; Hogan & Schmidt, 2002; Worden, 2002). Worden's (2002) work is particularly similar in that it indicates that bereaved individuals must work through distinct tasks to move beyond the most difficult parts of the grief process. However, the POT does not designate specific tasks the griever must undertake. Rather, experiences that are common among women in the process of maternal perinatal bereavement are highlighted and seen as milestones along the way. The specific barriers that a woman must push through vary according to each person's unique circumstances, but the overall movement, according to the POT, should be in a forward direction with the bereaved mother mustering enough energy and strength at various points to overcome her pain, whether this pain is the shock and angst associated with getting the news of the loss, or the pain associated with the re-emergence of grief on the anniversary of the loss years later.

According to the POT, there are many painful milestones along the path of maternal perinatal bereavement; it is the ability of the bereaved mother to muster the inner resources to push beyond the pain that determines what combination of possible outcomes she will experience. The POT illustrates that women push on when facing signs of loss and try to maintain hope; they push on when faced with the news of the baby's death and even try to support others. Eventually, they are able to propel themselves beyond their grief by taking the initiative to reach out for support and to overcome feelings of isolation. Even many years after the loss, when women experience periods of regrieving, they continue to push themselves beyond their pain through distraction, through the use of ritual, or by relying on faith traditions for comfort (Wright, 2010). In essence, pushing on is the manifestation of the griever's determination to survive the loss and live on despite the pain, integrating the loss into the fabric of their lives. Pushing on is evident in each category of the theory, as discussed in the following sections.

THE PROCESS OF MATERNAL PERINATAL BEREAVEMENT

According to the POT, there are seven components of the experience of perinatal bereavement. The first component is the core category, pushing on. Pushing on refers to the innate resilience of the bereaved mother that provides forward momentum through the grief process and is also evident in the other six components: experiencing the pregnancy, losing the baby, bearing the burden, working it through, coming to terms, and living a changed life. These components can be viewed as stages. Stage theories, in contrast to phase models, "posit discrete transitions from one kind of behavior and form of existence to another" (Williams, 2003, p. 273). Although grief is messy, complex, and difficult to adequately capture in writing or in a model, the strength of a stage model is that is presupposes that the grief trajectory progresses in an orderly fashion (Maciejewski, Zhang, Block, & Prigerson, 2007). Stage models have been widely accepted by clinicians because these models allow for the identification of normal grief trajectories. When normal grief trajectories can be identified, those who need greater support can be identified and referred to a specialist for further follow-up (Maciejewski et al., 2007).

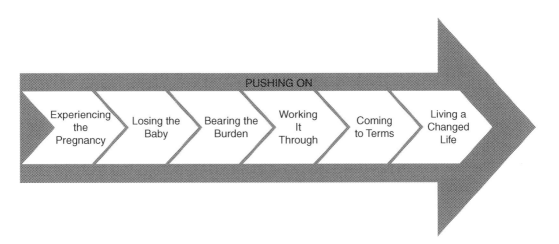

FIGURE 5.1 The Pushing On theory.

The POT includes six distinct stages that were identified through the grounded theory process. The processes within each stage may occur all at once, in an orderly fashion, or not at all for some women. However, the basic process of maternal perinatal bereavement, as depicted in Figure 5.1, includes the major turning points in the process of maternal perinatal bereavement, as described by women who have lived the experience (Wright, 2010). In the following sections, each of the stages is presented in chronological order to help organize the experience in an understandable way, knowing that the actual human experience may be much less organized and circumscriptive.

Experiencing the Pregnancy

The process of maternal perinatal bereavement begins with the experience of the pregnancy, the moment in time when women note the transition from pregnancy as a possibility to pregnancy as a reality. Factors that influence the pregnancy experience have been discussed in the literature, including history of previous pregnancy loss (Ockhuijsen, van den Hoogen, Boivin, Macklon, & de Boer, 2014), HIV status (Sanders, 2008), adolescent pregnancy (Black, Fleming, & Rome, 2012), and unplanned pregnancy (Gray, 2014). Like grief, the experience of pregnancy is influenced by numerous factors. Thus, it is important to note that the experience of pregnancy, as described in the POT, was derived from interviews with women who, for the most part, planned and wanted their pregnancies. Their experiences of pregnancy loss likely differed from the experiences of women who did not plan the pregnancy, had extenuating circumstances such as chronic disease, or experienced a crisis pregnancy. Experiencing the pregnancy, as described in the POT, involved three main dimensions: finding out about the pregnancy, developing a relationship, and prenatal mothering.

Finding out about the pregnancy was a moment in time that was crystallized in the women's memory and elicited myriad emotions such as relief, fear, ambivalence, anger, and others. Women's reactions to getting news of a pregnancy can be influenced by many factors including previous infertility, previous loss, number of living children, perceived financial stability, perceived ability to care for a child, and relationship status. Once the pregnancy is confirmed, a complex process of accepting or rejecting the pregnancy ensues. According to the POT, if the pregnancy is accepted and the woman commits to continuing the pregnancy, she begins to think that the pregnancy will end with a live birth, and she begins to form an emotional attachment to the anticipated baby (Wright, 2010).

Developing a relationship occurs through coming to know the baby by seeing ultrasound images, hearing sounds of the baby's heartbeat, and feeling fetal movement (Black, 1992; Righetti, Dell'Avanzo, Grigio, & Nicolini, 2005). Women commonly choose names and describe getting to know their babies' personalities. If the baby responds to her mother's voice or movement, the mother feels she is coming to know her baby, and that the baby is also coming to know her. Once a woman feels that an emotional connection has been formed between herself and her baby, she begins to develop the attributes of a mother, taking deliberate steps to ensure her baby's well-being (Wright, 2010).

Wright (2010) used the term *prenatal mothering* to describe the actions women take to ensure the safety and health of their babies. Women who are engaged in prenatal mothering are concerned about the effects of their own diets on their babies, take prenatal vitamins, keep prenatal appointments, record kick counts, and take steps to learn about maintaining a healthy pregnancy. Some researchers have described a similar process of "prenatal motherhood" (O'Leary, Warland, & Parker, 2011), which involves "a mother's intuitive knowledge of her baby" (p. 218) and facilitates protective behaviors.

Women routinely monitor their own physical symptoms during pregnancy (Wright, 2010). While self-monitoring is a normal and routine part of the pregnancy experience, it is often fueled by anxiety, which is also a normal part of the pregnancy experience (Theodorou & Spyrou, 2013). As a mother's level of anxiety increases, so too does the amount of her self-monitoring and the need to more frequent reassurance that the pregnancy is progressing well. This increased anxiety is especially true for women who experienced a prior loss because they often experience higher levels of anxiety during a subsequent pregnancy (Hutti, Armstrong, & Myers, 2011; Mills et al., 2014). Thus, it appears that women's internal drive to monitor a pregnancy occurs on a spectrum, with women who experienced a previous loss on the more extreme end. Diligent monitoring of the pregnancy sometimes allows women to recognize signs of trouble, but not always. The next stage of the POT, losing the baby, involves women's experiences of the actual loss.

Losing the Baby

Prior to confirmation that the loss had occurred, some women notice signs of trouble. They turn to a trusted person, such as a spouse, friend, or coworker, to help them interpret the signs. The response that they receive from the other person helps them to gauge the severity of their symptoms and determine whether it is time to contact a health care provider. Women also try to interpret the nonverbal communication of health care providers during appointments to determine whether the pregnancy is progressing well or if there is cause for alarm. For example, one woman in Wright's (2010) study explained, "The [ultrasound] technician . . . seemed very grumpy" and thought, "Well, . . . if she thought one of my babies had died, she wouldn't be grumpy" (Wright, 2010, p. 52). This example illustrates women's ability to remain hopeful until the news of the loss is actually delivered.

Getting the news of the loss from a health care provider is a moment crystallized in women's memories. Women can recall what the doctor was wearing, the tone of voice used, and other minute details. At that moment, women experience numbness, shock, and detachment (Rillstone & Hutchinson, 2001; Wright, 2010), which are common responses to the loss of a loved one (Hogan & DeSantis, 1992, 1996; Hogan et al., 1996; Lindemann, 1994). The protective cocoon of blunted emotions does not last very long, however, and women are quickly jarred into bearing the emotional and physical burden of the loss.

Bearing the Burden

The burdens involved in perinatal loss are numerous and occur over a period of time after the loss. One of the first burdens women encounter is being asked to make decisions about whether they want to hold the baby, have photos taken, obtain hand prints and footprints, and note who should be in the room. Women often feel overwhelmed by these choices because they are still reeling from the shock of the loss (Wright, 2010).

Slowly, the emotional burdens of the loss take hold and can include feelings of profound sadness, depression, crying, inability to sleep, lethargy, anger, self-blame, complicated grief, questioning why the loss occurred, and increased fear of death (Barr & Cacciatore, 2008; Kersting & Wagner, 2012; Sutan & Miskam, 2012; van den Akker, 2011; Wright, 2010). A potential for posttraumatic stress disorders has also been identified (Christiansen, Elklit, & Olff, 2013; Murphy et al., 2014). Intrusivity, the intrusion of unbidden thoughts into one's consciousness (Hogan, Greenfield, & Schmidt, 2001), is a component of posttraumatic stress disorder and is also a common experience after a loss. Intrusivity often plagues women after pregnancy loss and contributes to their emotional distress (Wright, 2010). Another aspect of perinatal bereavement that was particularly distressing was having to share the news of the loss with others.

Sharing the news of the loss was most often interconnected with comforting others (Wright, 2010). One woman described this feeling, saying, "I just felt like the burden was constantly on me, to make other people comfortable" (Wright, 2010, p. 58). Likewise, Wojnar, Swanson, and Adolfsson (2011) noted that sharing the news of the loss was a very difficult aspect of loss, which they referred to in their conceptual model as "going public." Although comforting others was considered burdensome by bereaved women, in the long run, supporting others may be helpful (Kaunonen, Tarkka, Paunonen, & Laippala, 1999) because sharing the pain of grief can lead to closer relationships with others (Avelin, Rådestad, Säflund, Wredling, & Erlandsson, 2013).

However, not all aspects of perinatal grief can be shared with others. For example, women reported physical symptoms such as phantom kicks, somnolence, a physical aching in the arms to hold a baby, and lactation in the weeks and months following the loss (Wright, 2010). In another study (Fenstermacher, 2014), lactation after pregnancy loss was described as "horrific" and the "worst pain ever" (p. 138). Physical manifestations of grief are an emerging area of study (Gudmundsdottir, 2009), but it seems clear that for perinatally bereaved women, physical symptoms of grief are complicated by recovery from both the pregnancy and the loss.

Physical healing after pregnancy loss occurs over a predictable period of time, but the amount of time that women's lives are disrupted by emotional symptoms of grief varies. Generally, women who experienced late pregnancy loss noted that they had moved beyond the worst of the pain by approximately 9 to 12 months after the loss, and those who experienced early pregnancy loss reported reaching this turning point sooner, by 3 to 6 months after the loss (Wright, 2010). However, findings regarding the length of time a woman may experience emotional distress after pregnancy loss are conflicting (Wright, 2011). In time, however, women recognize the toll grief takes on their lives and they take deliberate steps to work through the pain.

Working It Through

Working through the pain of grief takes time and effort. For those who experience pregnancy loss, the work of pushing oneself beyond the deepest part of bereavement involves searching for answers, reflecting, and seeking help (Wright, 2010). In contrast to many other types of losses, pregnancy loss often involves ambiguity regarding the cause. Without knowing a cause for the loss, women tend to turn inward and engage in self-blame, mentally reviewing their actions for lack of diligence, searching desperately for a reason for the loss (Wojnar et al., 2011; Wright, 2010). Very often, women seek answers online, sometimes seeking a better understanding of pregnancy loss through websites about loss, and sometimes seeking support and understanding from others who have experienced the same type of loss (Carlson et al., 2011; Gold, Boggs, Mugisha, & Palladino, 2012).

Taking into account all of the information they glean from varied sources, women begin to reflect on their loss, the repercussions of the loss for their families, and for their own future; women mentally engage in efforts to mitigate their pain. Reflection differs from intrusivity in that it is intentional, as women deliberately recall the experience of the loss with the intention of gaining a better understanding of their own grief and that of others. Through this process of mental review, women often consider ways to move forward, to evaluate relationships with others who were supportive and helpful, and those who were not (Wright, 2010).

It is during this period of reflection and self-appraisal that mementos are most beneficial. Mementos validate the life that was lost and enable women to maintain some connection with their babies. The importance of tangible reminders created by nursing staff has been addressed in the literature (Blood & Cacciatore, 2014b; Kavanaugh & Moro, 2006; McCreight, 2008). The POT helps to situate the meaning-making process that is facilitated, in part by reflection and mementos, within the context of the entire experience of the loss. Eventually, through this process of engaged remembrance, women slowly begin to come to terms with their experience of loss.

Coming to Terms

Coming to terms suggests that women acknowledge the loss and recognize that they must learn to live on, integrating the loss into their lives. However, the loss leaves behind an ache that might never completely abate (Dyson & While, 1998; Wright, 2010) and may emerge from time to time, particularly on the anniversary of the loss, the due date, or special days like Mothers' Day (Wojnar et al., 2011; Wright, 2010). In coming to terms with the loss, women engage in patterns of forgiveness that allow them to overcome feelings of self-blame and their feelings of anger toward others. Often, women find the strength to forgive others by releasing them from the responsibility to provide comfort, saying the others just do not understand what pregnancy loss is like (Wright, 2010).

In forgiving others and themselves, women are able to put aside some of the deep feelings of anger, sadness, and grief that they had been dealing with and they begin to engage again in their lives. To do this, they harness deep inner resources, willing themselves to move beyond the suffering. They refocus their energy on their other children, their spouses, and their jobs, and may eventually find meaning in their suffering (Blood & Cacciatore, 2014b; Fenstermacher, 2014; Sturrock & Louw, 2013; Wright, 2010).

Some women find meaning in their suffering by believing there was an unknowable reason for the loss and take heart in the old adage that "everything happens for a reason." For others, this point of view brings cold comfort. For them, construction of meaning is an ongoing process; the meaning of the loss changes as new life circumstances arise. For example, some women come to believe that the loss has to occur to make a space for a subsequent child, or because her life circumstances are not conducive to raising a child at the time of the loss (Wright, 2010). The process of living through the loss, taking stock, and finding meaning in suffering helps women to mature and see the world differently than they had prior to the loss.

Living a Changed Life

Experiencing pregnancy loss alters a woman's view of herself, her family, and the world around her. Like other forms of loss, pregnancy loss is clearly a turning point in a woman's life that is fixed in time and other events are discussed as occurring either before the loss or after the loss. After a loss, women may feel a longing and an emptiness that ebbs and flows, sometimes on significant days, but sometimes unexpectedly (Fenstermacher, 2014; Wojnar et al., 2011; Wright, 2010).

Women also perceive greater fragility of the human condition and fear other losses, such as the loss of a spouse, parents, or one of their other children, as well as increased personal fear of death (Barr & Cacciatore, 2008; Wright, 2010). This fear is often manifested as hypervigilance and overprotectiveness (Barr, 2006; Côté-Arsenault & Dombeck, 2001; Warland, O'Leary, McCutcheon, & Williamson, 2010; Wright, 2010). Hypervigilence, protectiveness, and insecurity can become embedded in a woman's parenting style and can permeate future pregnancies (O'Leary & Warland, 2012). This fear of loss is not limited to the fear of another loss through death; some mothers fear separation from their spouses due to the stress of the loss. One woman in Wright's (2010) study expressed this fear, stating, "the statistics, for a loss of a baby, and a successful marriage, um, not very good" (p. 65). This fear is not entirely unfounded, as recent research has indicated that pregnancy loss can have a negative impact on marriage (Gold, Sen, & Hayward, 2010; Kagami et al., 2012).

While the experience of pregnancy loss can have catastrophic effects on some aspects of women's lives, there may also be some positive effects (Wright, 2010). For example gaining a new perspective involves personal growth, which is a well-studied outcome of pregnancy loss (Black & Sandelowski, 2010; Black & Wright, 2012; Sansoni & Giaquinto, 2001). Specific changes in worldview that have been found to occur after perinatal loss include greater self-awareness and understanding of the fragility of life, a new understanding of loss and a greater ability to support others, a general sense of gratitude, and deeper emotional bonds with others (Kavanaugh & Hershberger, 2005; Sefton, 2007; St. John et al., 2006; Wright, 2010). Interestingly, only women's bonds with those who they perceived as helpful during their grief were strengthened (Wright, 2010). Although many women fear marital breakdown or even divorce, women who work through their grief with their spouses reported stronger marital relationships than they had prior to the loss (Avelin et al., 2013; Wright, 2010).

COMPARISON WITH OTHER MODELS

Since the development of the POT, two other models of perinatal bereavement have been published. In comparing the POT with these two models, many similarities are noted, which help support the validity of the POT. For example, Wojnar et al. (2011) took on the very complex task of developing a theoretical model based on data from three different phenomenological studies with a total of 42 women who had experienced miscarriage. The benefit of this approach is that it increases the diversity of the data in terms of geography, sexual orientation, and cultural background. The model indicates that after miscarriage, women share common experiences that include getting pregnant, coming to know, bleeding and cramping, losing and gaining, scooping it up, sharing the loss, feeling empty, going public, making memories, getting through it, resuming menses, and trying again (Wojnar et al., 2011). The overarching theme that connected these experiences was "we are not in control" (Wojnar et al., 2011, p. 544).

Wojnar et al.'s (2011) model has some features in common with the POT (see Table 5.1), but there are also some differences. For example, the overarching theme of "we are not in control" communicates women's feelings of "helplessness, powerlessness, and lack of control over sustaining pregnancy" (Wojnar et al., 2011, p. 544). In contrast, the core category of the POT, pushing on, emphasizes women's ability to control their emotional processes at various points in the bereavement experience and harness inner resources to move beyond their suffering.

TABLE 5.1 Comparison of Perinatal Bereavement Theories

WRIGHT (2010)	WOJNAR ET AL. (2011)	FENSTERMACHER (2014)
Experiencing the pregnancy	Getting pregnant	Denying and hesitating Getting ready for this whole new life
Losing the baby	Coming to know Bleeding and cramping	Suffering through the loss
Bearing the burden	Losing and gaining Scooping it up Feeling empty	All of that pain for nothing Mixed emotions going everywhere
Working it through	Sharing the loss Making memories	Reaching out for support
Coming to terms	Getting through it	Preserving the memory and maintaining relationship Searching for meaning and asking why
Living a changed life	Resuming menses Trying again	Gaining a new perspective on life

Another difference between the two models is that the POT was derived from interviews with women who had experienced pregnancy loss at any time during their pregnancy, either early or late. Wojnar et al.'s (2011) model is based on data obtained from women who had specifically experienced miscarriage. This difference does not appear to make a notable difference in the results because the two models share several similarities. An advantage of Wojnar et al.'s (2011) model is that it extends into women's experiences of trying to conceive again and captures women's struggles to muster the courage to try again despite their fears and misgivings. In the POT, personal growth is featured more prominently at the end of the process. Both models highlight the need for women to share their grief with others as a means to healing, and that feelings of isolation are part of the grief process. Additionally, both models note the importance of breaking the news to others and the need to make memories. A limitation common to both models is that they were derived from data shared by women who were racially and educationally similar. A newly developed grounded theory of perinatal loss as experienced by Black adolescents (Fenstermacher, 2014) helps to address gaps left by the other models.

The pathbreaking grounded theory, "enduring to gain perspective" (Fenstermacher, 2014, p. 135), was developed from data collected through interviews with eight Black urban adolescents who had experienced pregnancy loss in the 3 months prior to the interview. The data were analyzed according to Straussian grounded theory method and yielded eight themes: denying and hesitating, getting ready for this whole new life, all that pain for nothing, mixed emotions going everywhere, reaching out for support, preserving memory and maintaining relationship, searching for meaning and asking why, and gaining new perspective (Fenstermacher, 2014). The core category, enduring to gain perspective, indicates that there is movement across the phases from pain to growth. In this way, the model shares some similarities with the POT (see Table 5.1). Other similarities between the models include the notion that expectant mothers, regardless of their age, reach a point in the pregnancy when they accept it and start to prepare for motherhood. This acceptance is evident in the phase of getting ready for a whole new life (Fenstermacher, 2014). Similar to both the POT and Wojnar et al.'s (2011) model is the notion that bereaved mothers reach out for support after loss, take steps to preserve the memory of their babies, and search for meaning in their grief. Also, like the POT, Fenstermacher (2014) noted that the experience of loss fueled a change in perspective on life that included a deeper appreciation for family and friends.

Some new dimensions of perinatal bereavement that Fenstermacher (2014) found were that the adolescents felt unprepared to monitor their symptoms and often misread signs of trouble for illness. This unpreparedness led them to delay seeking care. Further, when they arrived at the hospital, the participants believed that they received very little information about their losses or what would happen after the loss, such as lactation (Fenstermacher, 2014). Also, whereas the women in Wright's (2010) study attended support groups, sought information online, or sought support from their friends, family members, or spouses, the adolescents in Fenstermacher's study reported that they felt out of place at support group meetings because they were in the minority as unmarried Black adolescents. This feeling out of place led them to seek support primarily from other women in their families. Like the participants in previous studies, they also appreciated the support that was provided through hospital bereavement services (Fenstermacher, 2014).

Fenstermacher (2014) also pointed out the role of time in the enduring to gain perspective model, indicating that time was "integral to the bereavement process" (p. 14). The adolescents in Fenstermacher's study explained that at 12 weeks postloss they had reached a turning point and were able to talk about the loss with less of an emotional response. Wright (2010) also noted that at 3 to 6 months after the loss, women who had experienced early losses had begun to turn a corner in their grief, but those who experienced losses later in pregnancy took longer to reach this point, often until 9 to 12 months after the loss.

Interestingly, there is a significant difference between the POT and the other two models in that the POT suggests that women need to summon inner strength to push past the pain of the grief. The other models suggest that women endure the pain and that they are not in control of the process (Fenstermacher, 2014; Wojnar et al., 2011). This difference may result from different cultural or ethnic viewpoints on the part of the participants. In Wright's (2010) study, the participants were mostly from northeastern Pennsylvania, descendants of European immigrants who sought work in the local coal mining industry decades earlier. The values of hard work and self-sufficiency are deeply embedded in their psyche and underpin their approach to overcoming diversity (Dublin & Licht, 2005). Future research is needed to determine whether this variation will have a significant effect on the generalizability of the theory.

CLINICAL IMPLICATIONS OF THE POT

Because the POT provides a sweeping overview of the process of perinatal bereavement, it helps bring to light several clinical interventions that would be useful at different points in the grief process. For example, when a woman is pregnant, clinicians should pay close attention to the words she uses when discussing her pregnancy. If the woman uses a name, refers to her "baby," or describes this pregnancy as a sister, brother, or grandchild, she is indicating that she has developed a relationship and is taking steps to mother her baby (Wright, 2010).

Behaviors associated with prenatal mothering, such as changing unhealthy habits and monitoring the pregnancy, suggest that a woman is taking steps to provide a good intrauterine life for her baby. Therefore, she may be caught off guard when a pregnancy ends unexpectedly. In an attempt to figure out what went wrong, she may mentally review her actions to determine whether she missed some sign of trouble or engaged in some risky behavior. Such analysis can lead to self-blame and recrimination. To counter these sentiments, when breaking the news of the loss, it may be helpful for health care providers to reassure women that the loss was not their fault and the cause of loss is often undetermined. As an example of how helpful this simple approach can be, one woman in Wright's (2010, p. 71) study stated, "The doctor said it wasn't my fault, I didn't do it, um, so yeah, she definitely helped me." Another mother noted,

> One of the first things the nurse said, like, "Don't think it was your fault, you didn't do anything," and to know that there was something that was like, from the moment of conception, this baby was just destined to be the way she was, it was, it was something that was just taken out of my hands and it helped so much, like, to know that. (Wright, 2010, p. 71)

Other strategies for breaking bad news have been discussed at length in the literature. Use of these strategies is particularly important because getting the news of the loss is crystallized in women's memory forever and affects her perception of the loss experience (Wright, 2010). Thus, when bad news must be shared, the patient should be afforded privacy in a room where she can take time to take in the news without interruptions. It should also have a telephone available so that she can reach out to other loved ones to share the news or seek support (Poddar, Tyagi, Hawkins, & Opemuy, 2011; Van den Berg, Vissenberg, & Goddijn, 2014). The provider must convey sympathy, provide time for discussion and questions, allow the patient to take in the information, and seek verification as needed (Davenport & Schopp, 2011; Harrison & Walling, 2010). In the case of pregnancy loss, specifically, seeking verification of the loss is especially crucial because women have reported a need to be sure that the loss had truly occurred before making any decisions about treatment (Limbo, Glasser, & Sundram, 2014).

These approaches suggest that the actions and skill of the health care provider in sharing the news of the loss can have a positive effect on how patients perceive and deal with their situation. However, Morse (2011) presented a very thorough and thoughtful analysis of how bad news is perceived by the patient, which can help illuminate providers' approach. Health care providers should be aware that when a woman seeks care for suspicions of trouble with a pregnancy, she has already noted changes internally and discussed them with a trusted person (Wright, 2010). Through this process of discernment, she has already determined there is possible cause for alarm. The suspicion that something could be wrong is accompanied by the need for confirmation (Morse, 2011). Thus, when a woman presents with signs that her pregnancy is not progressing well, the health care provider must acknowledge that the woman already suspects that there is something wrong and then confirm her fears. A provider approaching the conversation from this perspective might begin with, "When you thought you noticed signs that the baby had stopped moving, you were right about that." Such an approach acknowledges the mother's efforts to monitor her pregnancy, allowing her to be confident of her ability, despite the negative outcome.

When breaking the news to unsuspecting women about a loss, the provider should understand that prior to breaking the news in words, they had already communicated concern through posture, facial expression, and even nervous habits (Morse, 2011). Wright (2010) noted that women studied the faces of health care providers for signs of concern but sometimes misinterpreted providers' nonverbal communication, maintaining hope until the news of the loss was shared verbally. The emotional sequelae that unfold after women hear the news of the loss may be difficult for providers to witness. However, knowledge of women's possible reactions, which can range from ambivalence to severe distress, can help providers offer useful and genuine support and appropriate referrals, as needed. In particular, the provider should be ready to access the services of a social worker or chaplain for the patient, and arrange for bereavement support and follow-up (Harrison & Walling, 2010).

Supportive interventions in the clinical setting, particularly in the inpatient setting, have been systematically studied over the course of the past 30 years and best practices have been established (Limbo, 2012). Interestingly, the POT indicates that at the time of the loss, women viewed decisions regarding care of the deceased baby and mementos as a distinct burden. In reflection, women appreciated those mementos and the time that they had spent with their babies. These seemingly paradoxical implications of the POT are understandable within the context of current literature. The POT provides a framework for working with bereaved mothers, both immediately after a loss and in the ensuing weeks and months.

At the time of the loss, bereaved mothers may experience shock, numbness, and other signs of grief (Warland et al., 2010; Wright, 2010). Therefore, health care providers should be cautious in their approach when presenting options to newly bereaved mothers, knowing that these women may need time to consider their choices and that they may change their minds (Limbo, 2012). To prepare staff members for working with perinatally bereaved families, education on relationship-based approaches to perinatal care is essential (Limbo, 2012) because it encourages the development of a supportive, trusting relationship between the health care provider and the family. Further, this approach to clinical care after perinatal loss necessarily involves respect for the individual's values and cultural and religious traditions (Warland & Davis, 2011). Situating these interactions within the entire context of the experience of the loss may help health care providers more fully embrace the magnitude of their actions on the experience of the loss for bereaved women.

The POT also helps to explicate the importance of mementos in the grief process. Situating the current clinical practice of making mementos helps clinicians to understand that these interventions are not only helpful, but also that they specifically help women at a certain point in the grief process to gain a deeper understanding of their loss and to move forward. Klass (1996) noted that after the loss of a child, parents must work toward reintegration of a deceased child into their psychic and social worlds. For perinatally bereaved women, mementos seem to be a tangible touchpoint for reconnecting with the loss experience and integrating it into their present realities. Therefore, creating mementos, with the consent of the bereaved mother, is a clinical intervention that mothers increasingly appreciate as they journey through their grief, even if they feel that being asked whether they want them is a burden at the time of the loss.

One recommendation for easing the burden of decision making is to create mementos in the office setting with each office visit. For example, clinicians can ask at each prenatal visit if the mother would like to record the heartbeat on her phone after the clinician finds the heartbeat with the Doppler. In the event of a loss later in the pregnancy, the mother will have a recording of the heartbeat that she can transfer to a book, a movie, or even a stuffed animal. Others mementos may include ultrasound images, a copy of the confirmatory lab results, or even the disposable measuring tape used to measure fundal height, marked with the date and measurement. When later losses occur in inpatient settings, interventions such as offering the baby to parents to see and hold (Warland & Davis, 2011), taking photos of the baby (Blood & Cacciatore, 2014a), creating "proof of life" certificates (Johnson & Langford, 2010), making memory boxes (Capitulo, 2005), consulting palliative care or perinatal hospice as appropriate (Geller, Psaros, & Kornfield, 2010; Limbo & Lathrop, 2014), and coordinating bereavement services and appropriate follow-up are all evidence-based recommendations that have been cited as helpful (Harrison & Walling, 2010).

Women have a desire for professional follow-up and a need to connect with others after perinatal loss (Wright, 2010). Support can be garnered through formal resources, such as a bereavement team, or informally through support groups, close friends, family members, and spouses. Knowing that when women reach out for support and do not receive it relationships can be damaged, health care professionals have a role in teaching women how to communicate their need for support to others and how to respond to others when their needs are not met or when others do not respond appropriately (Wright, 2010). This preparation may be crucial in helping women to maintain relationships with loved ones who do not or cannot provide adequate support.

Helping to prepare women to deal with feelings of isolation; lack of support; difficult days, such as the anniversary of the loss; and potentially difficult social situations should be part of professional follow-up care (Wright, 2010). Also, for those professionals who work with bereaved women through support groups or other bereavement support programs, it is important to recognize that indicators of continuing bonds are a normal part of the perinatal bereavement process and may be manifested by participation in events such as annual walks to remember, the planting of a tree, dedication of a bench, or care of a grave (Murphy & Thomas, 2013). Helping to draw attention to positive outcomes of grief, such as gaining a greater appreciation for loved ones and other signs of personal growth (Black & Sandelowski, 2010; Black & Wright, 2012), will help women to recognize the progress they have made through the grief process. In these interventions with bereaved parents, the value of the POT in outlining the typical trajectory of perinatal bereavement helps providers to recognize when women are following the usual path of grief and when they may need additional support.

DISCUSSION

This chapter provides an overview of the process of maternal perinatal bereavement, as represented by the POT. Development of the POT flows from the natural progression of the field of perinatal bereavement and also answers the call for new gender-sensitive theories in the field of women's health (Im & Meleis, 2011). Because this substantive theory was discovered through the grounded theory method, it is expected to ring true for others who have experienced such a loss and should also be applicable in clinical practice (Glaser, 1998). The POT bears many similarities to other models of perinatal bereavement and is congruent with findings in the extant literature. However, it adds several new insights into perinatal loss.

One important new insight offered by the POT is that the process of maternal–fetal bonding can occur very early in pregnancy, even as early as the moment a woman finds out that she is pregnant (Wright, 2010). This finding challenges earlier presumptions that maternal attachment may not begin until quickening (Rubin, 1984) or until hearing a heartbeat and seeing ultrasound images (Righetti et al., 2005). Thus, the POT helps to elucidate the private yet truncated relationship between mother and baby in utero. This understanding, situated within the greater context of the process of maternal perinatal bereavement, is consistent with decades of research indicating that women can experience profound grief after perinatal loss, even if the loss occurs quite early in the pregnancy.

The POT also helps to situate the experience of pregnancy loss within extant literature on grief and supports previously discovered insights into grief and loss, such as the notion that personal growth results from working through the grief process (Black & Sandelowski, 2010; Black & Wright, 2012). New dimensions of personal growth relative to perinatal bereavement captured in the POT include gaining emotional strength, developing closer relationships with spouses and others, and maturity (Black & Wright, 2012). The process of finding meaning in loss involves deep reflection and integration of the loss into other aspects of one's life (Neimeyer, 2011; Wright, 2010).

The importance of mementos in the process of meaning making is also explicated by the POT. The extant literature made it clear that parents cherished mementos and that these items had a role in healing after loss, but the mechanism by which that occurred had not been previously elucidated. The POT supports the need for clinicians to understand the rationale that underpins the clinical interventions they recommend to bereaved mothers. In this way, clinicians may be more dedicated to using relationship-based interventions during these meaningful moments and can share with women the reasons that mementos may be helpful to them in the future.

Despite its strengths, the POT has several limitations that must be considered. It was developed through interviews with women who were, for the most part, White and married. With few exceptions, the participants had planned their pregnancies (Wright, 2010). Additionally, most of the participants held strong religious beliefs, which is reflective of the geographic area in which the study was conducted. The women's religious beliefs may have amplified their responses to pregnancy loss because of their deeply rooted beliefs in the sanctity of life. Women who hold more secular views may not have reported such strong responses based on their own worldviews. Likewise, there is some risk that the theory magnifies the significance of the loss in some ways because the women who chose to participate in the study on which the theory is based self-selected and were likely emotionally invested in their experience of loss.

CONCLUSION

The development of the POT represents a contribution that helps to unify extant findings regarding women's experiences of perinatal loss. Use of the grounded theory method allowed for the development of a new theory that is based on the words of the women who lived the experience of perinatal loss. Because of its foundation, validity is inherent in the theory. Further, the state of the science is such that the concepts of the theory were validated through comparison with the extant research findings. In fact, qualitative inquiry that led to the development of two other theoretical models resulted in remarkably similar findings, indicating that there are commonalities in the experience of pregnancy loss and the process of maternal perinatal bereavement is becoming increasingly clear through research.

All three of the theoretical frameworks that have been discussed (Fenstermacher, 2014; Wojnar et al., 2011; Wright, 2010) are rooted in the words of the women who lived the experience of pregnancy loss. The model developed by Wojnar et al. (2011) focuses more heavily on the experience of miscarriage and may be more appropriate for framing future studies on early loss. Fenstermacher's (2014) model may be useful for future studies of pregnancy loss among adolescents or minority women. The POT may be most appropriate to frame studies of how women move through the grief process and whether interventions can be useful at certain points to facilitate progress. Another excellent contribution to the field of perinatal bereavement studies would be to use these three theories as the basis for the development of a meta-theory.

Future research specific to the POT could include determining whether the POT accurately depicts the process of maternal perinatal bereavement through instrument development and testing. Because the POT indicates that the overall process of maternal perinatal bereavement is the same regardless of gestational age at the time of loss, theory testing could include a comparison of grief responses between those who had earlier losses and those who had later losses. Also, the POT illustrates that there is a relationship between acceptance of a pregnancy and a grief response if a loss occurs. This hypothesized relationship between these two variables should be studied more carefully through longitudinal design.

The POT provides a framework for understanding the experience of pregnancy loss, which echoes many elements of the extant literature as well as other models of perinatal bereavement. Because it offers a platform for a common understanding of pregnancy loss, the theory can be used to frame clinical interventions, situating them within the larger context of the process of maternal perinatal bereavement. It is currently being used as a guiding theory for a pregnancy loss support group and is working well (Wright, Shea, & Gallagher, 2014).

The next logical step would be to determine the extent to which the theory represents the reality of perinatal bereavement and whether the stages are distinct and follow the proposed pattern. Once this determination is made, interventions can be developed to ease the transition from stage to stage and to prevent women from becoming mired in their grief. Such research would help to propel the field toward evidence-based clinical interventions that could help alleviate the grief associated with pregnancy loss.

CASE STUDY

Aria is 30 years old. She and her husband are Jewish and have five living children. Three months ago, Aria experienced the loss of a pregnancy at 22 weeks. She explains that she cries quite often and sometimes locks herself in the bathroom so that her children do not see her cry. She has an ultrasound photo of the baby that she says makes her feel closer to the baby. She also states that she feels that her husband does not understand her grief but tries to be supportive "in his own way." She is worried that she is not recovering well from the loss and is seeking advice.

FOCUS QUESTIONS

1. Based on the POT, is there any concern about how Aria is progressing through her grief?
2. In terms of support, what questions should you ask? What resources could you offer?
3. How would you respond to Aria based on the information in the case study?
4. Based on the POT, might Aria's relationship with her living children be changed due to her loss?

REFERENCES

Avelin, P., Rådestad, I., Säflund, K., Wredling, R., & Erlandsson, K. (2013). Parental grief and relationships after the loss of a stillborn baby. *Midwifery, 29*, 668–673. Retrieved from http://dx.doi.org/10.1016/j.midw.2012.06.007

Barr, P. (2006). Relation between grief and subsequent pregnancy status 13 months after perinatal bereavement. *Journal of Perinatal Medicine, 34*, 207–211. Retrieved from http://dx.doi.org/10.1515/JPM.2006.036

Barr, P., & Cacciatore, J. (2008). Personal fear of death and grief in bereaved mothers. *Death Studies, 32*, 445–460. Retrieved from http://dx.doi.org/10.1080/07481180801974752

Bennett, S. M., Litz, B. T., Maguen, S., & Ehrenreich, J. T. (2008). An exploratory study of the psychological impact and clinical care of perinatal loss. *Journal of Loss & Trauma, 13*, 485–510. Retrieved from http://dx.doi.org/10.1080/15325020802171268

Benoliel, J. Q. (2001). Expanding knowledge about women through grounded theory: Introduction to the collection. *Health Care for Women International, 22*, 7–9. Retrieved from http://dx.doi.org/10.1080/073993301300003045

Black, A. Y., Fleming, N. A., & Rome, E. S. (2012). Pregnancy in adolescents. *Adolescent Medicine: State of the Art Reviews, 23*, 123–138. Retrieved from http://www2.aap.org/sections/adolescenthealth/amstars.cfm

Black, B. P., & Sandelowski, M. (2010). Personal growth after severe fetal diagnosis. *Western Journal of Nursing Research, 32*, 1011–1030. Retrieved from http://dx.doi.org/10.1177/0193945910371215

Black, B. P., & Wright, P. M. (2012). Posttraumatic growth and transformation as outcomes of perinatal loss. *Illness, Crisis, & Loss, 20*, 225–237. Retrieved from http://dx.doi.org/10.2190/IL.20.3.b

Black, R. B. (1992). Seeing the baby: The impact of ultrasound technology. *Journal of Genetic Counseling, 1*, 45–54. Retrieved from http://dx.doi.org/10.1007/BF00960084

Blood, C., & Cacciatore, J. (2014a). Best practice in bereavement photography after perinatal death: Qualitative analysis with 104 parents. *BMC Psychology, 2*, 1–10. Retrieved from http://dx.doi.org/10.1186/2050-7283-2-15

Blood, C., & Cacciatore, J. (2014b). Parental grief and memento mori photography: Narrative, meaning, culture, and context. *Death Studies, 38*, 224–233. Retrieved from http://dx.doi.org/10.1080/07481187.2013.788584

Cacciatore, J., Schnebly, S., & Froen, J. F. (2009). The effects of social support on maternal anxiety and depression after stillbirth. *Health and Social Care in the Community, 17,* 167–176. Retrieved from http://dx.doi.org/10.1111/j.1365-2524.2008.00814.x

Capitulo, K. L. (2005). Evidence for healing interventions with perinatal bereavement. *MCN, The American Journal of Maternal Child Nursing, 30,* 389–396. Retrieved from http://dx.doi.org/10.1097/00005721-200511000-00007

Carlson, R., Lammert, C., & O'Leary, J. M. (2011). The evolution of group and online support for families who have experienced perinatal or neonatal loss. *Illness, Crisis, & Loss, 20,* 275–293. Retrieved from http://dx.doi.org/10.2190/IL.20.3.e

Christiansen, D. M., Elklit, A., & Olff, M. (2013). Parents bereaved by infant death: PTSD symptoms up to 18 years after the loss. *General Hospital Psychiatry, 35,* 605–611. Retrieved from http://dx.doi.org/10.1016/j.genhosppsych.2013.06.006

Côté-Arsenault, D., & Dombeck, M.-T. B. (2001). Maternal assignment of fetal personhood to a previous pregnancy loss: Relationship to anxiety in the current pregnancy. *Health Care for Women International, 22,* 649–665. Retrieved from http://dx.doi.org/10.1080/07399330127171

Cowchock, F. S., Lasker, J. N., Toedter, L. J., Skumanich, S. A., & Koenig, H. G. (2010). Religious beliefs affect grieving after pregnancy loss. *Journal of Religion & Health, 49,* 485–497. Retrieved from http://dx.doi.org/10.1007/s10943-009-9277-3

Davenport, L., & Schopp, G. (2011). Breaking bad news: Communication skills for difficult conversations. *Journal of the American Academy of Physician Assistants, 24,* 46–50. Retrieved from http://dx.doi.org/10.1097/01720610-201102000-00008

Dublin, T., & Licht, W. (2005). *The face of decline: The Pennsylvania anthracite region in the twentieth century.* Ithaca, NY: Cornell University Press.

Dyson, L., & While, A. (1998). The long shadow of perinatal bereavement. *British Journal of Community Nursing, 3,* 432–439. Retrieved from http://dx.doi.org/10.12968/bjcn.1998.3.9.7183

Fenstermacher, K. H. (2014). Enduring to gain perspective: A grounded theory study of the experience of perinatal bereavement in Black adolescents. *Research in Nursing & Health, 37,* 135–143. Retrieved from http://dx.doi.org/10.1002/nur.21583

Freud, S. (1957). Mourning and melancholia. In J. Strachey (Ed.), *The standard edition of the complete psychological works of Sigmund Freud* (Vol. 14, pp. 237–260). London, England: Hogarth Press and Institute for Psychoanalysis. (Original work published in 1917.)

Geller, P. A., Psaros, C., & Kornfield, S. L. (2010). Satisfaction with pregnancy loss aftercare: Are women getting what they want? *Archives of Women's Mental Health, 13,* 111–124. Retrieved from http://dx.doi.org/10.1007/s00737-010-0147-5

Glaser, B. G. (1992). *Basics of grounded theory analysis: Emergence vs. forcing.* Mill Valley, CA: Sociology Press.

Glaser, B. G. (1998). *Doing grounded theory: Issues and discussions.* Mill Valley, CA: Sociology Press.

Glaser, B. G., & Strauss, A. L. (1967). *The discovery of grounded theory: Strategies for qualitative research.* Hawthorne, NY: Aldine.

Gold, K. J., Boggs, M. E., Mugisha, E., & Palladino, C. L. (2012). Internet message boards for pregnancy loss: Who's online and why? *Women's Health Issues, 22,* e67–e72. Retrieved from http://dx.doi.org/10.1016/j.whi.2011.07.006

Gold, K. J., Sen, A., & Hayward, R. A. (2010). Marriage and cohabitation outcomes after pregnancy loss. *Pediatrics, 125,* e1202–e1207. Retrieved from http://dx.doi.org/10.1542/peds.2009-3081

Gray, J. B. (2014). The social support process in unplanned pregnancy. *Journal of Communication in Healthcare, 7,* 137–146. Retrieved from http://dx.doi.org/10.1179/1753807614Y.0000000054

Gudmundsdottir, M. (2009). Embodied grief: Bereaved parents' narratives of their suffering body. *Omega: Journal of Death and Dying, 59,* 253–269. Retrieved from http://dx.doi.org/10.2190/OM.59.3.e

Harrison, M. E., & Walling, A. (2010). What do we know about giving bad news? A review. *Clinical Pediatrics, 49,* 619–626. Retrieved from http://dx.doi.org/10.1177/0009922810361380

Hogan, N. S., & DeSantis, L. (1992). Adolescent sibling bereavement: An ongoing attachment. *Qualitative Health Research, 2,* 159–177. Retrieved from http://dx.doi.org/10.1177/104973239200200204

Hogan, N. S., & DeSantis, L. (1996). Basic constructs of a theory of adolescent sibling bereavement. In D. Klass, P. R. Silverman, & S. L. Nickman (Eds.), *Continuing bonds: New understandings of grief* (pp. 235–254). Philadelphia, PA: Taylor & Francis.

Hogan, N. S., Greenfield, D. B., & Schmidt, L. A. (2001). The development and validation of the Hogan Grief Reaction Checklist. *Death Studies, 25,* 1–32. Retrieved from http://dx.doi.org/10.1080/07481180125831

Hogan, N. S., Morse, J. M., & Tasón, M. C. (1996). Toward an experiential theory of bereavement. *Omega: Journal of Death and Dying, 33,* 43–65. Retrieved from http://dx.doi.org/10.2190/GU3X-JWV0-AG6G-21FX

Hogan, N. S., & Schmidt, L. A. (2002). Testing the grief to personal growth model using structural equation modeling. *Death Studies, 26,* 615–634. Retrieved from http://dx.doi.org/10.1080/07481180290088338

Hutti, M. H. (1986). An exploratory study of the miscarriage experience. *Health Care for Women International, 7,* 371–389. http://dx.doi.org/10.1080/07399338609515750

Hutti, M. H., Armstrong, D., & Myers, J. (2011). Healthcare utilization in the pregnancy following a perinatal loss. *MCN, The American Journal of Maternal Child Nursing, 36,* 104–111. Retrieved from http://dx.doi.org/10.1097/NMC.0b013e3182057335

Im, E.-O., & Meleis, A. I. (2011). An international imperative for gender-sensitive theories in women's health. *Journal of Nursing Scholarship, 33,* 309–314. Retrieved from http://dx.doi.org/10.1111/j.1547-5069.2001.00309.x

Jansson, C., & Adolfsson, A. (2011). Application of "Swanson's middle range caring theory" in Sweden after miscarriage. *International Journal of Clinical Medicine, 2,* 102–109. Retrieved from http://dx.doi.org/10.4236/ijcm.2011.22021

Johnson, O., & Langford, R. W. (2010). Proof of life: A protocol for pregnant women who experience pre-20-week perinatal loss. *Critical Care Nursing Quarterly, 33,* 204–211. Retrieved from http://dx.doi.org/10.1097/CNQ.0b013e3181e65f3b

Kagami, M., Maruyama, T., Koizumi, T., Miyazaki, K., Nishikawa-Uchida, S., Oda, H., . . . Yoshimura, Y. (2012). Psychological adjustment and psychological stress among Japanese couples with a history of recurrent pregnancy loss. *Human Reproduction, 27,* 787–794. Retrieved from http://dx.doi.org/10.1093/humrep/der441

Kaunonen, M., Tarkka, M.-T., Paunonen, M., & Laippala, P. (1999). Grief and social support after the death of a spouse. *Journal of Advanced Nursing, 30,* 1304–1311. Retrieved from http://dx.doi.org/10.1046/j.1365-2648.1999.01220.x

Kavanaugh, K., & Hershberger, P. (2005). Perinatal loss in low-income African American parents. *Journal of Obstetric, Gynecologic, & Neonatal Nursing, 34,* 595–605. Retrieved from http://dx.doi.org/10.1177/0884217505280000

Kavanaugh, K., & Moro, T. (2006). Supporting parents after stillborn or newborn death: There is much that nurses can do. *American Journal of Nursing, 106*(9), 74–79. Retrieved from http://dx.doi.org/10.1097/00000446-200609000-00037

Kersting, A., & Wagner, B. (2012). Complicated grief after perinatal loss. *Dialogues in Clinical Neuroscience, 14,* 187–194. Retrieved from http://www.dialogues-cns.org

Klass, D. (1996). The deceased child in the psychic and social worlds of bereaved parents during the resolution of grief. In D. Klass, P. R. Silverman, & S. L. Nickman (Eds.), *Continuing binds: New understandings of grief* (pp. 199–216). Philadelphia, PA: Taylor & Francis.

Lazarus, R. S., & Folkman, S. (1984). *Stress, appraisal, and coping.* New York, NY: Springer.

Limbo, R. (2012). Caring for families experiencing stillbirth: A unified position statement on contact with the baby. *Illness, Crisis, & Loss, 20,* 295–298. Retrieved from http://dx.doi.org/10.2190/IL.20.3.f

Limbo, R., Glasser, J. K., & Sundram, M. E. (2014). "Being sure": Women's experience with inevitable miscarriage. *MCN, The American Journal of Maternal Child Nursing, 39,* 165–174. Retrieved from http://dx.doi.org/10.1097/NMC.0000000000000027

Limbo, R., & Lathrop, A. (2014). Caregiving in mothers' narratives of perinatal hospice. *Illness, Crisis, & Loss, 22,* 43–65. Retrieved from http://dx.doi.org/10.2190/IL.22.1.e

Limbo, R. & Vinge, D. J. (1990). When a baby dies: Miscarriage, stillbirth, and newborn death. *The Caregiver Journal, 7,* 28–37. Retrieved from http://dx.doi.org/10.1080/1077842X.1990.10781573

Lindemann, E. (1994). Symptomatology and management of grief [Special section]. *American Journal of Psychiatry, 151,* 155–160. (Original work published in 1944.) Retrieved from http://ajp.psychiatryonline.org

Maciejewski, P. K., Zhang, B., Block, S. D., & Prigerson, H. G. (2007). An empirical examination of the stage theory of grief. *Journal of the American Medical Association, 297,* 716–723. Retrieved from http://dx.doi.org/10.1001/jama.297.7.716

Mann, J. R., Mannan, J., Quiñones, L. A., Palmer, A. A., & Torres, M. (2010). Religion, spirituality, social support, and perceived stress in pregnant and postpartum Hispanic women. *Journal of Obstetric, Gynecologic, and Neonatal Nursing, 39,* 645–657. Retrieved from http://dx.doi.org/10.1111/j.1552-6909.2010.01188.x

McCreight, B. S. (2008). Perinatal loss: A qualitative study in Northern Ireland. *Omega: Journal of Death and Dying, 57,* 1–19. Retrieved from http://dx.doi.org/10.2190/OM.57.1.a

Mills, T. A., Ricklesford, C., Cooke, A., Heazell, A. E. P., Whitworth, M., & Lavender, T. (2014). Parents' experiences and expectations of care in pregnancy after stillbirth or neonatal heath: A metasynthesis. *BJOG: An International Journal of Obstetrics & Gynaecology, 121,* 943–950. Retrieved from http://dx.doi.org/10.1111/1471-0528.12656

Morse, J. (2011). Hearing bad news. *Journal of Medical Humanities, 32,* 187–211. Retrieved from http://dx.doi.org/10.1007/s10912-011-9138-4

Murphy, S., Shevlin, M., & Elklit, A. (2014). Psychological consequences of pregnancy loss and infant death in a sample of bereaved parents. *Journal of Loss & Trauma, 19,* 56–69. Retrieved from http://dx.doi.org/10.1080/15325024.2012.735531

Murphy, S., & Thomas, H. (2013). Stillbirth and loss: Family practices and display. *Sociological Research Online, 18*(1), Art. No. 2. Retrieved from http://dx.doi.org/10.5153/sro.2889

Neimeyer, R. A. (2011). Reconstructing meaning in bereavement. In M. Watson & D. W. Kissane (Eds.), *Handbook of psychotherapy in cancer care* (pp. 247–257). Hoboken, NJ: Wiley-Blackwell.

Ockhuijsen, H. D. L.,van den Hoogen, A., Boivin, J., Macklon, N. S., & de Boer, F. (2014). Pregnancy after miscarriage: Balancing between loss of control and searching for control. *Research in Nursing and Health, 37*, 267–275. Retrieved from http://dx.doi .org/10.1002/nur.21610

O'Leary, J., & Warland, J. (2012). Intentional parenting of children born after a perinatal loss. *Journal of Loss & Trauma, 17*, 137–157. Retrieved from http://dx.doi.org/10.108 0/15325024.2011.595297

O'Leary, J., Warland, J., & Parker, L. (2011). Prenatal parenthood. *Journal of Perinatal Education, 20*, 218–220. Retrieved from http://dx.doi.org/10.1891/1058-1243.20.4.218

Poddar, A., Tyagi, J., Hawkins, E., & Opemuy, I. (2011). Standards of care provided by early pregnancy assessment units (EPAU): A UK-wide survey. *Journal of Obsterics & Gynecology, 31*, 640–644. Retrieved from http://dx.doi.org/10.3109/01443615.2011. 593650

Righetti, P. L., Dell'Avanzo, M., Grigio, M., & Nicolini, U. (2005). Maternal/paternal antenatal attachment and fourth-dimensional ultrasound technique: A preliminary report. *British Journal of Psychology, 96*, 129–137. Retrieved from http://dx.doi .org/10.1348/000712604X15518

Rillstone, P., & Hutchinson, S. A. (2001). Managing the reemergence of anguish: Pregnancy after a loss due to anomalies. *Journal of Obstetric, Gynecologic, and Neonatal Nursing, 30*, 291–298. Retrieved from http://dx.doi.org/10.1111/j.1552-6909.2001 .tb01547.x

Rubin, R. (1984). *Maternal identity and the maternal experience.* New York, NY: Springer.

Sanders, L. B. (2008). Women's voices: The lived experience of pregnancy and mother-hood after diagnosis with HIV. *Journal of the Association of Nurses in AIDS Care, 19*, 47–57. Retrieved from http://dx.doi.org/10.1016/j.jana.2007.10.002

Sansoni, J., & Giaquinto, A. (W. S. Blanchard, Trans.). (2001). Grief of parents for a pre-born child loss [in Italian]. *Professioni Infermieristiche, 54*(1), 3–18. Retrieved from http://profinf.net/pro/index.php/pi

Sefton, M. (2007). Grief analysis of adolescents experiencing an early miscar-riage. *Hispanic Health Care International, 5*, 13–20. Retrieved from http://dx.doi .org/10.1891/154041507780851897

St. John, A., Cooke, M., & Goopy, S. (2006). Shrouds of silence: Three women's stories of prenatal loss. *Australian Journal of Advanced Nursing, 23*(3), 8–12. Retrieved from http://www.ajan.com.au

Sturrock, C., & Louw, J. (2013). Meaning-making after neonatal death: Narratives of Xhosa-speaking women in South Africa. *Death Studies, 37*, 569–588. Retrieved from http://dx.doi.org/10.1080/07481187.2012.673534

Sutan, R., & Miskam, H. M. (2012). Psychological impact of perinatal loss among Muslim women. *BMC Women's Health, 12*, 1–9. Retrieved from http://dx.doi .org/10.1186/1472-6874-12-15

Swanson, K. M. (1991). Empirical development of a middle range theory of caring. *Nursing Research, 40*, 161–166. Retrieved from http://dx.doi.org/10.1097/00006199 -199105000-00008

Swanson, K. M. (2000). Predicting depressive symptoms after miscarriage: A path analysis based on the Lazarus paradigm. *Journal of Women's Health & Gender-Based Medicine, 9*, 191–206. Retrieved from http://dx.doi.org/10.1089/152460900318696

Swanson-Kauffman, K. M. (1986). A combined qualitative methodology for nursing research. *Advances in Nursing Science, 83*(3), 58–69. Retrieved from http://dx.doi .org/10.1097/00012272-198604000-00008

Theodorou, E., & Spyrou, S. (2013). Motherhood in utero: Consuming away anxiety. *Journal of Consumer Culture, 13,* 79–96. Retrieved from http://dx.doi .org/10.1177/1469540513480163

Toedter, L. J., Lasker, J. N., & Alhadeff, J. M. (1988). The Perinatal Grief Scale: Development and initial validation. *American Journal of Orthopsychiatry, 58,* 435–449. Retrieved from http://dx.doi.org/10.1111/j.1939-0025.1988.tb01604.x

Toffol, E., Koponen, P., & Partonen, T. (2013). Miscarriage and mental health: Results of two population-based studies. *Psychiatry Research, 205,* 151–158. Retrieved from http://dx.doi.org/10.1016/j.psychres.2012.08.029

van den Akker, O. B. A. (2011). The psychological and social consequences of miscarriage. *Expert Review of Obstetrics & Gynecology, 6,* 295–304. Retrieved from http:// dx.doi.org/10.1586/eog.11.14

Van den Berg, M. M. J., Vissenberg, R., & Goddijn, M. (2014). Recurrent miscarriage clinics. *Obstetric & Gynecology Clinics of North America, 41,* 145–155. Retrieved from http://dx.doi.org/10.1016/j.ogc.2013.10.010

Warland, J., & Davis, D. L. (2011). *Caring for families experiencing stillbirth: A unified position statement on contact with the baby, An international collaboration.* Retrieved from http://missfoundation.org/news/StillbirthContactwBaby_position_statement.pdf

Warland, J., O'Leary, J., McCutcheon, H., & Williamson, V. (2010). Parenting paradox: Parenting after infant loss, *Midwifery, 27,* e163–e169. Retrieved from http://dx.doi .org/10.1016/j.midw.2010.02.004

Williams, J. D. (2003). *Preparing to teach writing: Research, theory, and practice* (3rd ed.). Mahwah, NJ: Erlbaum.

Wojnar, D. M., Swanson, K. M., & Adolfsson, A.-S. (2011). Confronting the inevitable: A conceptual model of miscarriage for use in clinical practice and research. *Death Studies, 35,* 536–558. Retrieved from http://dx.doi.org/10.1080/07481187.2010.536 886

Worden, J. W. (2002). *Grief counseling and grief therapy: A handbook for the mental health practitioner* (3rd ed.). New York, NY: Springer.

Wright, P. M. (2010). *Pushing on: A grounded theory study of maternal perinatal bereavement* (Doctoral dissertation). Retrieved from ProQuest Dissertations and Theses database. (AAT No. 3404182)

Wright, P. M. (2011). Barriers to a comprehensive understanding of pregnancy loss. *Journal of Loss and Trauma, 16,* 1–12. Retrieved from http://dx.doi.org/10.1080/15 325024.2010.519298

Wright, P. M., Shea, D. M., & Gallagher, R. (2014). From seed to tree: Developing support for perinatally bereaved mothers. *Journal of Perinatal Education, 23,* 151–54. Retrieved from http://dx.doi.org/10.1891/1058-1243.23.3.151

CHAPTER 6

When the Unthinkable Happens: A Mindfulness Approach to Perinatal and Pediatric Death

Joanne Cacciatore

Compassion is hard because it requires the inner disposition to go with others to the place where they are weak, vulnerable, lonely, and broken. . .what we desire most is to do away with suffering by fleeing from it or finding a quick cure for it. So we ignore our greatest gift, which is our ability to enter into solidarity with those who suffer.

(Nouwen, 1981, p. 24)

Grief is a nearly universal response to the death of a loved one. And while a significant majority of mourners in the general population seem to cope well with loss, a minority of the bereaved experience an enlongation of grief that may also be associated with physical or mental health issues, particularly those experiencing traumatic grief. Traumatic grief results from deaths that are violent, sudden, due to human actions (Green, 2000), and child death (Rando, 1985), and it has been linked to a host of psychosocial and physical maladies (Badenhorst, Riches, Turton, & Hughes, 2006; Dyregrov & Matthiesen, 1991; Dyregrov, Nordanger, & Dyregrov, 2003; Rogers et al., 2008). Indeed, the death of a baby or child, in particular, is an excruciatingly painful experience for parents, siblings, and grandparents, and manifest in emotional, cognitive, existential, social, and physiological effects (Cacciatore, Lacasse, Lietz, & McPherson, 2013). This chapter explores traumatic grief and loss, discusses various treatments for it, and especially focuses on mindfulness-based interventions for specific use in traumatic grief with bereaved parents.

Traumatic grief, when treated at all, is often approached medico-psychopharmacologically and/or psychosocially. Some psychosocial approaches have strong empirical standing depending on the precise intervention and the population served. However, to date, pharmacologically based treatment of traumatic grief has not been identified as evidence-based, yet is overused as a first line of treatment (Cacciatore & Thieleman, 2012; Thieleman & Cacciatore, 2014a). This is particularly true in the case of perinatal death where nearly one in every four mothers is being pre-scribed psychiatric medication often within days after the loss (Lacasse & Cacciatore, 2014).

Traumatic grief appears relatively responsive to the psychosocial approach, particularly when it includes exposure elements, such as retell-ing the story of the loss, ritualization, and building tolerance to the emo-tions associated with loss. In addition, these methods offer a way to make symbolic contact with the deceased, such as through a guided encounter of memories, a dialogue, or writing letters. A focus on reconstructing meaning in the aftermath of a loss has also been shown to be an important element (Cacciatore & Flint, 2013a; Neimeyer & Currier, 2009). There is also some support for cognitive-behavioral-based approaches (Currier, Holland, & Neimeyer, 2010), though more studies are needed.

Overall, generalized psychotherapy for traumatic bereavement does not appear to be as efficacious as when it is used for other problems. This may be due, in part, to the finding that grief is a unique aspect of the human experience that, for some, may abate over time (Neimeyer & Currier, 2009). However, clinician discomfort and lack of specialized training in the field of traumatic death, especially the deaths of children, may also be a contributing factor to psychotherapy's limited efficacy (Capitulo, 2005).

More recently, Thieleman, Cacciatore, and Hill (2014) have presented evidence for a mindfulness-based, psychosocial approach for specific use in traumatic grief with bereaved parents. Outcomes from these preliminary data suggest that a mindfulness framework that fosters mindful provider feelings and behaviors (Table 6.1) known as ATTEND (attunement, trust, touch, egalitarianism, nuance, and death education, targeted toward both provider and client/patient; Cacciatore, 2010) shows reduced traumatic stress, anxiety, and depressive symptoms in grieving parents, even when controlling for time since loss. Thieleman and Cacciatore (2014b) also found this same mindfulness-based approach protected providers from secondary traumatic stress, reduced the likelihood of compassion fatigue, and signifi-cantly increased compassion satisfaction.

While there is no panacea, mindfulness-based interventions are empiri-cally promising in helping individuals cope better. Despite clinical skepti-cism about the potency of these interventions (partly due to the insufficient methodological quality of the research), research suggests that the utiliza-tion of mindfulness-based interventions should be considered an option for both patients/clients and providers dealing with perinatal/pediatric deaths

TABLE 6.1 ATTEND Framework

Attunement: mindful, responsive, empathic, deeply self-aware
Trust: active compassion, communicative, relationship-focused
Touch: therapeutic intimacy, reflexive, appropriate contact
Egalitarianism: shared decision making, humility, creativity
Nuance: individual and cultural sensitivity
Death education: psychoeducation and continuing provider education
Based on a foundation of provider self-care and compassion

because such interventions offer tangible therapeutic endpoints, they are noninvasive and low-cost, as well as offer a favorable risk–benefit ratio for patients/clients and providers. The purpose of this chapter is to review mindfulness-based interventions, data on their effectiveness, and ideas for future research.

MINDFULNESS APPROACHES

Mindfulness has been defined in several ways, such as (a) "the awareness that emerges through paying attention on purpose, in the present moment, and nonjudgmentally to the unfolding of experience moment by moment" (Kabat-Zinn, 2003, p. 145); (b) "awareness of present experience with acceptance" (Germer, 2006, p. 7); (c) a "receptive attention to and awareness of present events and experience" (Brown, Ryan, & Creswell, 2007, p. 212); (d) the self-regulation of attention with an attitude of "curiosity, openness, and acceptance" (Bishop, Lau, Shapiro, Carlson, Anderson, & Carmody, 2004, p. 232); (e) "the repeated practice of divided sustained bare attention and awareness" (Rapgay & Bystrisky, 2009, p. 152); and (f) a "unique behavioral technique involving the cultivation of non-judgmental, non-reactive, meta-cognitive awareness of present-moment experience" (Garland & Gaylord, 2009, p. 3).

Traditionally a core component of Buddhist and Judeo-Christian mystic practice, mindfulness can also be viewed secularly as "an inherent human capacity" that exists across and outside of any specific religious practice, one that allows individuals to approach and accept some degree of suffering as part of the human condition (Kabat-Zinn, 2003, p. 146). In the Pali language spoken in ancient India, the connotation of mindfulness was awareness, attention, and remembering (Chiesa & Malinowski, 2011; Germer, 2006).

Western culture's interest in mindfulness has grown exponentially over the past 50 years, and practices have been integrated into a variety of general, psychotherapeutic treatment approaches including acceptance and commitment therapy (ACT), dialectical behavioral therapy (DBT), mindfulness-based cognitive therapy (MBCT), and mindfulness-based stress reduction (MBSR; Baer & Krietemeyer, 2006).

MBSR and MBCT, specifically, have been used successfully to treat anxiety (Koszycki, Benger, Shlik, & Bradwejn, 2007), depression and recurrent depression (Kenny & Williams, 2007), eating disorders (Kristeller, Baer, & Quillian-Wolever, 2006), chronic pain (Kabat-Zinn, 1982), insomnia (Heidenreich, Tuin, Pflug, Michal, & Michalak, 2006), substance abuse (Bowen et al., 2006), and domestic violence (Silva, 2007). There are also many studies that demonstrate improvements in chronic health conditions such as cardiovascular disease. One randomized controlled trial found that MBSR reduced systolic and diastolic blood pressure and heart rate for hypertensive individuals (Manikonda et al., 2008).

Mindfulness-Based Stress Reduction (MBSR)

MBSR was initially developed as a secular, group-based program designed to treat patients with chronic pain (Ospina et al., 2007; Shigaki, Glass, & Schopp, 2006). By 1998, more than 200 U.S. clinics and hospitals were offering MBSR programs (Majumdar et al., 2002), typically administered over an 8-week period with weekly 2.5-hour sessions and daily home meditation practice, culminating in a 7.5-hour meditation retreat (Ott, Norris, & Bauer-Wu, 2006; Shennan, Payne, & Fenlon, 2011). In addition to providing education on stress and coping, core components of the MBSR program include a combination of deep self-awareness of bodily sensations, sitting and walking meditation, and yoga (Ledesma & Kumano, 2009). MBSR is the most commonly cited form of mindfulness-based intervention in clinical trials (Shennan et al., 2011). One randomized controlled trial of MBSR demonstrated significant mood improvement, increased quality of life, and higher functioning in clients with generalized anxiety disorder (Koszycki et al., 2007).

Mindfulness-Based Cognitive Therapy (MBCT)

MBCT was originally developed to treat depression, relapse, and recurrence. MBCT combines aspects of MBSR with aspects of cognitive therapy. Often, clinicians employ the 3-minute breathing space exercise (Ospina et al., 2007; Shennan et al., 2011), wherein clients learn to sit quietly for 3 full minutes while focusing on the breath. While traditional cognitive behavioral therapy

(CBT) teaches clients to replace maladaptive thought patterns with adaptive thought patterns, MBCT helps clients cultivate a tolerance for maladaptive thoughts, observing them objectively without reaction, akin to exposure and desensitization techniques (Shigaki et al., 2006). Specifically, MBCT helps clients become aware of their own negative thoughts that often trigger negative episodic feelings. Rather than avoiding or repressing the negative thoughts, they generate awareness around their emotion and cognitive processing (Brown et al., 2007; Chiesa & Malinowski, 2011). Such a perspective has been described as a state of self-observation that introduces a gap between one's perception and response to stimuli in stressful situations (Bishop et al., 2004). Shapiro, Carlson, Astin, and Freedman (2006) note that "the capacity to dispassionately observe or witness the contents of one's consciousness—enables a person to experience even very strong emotions with greater objectivity and less reactivity" (p. 381).

In two randomized controlled trials (Ma & Teasdale, 2004; Teasdale et al., 2000), MBCT was found to cut the risk of depressive relapse in half for high-risk clients with a history of three or more previous depressive episodes when compared to the treatment as usual (TAU) group, assessed over a 1-year follow-up period. These results were independently replicated in a subsequent randomized controlled trial (Godfrin & van Heeringen, 2010) and have been replicated by others as well (e.g., Kuyken et al., 2008; Segal et al., 2010).

Another randomized controlled trial found MBCT more effective, and cost less, than antidepressants in preventing depressive relapse in those with three or more depressive episodes. In addition, MBCT was more effective in improving physical and psychological components of quality of life and in reducing residual symptoms of depression as well as psychiatric comorbidity (Kuyken et al., 2008). Seventy-five percent of participants in the MBCT group were able to successfully discontinue psychiatric medications (Kuyken et al., 2008). In a later study (Segal et al., 2010), MBCT was found to be as effective as psychiatric medications, overall, in preventing relapse in depression. These findings are significant given that many individuals who are at risk of depressive relapse do not wish to continue taking medications for a variety of personal and health reasons (Segal et al., 2010). MBCT has thus been shown to be an effective nonpharmacological alternative for the prevention of relapse in depression.

One randomized controlled pilot study (Barnhofer et al., 2009) found that MBCT reduced symptoms of depression from severe to mild in currently symptomatic patients, while there was no such change in the TAU group. There is also preliminary evidence that MBCT may be effective for anxiety, which also affects many traumatically bereaved individuals. One randomized pilot study found moderate to high effect sizes for MBCT in treating social phobia in young adults, similar to results from CBT (Piet,

Hougaard, Hecksher, & Rosenberg, 2010). MBCT has also shown promise in a pilot randomized controlled trial for increasing sleep quality and decreasing mood disturbances (Britton, Haynes, Fridel, & Bootzin, 2010), common concerns in traumatic grief. Because those who are traumatically bereaved also often report symptoms of traumatic stress, such as hypervigilance, experiential avoidance, and intrusive thoughts, as well as depressive and anxious symptoms, there has been a recent burgeoning interest in evaluating integrative approaches such as mindfulness-based models for grief.

Using Mindfulness With Grief

Though more research beyond these preliminary data is needed, mindfulness-based approaches such as MBCT and MBSR may also be effective in treating traumatic grief-related distress in grieving parents. One novel approach to traumatic grief specifically has been proposed in the literature and preliminary data are promising. Using the ATTEND model in therapeutic practice, Thieleman et al. (2014) fostered provider/client mindfulness successfully throughout sessions by teaching mind–body awareness exercises; teaching clients to notice thoughts, sensations, and emotions without judgment; using intentional silence and pause; and suggesting awareness journaling and meditation exercises. In addition, providers commit to their own mindfulness and/or meditation practice at home. These methods, both highly efficient and cost-effective, seem to protect grieving parents, and the providers and volunteers who serve them, from the enduring and deleterious effects of traumatic and secondary traumatic grief (Cacciatore, Thieleman, et al., 2013; Thieleman & Cacciatore, 2014b; Thieleman et al., 2014).

Like other mindfulness-based approaches, these practices increase emotional regulation by helping both patients/clients and clinicians respond rather than react habitually, cultivate greater self-awareness (Cacciatore, Thieleman, et al., 2013), and deepen the nature of therapeutic intimacy through attunement (Cacciatore, 2010; Cacciatore & Flint, 2012a). Clinicians themselves model nonjudgmental acceptance and active self/other compassion, and this milieu creates a safe environment for clients/patients. One double-blind randomized controlled trial found that, even when *only the provider practiced mindfulness* meditation, the results for clients whose provider practiced had significant symptom relief compared to nonpracticing providers (Grepmair et al., 2007).

This may be, in part, because providers who practice mindfulness engage in deepened empathy, are more actively compassionate, and are more attuned to clients. They have an enhanced ability to remain present through traumatic recollection, all of which can help strengthen intimacy and trust in the therapeutic relationship (Thieleman, Cacciatore, & Hill, 2014). Indeed,

Shapiro et al. (1998) found that medical students experienced a significant increase in core empathy with a concomitant reduction in anxiety and depression when compared to a control group as part of a randomized controlled trial on mindfulness practice in medical school. The team found that mindfulness reduces self-criticism and avoidance behaviors, and improves life satisfaction and self-compassion. Consistent with these findings, Thieleman and Cacciatore (2014b) also found that a mindfulness approach to traumatic grief, when practiced by providers who are identified as high-risk, is protective against provider burnout and compassion fatigue, while improving compassion satisfaction. Mindfulness practices with bereaved parents appear to result in better outcomes and reduced risk for patients/clients, as well as increased provider satisfaction, esteem, and compassion for self and other (Cacciatore & Flint, 2012a; Grepmair et al., 2007; Thieleman & Cacciatore, 2014b).

Mindfulness and Being With What Is

One major concept in mindfulness practice is radical acceptance and normalization of the neverending fluctuations of human emotions (Baer, 2003), which are particularly salient with suffering. In this context, bereaved parents' experiences are, thus, viewed as normal reactions to painful losses and are to be treated with the utmost care and compassion. In contrast, traditional medical pedagogy has maintained antipodean views in response to trauma and suffering: The first view is to "respond to suffering with objectivity and detachment," purportedly to avoid provider exhaustion and to ensure that medical decisions are made with objectivity. This approach has been strongly criticized in the literature for increasing the risk of pathologizing bereaved parents and others traumatically bereaved, leading to premature and overly aggressive pharmacological treatment of grief (Dowrick & Frances, 2013; Lacasse & Cacciatore, 2014; Thieleman & Cacciatore, 2014a; Wakefield, 2012).

The other admonition is for providers to "form bonds of compassionate solidarity with [patients]" (Coulehan, 2009, p. 585). This is consistent with mindfulness-based approaches that seem to promote humility and compassion (Cacciatore, 2010), suffering *with* the other, as virtues worthy of cultivation in both mental health and medical care. These traits seem to ameliorate emotional angst and long-term negative outcomes for clients/patients and providers (Coulehan, 2009; Thieleman & Cacciatore, 2014b). Over time, the intensity and frequency of traumatic grief symptoms become less debilitating and mourners are better able to not only tolerate their experiences of suffering, but also cope more effectively. Mindfulness practices prepare clinicians to be with what is, and this state may reduce symptoms and improve client awareness of and tolerance for painful emotions, coping skills, and overall well-being, all in the client's own time (Cacciatore & Flint, 2012a).

MEDITATION

Of all mindfulness practices, one of the most cost-effective strategies to help providers working with bereaved parents is meditation. That is, meditation, or contemplative practices, on the part of the *provider*.

The word *meditation* derives from Latin's *meditari* "to engage in contemplation or reflection," the same root as the word *medicine* (Hussain & Bhushan, 2010). Meditation practices are largely rooted in ancient spiritual traditions practiced as many as 5,000 years ago (Chiesa & Malinowski, 2011), and are thus found in cultures throughout the world (Fortney & Taylor, 2010). Over the past 40 years, both secular and spiritual forms of meditation have interested clinicians, researchers, and the general public in Western countries as a means to alleviate health-related problems and to attain or maintain general wellness (Ospina et al., 2008). The U.S. Agency for Healthcare Research and Quality (AHRQ) identified five major categories of contemplative practice: (a) mantra meditation, (b) yoga, (c) qigong, (d) tai chi, and (e) mindfulness meditation (Ospina et al., 2007; see Table 6.2). One national survey found that 31% of hospitals treating cancer patients offered meditation as an outpatient service (Ananth, 2011), primarily due to patient demand, while citing budgetary constraints (70%) and lack of evidence-based studies (40%) as the two most significant barriers for implementation (Ananth, 2011). However, little could be found on provider practice instruction in hospitals and agencies.

Still, there is a strong argument that practice decisions should be based on factors that include "client preferences and values, situational circumstances,

TABLE 6.2 Sit Instructions

Focused Meditation Practice

1. Get in a comfortable position either sitting in a chair or sitting on a cushion.

2. Place your tongue at the roof of your mouth behind your teeth and press slightly.

3. Gently close your eyes and take three long, slow, deep breaths.

4. Focus all your attention on the ambient sound in the room. You may hear your own breath, the buzzing of lights, ticking of clocks, passing of cars. All these sounds are fine. Just listen deeper and deeper and deeper.

5. If your mind wanders from the sound, just notice the wandering and gently bring your mind back to the sound.

6. Do this exercise for 15 to 30 minutes over the course of 2 weeks. Record, in a daily journal, anything you notice and/or feel about this experience.

professional ethics, the practitioner's existing skills, and available resources" (Thyer & Myers, 2010, p. 8). Because of the ease of implementation, meditation practice may decrease the financial burden for patients and health care providers in that they are noninvasive, low-cost, and have a favorable risk–benefit ratio (Carlson & Bultz, 2008; Elkins, Fisher, & Johnson, 2010; Maizes, Rakel, & Niemiec 2009; Schaub, 2011; Wesa, 2008). Future research that explores psychological efficacy, physiological and cognitive outcomes, and specific benefit for client/patient traumatic stress and secondary stress for providers balanced against cost–benefit ratio may encourage health insurance providers to realize the financial imperative for these practices (Shigaki et al., 2006).

CONCERNS ABOUT THE MINDFULNESS APPROACH TO TRAUMATIC GRIEF

Despite clinical skepticism about the potency of these interventions (partly due to the dearth of research, lack of funding, and difficulty executing randomized controlled trials), preliminary research suggests that the utilization of mindfulness-based interventions should be considered an option for both patients/clients and providers dealing with perinatal/pediatric deaths because such interventions offer tangible therapeutic endpoints, are noninvasive and low-cost, and provide a highly favorable risk–benefit ratio. Yet, many mental health and medical providers may not be familiar with mindfulness-based approaches to physical, social, or psychological health, despite the fact that these skills "can be cultivated by anyone" (Germer, 2006, p. 5). Administrative teams may not recognize the long-term benefits of mindfulness practices for providers and the potentiality for clients/patients.

Yet, health care professionals who encounter death are particularly vulnerable to depression, anxiety, anger, helplessness (Coulehan, 2009; West et al., 2009), lethargy, intrusive thoughts, and nightmares. Emotional exhaustion and compassion fatigue are not uncommon experiences for physicians, nurses, social workers, and even clergy, particularly when faced with sudden and traumatic deaths, especially the death of a child. These psychological effects may greatly impact the quality of care providers are able to offer patients. Research suggests that a compassionate, mindful presence in the midst of the traumatic loss helps moderate long-term, negative psychiatric sequelae for providers, and this may provide siginficant benefit to administrators. Providers who practice mindfulness-based interventions suffer compassion fatigue less often and are more empathic with clients, reducing the effects of trauma and, perhaps, improving the provider–patient relationship and patient satisfaction (Krasner et al., 2009; Thieleman & Cacciatore, 2014a, 2014b; West et al., 2009).

CONCLUSION

Interest has been piqued in mindfulness practices among providers serving bereaved parents and the bereaved themselves. Despite the medical community's initial skepticism about the potency of these interventions, preliminary data suggest these methods present less potential harm, are more cost-effective, and may be highly effacious in helping bereaved parents, and they may also be protective for providers who are at high risk of negative psychological outcomes. Future research can be improved with more randamized controlled trials in the bereaved parent population and by utilizing mixed methods to account for the interdependent biological mechanisms and contextual health behaviors that are integral to outcomes.

CASE STUDY

Shawnice is a 29-year-old patient who experienced the death of a baby at 34 weeks gestation. She reports that her baby died 3 months ago and she feels very anxious and tearful throughout the day. She notes that certain experiences trigger these episodes, especially seeing a baby or hearing other people talk badly about their children. Shawnice participates in a perinatal bereavement support group and also receives individual psychotherapy.

FOCUS QUESTIONS

1. How could mindfulness-based approaches complement the supportive measures that Shawnice is receiving?
2. What are the benefits of mindfulness-based interventions?
3. How would you identify practitioners in Shawnice's community who are skilled in using mindfulness approaches with someone who experienced a traumatic death?
4. How would you determine that mindfulness-based interventions were effective for Shawnice?

REFERENCES

Ananth, S. (2011). 2010 Complementary and alternative medicine survey of hospitals. *Samueli Institute.* Retrieved from http://www.siib.org/news/36-SIIB.html

Badenhorst, W., Riches, S., Turton, P., & Hughes, P. (2006). The psychological effects of stillbirth and neonatal death on fathers: Systematic review. *Journal of Psychosomatic Obstetrics & Gynecology, 27*(4), 245–256.

Baer, R. A. (2003). Mindfulness training as a clinical intervention: A conceptual and empirical review. *Clinical Psychology: Science and Practice, 10*(2), 125–143.

Baer, R. A., & Krietemeyer, J. (2006). Overview of mindfulness- and acceptance-based treatment approaches. In R. A. Baer (Ed.), *Mindfulness-based treatment approaches: Clinician's guide to evidence base and applications* (pp. 3–27). San Diego, CA: Elsevier.

Barnhofer, T., Crane, C., Hargus, E., Amarasinghe, M., Winder, R., & Williams, J. M. G. (2009). Mindfulness-based cognitive therapy as a treatment for chronic depression: A preliminary study. *Behaviour Research and Therapy, 47*(5), 366–373.

Bishop, S. R., Lau, M., Shapiro, S., Carlson, L., Anderson, N. D., & Carmody, J. (2004). Mindfulness: A proposed operational definition. *Clinical Psychology: Science and Practice, 11*(3), 230–241. doi:10.1093/clipsy.bph077

Bowen, S., Witkiewitz, K., Dillworth, T., Chawla, N., Simpson, T. L., & Ostafin, B. (2006). Mindfulness meditation and substance use in an incarcerated population. *Psychology of Addictive Behaviors, 20*(2), 343–347.

Britton, W. B., Haynes, P. L., Fridel, K. W., & Bootzin, R. R. (2010). Polysomnographic and subjective profiles of sleep continuity before and after mindfulness-based cognitive therapy in partially remitted depression. *Psychosomatic Medicine, 72*(6), 539–548.

Brown, K. W., Ryan, R. M., & Creswell, J. D. (2007). Mindfulness: Theoretical foundations and evidence for its salutary effects. *Psychological Inquiry, 18*(4), 211–237.

Cacciatore, J. (2010). Stillbirth: Clinical recommendations for care in the era of evidence-based medicine. *Clinical Obstetrics and Gynecology, 53*(3), 691–699.

Cacciatore, J., & Flint, M. (2012a). ATTEND: A mindfulness-based bereavement care model. *Death Studies, 36*(1), 61–82.

Cacciatore, J., & Flint, M. (2012b). Mediating grief: Postmortem ritualization after a child's death. *Journal of Loss and Trauma, 17*(2), 158–172.

Cacciatore, J., & Thieleman, K. (2012). The use of psychiatric medications in treating acute traumatic bereavement: A case series. *Journal of Loss and Trauma, 17*(6), 557–579.

Cacciatore, J., Lacasse, J. R., Lietz, C., & McPherson, J. (2013). A parent's TEARS: Primary results from the traumatic experiences and resiliency study. *Omega Journal of Death and Dying, 68*(3), 183–205.

Cacciatore, J., Thieleman, K., Osborn, J., & Orlowski, K. (2013). Of the soul and suffering: Mindfulness-based interventions and bereavement. *Clinical Social Work Journal, 42*(3), 269–281.

Capitulo, K. L. (2005). Evidence for healing interventions with perinatal bereavement. *American Journal of Maternal-Child Nursing, 30*(6), 389–396.

Carlson, L. E., & Bultz, B. D. (2008) Mind–body interventions in oncology. *Current Treatment Options in Oncology, 9*, 127–134.

Chiesa, A., & Malinowski, P. (2011). Mindfulness-based approaches: Are they all the same? *Journal of Clinical Psychology, 67*(4), 404–424.

Coulehan, J. (2009). Compassionate solidarity: Suffering, poetry, and medicine. *Perspectives in Biology and Medicine, 52*(4), 585–603.

Currier, J. M., Holland, J. M., & Neimeyer, R. A. (2010). Do CBT-based interventions alleviate distress following bereavement? A review of the current evidence. *International Journal of Cognitive Therapy, 3*(1), 77–93.

Dowrick, C., & Frances, A. (2013). Medicalising unhappiness: New classification of depression risks more patients being put on drug treatment. *British Medical Journal, 347*, f7140.

Dyregrov, A., & Matthiesen, S. B. (1991). Parental grief following the death of an infant—a follow-up over one year. *Scandinavian Journal of Psychology, 32*(3), 193–207.

Dyregrov, K., Nordanger, D., & Dyregrov, A. (2003). Predictors of psychosocial distress after suicide, SIDS, and accidents. *Death Studies, 27*(2), 143–165.

Elkins, G., Fisher, W., & Johnson, A. (2010). Mind–body therapies in integrative oncology. *Current Treatment Options in Oncology, 11*, 128–140.

Fortney, L., & Taylor, M. (2010). Meditation in medical practice: A review of the evidence and practice. *Primary Care, 37*(1), 81–90.

Garland, E., & Gaylord, S. (2009). Envisioning a future contemplative science of mindfulness: Fruitful methods and new content for the next wave of research. *Complementary Health Practice Review, 14*(1), 3–9.

Germer, C. K. (2006). What is mindfulness? In C. K Germer, R. D. Siegel, & P. R. Fulton (Ed.), *Mindfulness & psychotherapy* (pp. 3–16). New York, NY: The Guilford Press.

Godfrin, K. A., & van Heeringen, C. (2010). The effects of mindfulness-based cognitive therapy on recurrence of depressive episodes, mental health and quality of life: A randomized controlled study. *Behaviour Research and Therapy, 48*(8), 738–746.

Green, B. L. (2000). Traumatic loss: Conceptual and empirical links between trauma and bereavement. *Journal of Personal and Interpersonal Loss, 5*(1), 1–17.

Grepmair, L., Mitterlehner, F., Loew, T., Bachler, E., Rother, W., & Nickel, M. (2007). Promoting mindfulness in psychotherapists in training influences the treatment results of their patients: A randomized, double-blind, controlled study. *Psychotherapy and Psychosomatics, 76*(6), 332–338.

Heidenreich, T., Tuin, I., Pflug, B., Michal, M., & Michalak, J. (2006). Mindfulness-based cognitive therapy for insomnia: A pilot study. *Psychotherapy and Psychosomatics, 75*, 188–189.

Hussain, D., & Bhushan, B. (2010). Psychology of meditation and health: Present status and future directions. *International Journal of Psychology and Psychological Therapy, 10*(3), 439–451.

Kabat-Zinn, J. (1982). An outpatient program in behavioral medicine for chronic pain patients based on the practice of mindfulness meditation: Theoretical considerations and preliminary results. *General Hospital Psychiatry, 4*(1), 33–47.

Kabat-Zinn, J. (2003). Mindfulness-based interventions in context: Past, present, and future. *Clinical Psychology: Science and Practice, 10*(2), 144–156.

Kenny, M., & Williams, J. M. (2007). Treatment resistant depressed patients show good response to mindfulness-based cognitive therapy. *Behavior Research and Therapy, 45*, 617–625.

Koszycki, D., Benger, M., Shlik, J., & Bradwejn, J. (2007). Randomized trail of meditation based stress reduction program in generalized social anxiety disorder. *Behavior Research and Therapy, 45*, 2517–2525.

Krasner, M., Epstein, R., Beckman, H., Suchman, A., Chapman, B., Mooney, C. J., & Quill, T. E. (2009). Association of an education program in mindful communication with burnout, empathy, and attitudes among primary care physicians. *Journal of the American Medical Association, 302*(12), 1284–1293.

Kristeller, J. L., Baer, R. A., & Quillian-Wolever, R. (2006). Mindfulness-based approaches to eating disorders. In R. Baer (Ed.), *Mindfulness-based treatment approaches: Clinician's guide to evidence base and applications* (pp. 75–91). New York, NY: Academic Press.

Kuyken, W., Byford, S., Taylor, R. S., Watkins, E., Holden, E., & White, K. (2008). Mindfulness-based cognitive therapy to prevent relapse in recurrent depression. *Journal of Consulting Clinical Psychology, 76*(6), 966–978. doi:10.1037/a0013786

Lacasse, J., & Cacciatore, J. (2014). TEARS: A retrospective, observational study of psychiatric medication in treating bereaved mothers. *Death Studies, 38,* 589–596.

Ledesma, D., & Kumano, H. (2009). Mindfulness-based stress reduction and cancer: A meta-analysis. *Psycho-Oncology, 18*(6), 571–579.

Ma, S. H., & Teasdale, J. D. (2004). Mindfulness-based cognitive therapy for depression: Replication and exploration of differential relapse prevention effects. *Journal of Consulting and Clinical Psychology, 72*(1), 31–40.

Maizes, V., Rakel, D., & Niemiec, C. (2009). Integrative medicine and patient-centered care. *Explore, 5*(5), 277–289.

Majumdar, M., Grossman, P., Dietz-Waschkowski, B., Kersig, S., & Walach, H. (2002). Does mindfulness meditation contribute to health? Outcome evaluation of a German sample. *Journal of Alternative and Complementary Medicine. 8*(6), 719–730.

Manikonda, J. P., Stork, S. S., Togel, S. S., Lobmuller, A. A., Grunberg, I. I., Bedel, S. S., & Voelker, W. W., (2008). Contemplative meditation reduces ambulatory blood pressure and stress-induced hypertension: A randomized pilot trial. *Journal of Human Hypertension, 22,* 138–140.

Neimeyer, R. A., & Currier, J. M. (2009). Grief therapy: Evidence of efficacy and emerging directions. *Current Directions in Psychological Science, 18*(6), 352–356.

Nouwen, H. (1981). *The way of the heart.* New York, NY: Ballantine Books.

Ospina, M. B., Bond, K., Karkhaneh, M., Buscemi, N., Dryden, D. M., Barnes, V.,. . . Shannahoff-Khalsa, D. (2008). Clinical trials of meditation practices in health care: Characteristics and quality. *The Journal of Alternative and Complementary Medicine, 14*(10), 1199–1213.

Ospina, M. B., Bond, T. K., Karkhaneh, M., Tjosvold, L., Vandermeer, B., Liang, Y.,. . . Klassen, T. P. (2007). *Meditation practices for health: State of the research. Evidence Report/ Technology Assessment No. 155.* (Prepared by the University of Alberta Evidence-Based Practice Center Under Contract No. 290-02-0023.). Rockville, MD: Agency for Healthcare Research and Quality.

Ott, M. J., Norris, R. L., & Bauer-Wu, S. M. (2006). Mindfulness meditation for oncology patients: A discussion and critical review. *Integrative Cancer Therapies, 5*(2), 98–108.

Piet, J., Hougaard, E., Hecksher, M. S., & Rosenberg, N. K. (2010). A randomized pilot study of mindfulness-based cognitive therapy and group cognitive-behavioral therapy for young adults with social phobia. *Scandinavian Journal of Psychology, 51*(5), 403–410.

Rando, T. A. (1985). Bereaved parents: Particular difficulties, unique factors, and treatment issues. *Social Work, 30*(1), 19–23.

Rapgay, L. & Bystrisky, A. (2009). Classical mindfulness: An introduction to its theory and practice for clinical application. *Annals of the New York Academy of Sciences, 1172*(1), 148–162.

Rogers, C. H., Floyd, F. J., Seltzer, M. M., Greenberg, J., & Hong, J. (2008). Long-term effects of the death of a child on parents' adjustment in midlife. *Journal of Family Psychology, 22*(2), 203–211.

Schaub, R. (2011). Clinical meditation teacher: A new role for health professionals. *Journal of Evidence-Based Complementary & Alternative Medicine, 16*(2), 145–148.

Segal, Z. V., Bieling, P., Young, T., MacQueen, G., Cooke, R., Martin, L., . . . Levitan, R. D. (2010). Antidepressant monotherapy vs sequential pharmacotherapy and mindfulness-based cognitive therapy, or placebo, for relapse prophylaxis in recurrent depression. *Archives of General Psychiatry, 67*(12), 1256–1264.

Shapiro, S. L., Carlson, L. E., Astin, J. A., & Freedman, B. (2006). Mechanisms of mindfulness. *Journal of Clinical Psychology, 62*(3), 373–386.

Shapiro, S. L., Schwartz, G. E., & Bonner, G. (1998). Effects of mindfulness-based stress reduction on medical and premedical students. *Journal of Behavioral Medicine, 21*(6), 581–599.

Shennan, C., Payne, S., & Fenlon, D. (2011). What is the evidence for the use of mindfulness-based interventions in cancer care? A review. *Psycho-Oncology, 20*(7), 681–697.

Shigaki, C. L., Glass, B., & Schopp, L. H. (2006). Mindfulness-based stress reduction in medical settings. *Journal of Clinical Psychology in Medical Settings, 13*(3), 209–215.

Silva, J. (2007). Mindfulness-based CBT for the reduction of anger in married men. *Dissertation Abstracts International: The Sciences and Engineering, 68*(3B), 1945.

Teasdale, J. D., Segal, Z. V., Williams, J. M. G., Ridgeway, V. A., Soulsby, J. M., & Lau, M. A. (2000). Prevention of relapse/recurrence in major depression by mindfulness-based cognitive therapy. *Journal of Consulting and Clinical Psychology, 68*(4), 615–623.

Thieleman, K., & Cacciatore, J. (2014a). When a child dies: A critical analysis of grief-related controversies in the *DSM-5. Research on Social Work Practice, 24*(1), 114–122.

Thieleman, K., & Cacciatore, J. (2014b). A witness to suffering: Mindfulness and compassion fatigue amongst traumatic bereavement volunteers and professionals. *Social Work, 59*(1), 34–41.

Thieleman, K., Cacciatore, J., & Hill, T. W. (2014). Traumatic bereavement and mindfulness: A preliminary study of mental health outcomes using the ATTEND model. *Clinical Social Work Journal, 42*(3), 260–268.

Thyer, B. A., & Myers, L. L. (2010). The quest for evidence-based practice: A view from the United States. *Journal of Social Work, 11*(1), 8–25.

Wakefield, J. C. (2012). Should prolonged grief be reclassified as a mental disorder in *DSM-5*?: Reconsidering the empirical and conceptual arguments for complicated grief disorder. *Journal of Nervous and Mental Disease, 200*(6), 499–511.

Wesa, K. (2008). Integrative oncology: Complementary therapies for cancer survivors. *Hematology/Oncology Clinics of North America, 22*(2), 343–353.

West, C., Tan, A. D., Habermann, T. M., Sloan, J. A., & Shanafelt, T. D. (2009). Association of resident fatigue and distress with perceived medical errors. *JAMA, 302*(12), 1294–1300.

CHAPTER 7

Complicated Grief and Perinatal Loss

Patricia Moyle Wright

*U*nexpected loss during pregnancy often results in myriad emotions that can range from ambivalence to devastation. Grief reactions often involve anxiety, guilt and self-blame, depressive symptoms, persistent sadness, and longing. For most perinatally bereaved women, grief symptoms will dissipate gradually over the course of a year, sometimes less (Wright, 2010). For some, however, moving beyond the darkest part of the grief is a great challenge. Some women experience very severe and persistent symptoms, which include prolonged grief, intense longing, and persistent sadness, that interfere with their daily lives. For these women, perinatal grief does not run its normal course and may be considered to be complicated.

Complicated grief (CG) has garnered significant attention in the grief literature over the past few years. The notion that grief symptoms can become so severe as to rise to the level of pathology has been hotly debated. CG has been viewed as an aberrant pathway by some researchers (Horowitz et al., 2003; Prigerson et al., 1997; Shear & Shair, 2005). Others question whether the symptoms associated with CG are actually dimensions of the normal grief process (Hogan, Worden, & Schmidt, 2004; Stroebe et al., 2000). Despite the ongoing controversy, the empirical evidence on CG that has been gathered in the past decade has garnered significant attention among grief researchers. An ever-growing cadre of researchers has worked diligently to conduct rigorous research to uncover the dimensions of grief and its course. This work has led to widespread acceptance of the concept of CG. Research has been conducted on the incidence and manifestations of CG in various bereaved groups, including perinatally bereaved mothers. The literature has been focused on the development of criteria to identify CG, support for and opposition to inclusion of the CG criteria in the *Diagnostic and Statistical Manual of Mental Disorders, Fifth Edition (DSM-5)*, and treatment options for CG.

The research that has been conducted on CG thus far supports the notion that CG can manifest following any significant loss in a person's life. The risk for CG after pregnancy loss, specifically, has been the subject of only limited research. The consequences of pregnancy loss are varied and often prolonged, which may predispose women to CG. This chapter provides an overview of the general literature on CG and on CG as it relates to women's experiences of perinatal loss. Treatment considerations are also reviewed and implications for future research are explored. Of note, CG and prolonged grief have recently been equated in the literature (Shear, 2015), but there has been about this linkage (Rando, 2013). For the purposes of this chapter, the term *complicated grief* (CG) is used because this is the term that has been used most frequently with regard to reactions to perinatal loss.

DEFINING CG

CG, as its name implies, differs from the expected grief trajectory. Typically, grief ensues after a significant loss and involves searching and yearning, feelings of sadness, anxiety, depression, and emotional pain (Lichtenthal, Cruess, & Prigerson, 2004; Parkes, 2014). Physical aspects of grief have also been reported (Fenstermacher, 2014; Thieleman & Cacciatore, 2013; Wright, 2010). Such responses to grief are expected and can be sometimes very intense. However, in the normal course of grief, symptoms are expected to gradually decrease over time. By roughly 6 months after a loss, it is expected that the bereft individual will be able to begin to re-engage in life and assume many of his or her usual activities (Moore, 2011). There is variation on this time frame and it is well known that waves of regrieving can occur, often unexpectedly, and can be very intense (Shear, 2015), but these reoccurrences of emotional suffering are expected to be short-lived, temporary setbacks in an otherwise forward-moving process.

However, the usual course of grief is not experienced by every bereaved individual. For some, grief can be absent, delayed, or prolonged. Such variations are generally thought to be related to the relationship the survivor had with the deceased and the survivor's coping patterns (Christiansen, Elklit, & Olff, 2013). For those with inadequate coping ability and poor support, adjustment after loss is more challenging and other issues, such as depression, may arise (Parkes, 2014). Pre-existing mental health disorders may become exacerbated (Shear et al., 2011). Even in the absence of pre-existing conditions, traumatic losses can predispose individuals to very severe grief responses. Some bereaved individuals may even exhibit symptoms of posttraumatic stress disorder (PTSD), which can include reliving the experience, avoidance behaviors, and arousal (Christiansen et al., 2013). Still others respond to loss in ways that do not fit with the atypical grief patterns that have already been identified. Roughly 2% to 3% of bereaved individuals experience symptom clusters that are indicative of CG reactions (Shear, 2015). Estimates are higher (10%–20%) for those who lose a romantic partner or a child (Shear, 2015; Shear et al., 2011).

CG is defined as a prolonged, abnormal response to loss that impairs participation with usual daily activities (Prigerson et al., 1995; Stroebe, Schut, & van den Bout, 2013). It involves chronic and excessive grief reactions that are characterized by longing, strong yearning, preoccupying thoughts about the deceased person, hallucinations, intrusive thoughts about the decreased, disturbed sleep, avoidance of people or places that could trigger grief, and failure to adapt to the loss (Horowitz et al., 2003; Prigerson et al., 1996; Shear, 2015; Worden, 1991).

Some key factors predispose individuals to CG, including history of mental health issues (Horowitz et al., 2003); neurophysiological alterations that cause dysregulation of emotional responses (Shear, 2015); sudden, violent, or traumatic loss; loss of a baby; or preventable loss (Rando, 1986). Consequences associated with CG have also been identified and include suicidality, heart disease (Prigerson et al., 1996), increased systolic blood pressure, cancer, changes in addictive behaviors, depression, anxiety, hospitalization, accidents (Lichtenthal, Cruess, & Prigerson, 2004), altered neuroendocrine and immune responses (Buckley et al., 2012), and disturbed sleep (Shear, 2015). Given the sheer number of negative consequences associated with CG and that some are especially dire and life-threatening, researchers have forwarded the movement to recognize CG as a unique mental health issue that should be diagnosed and treated (Horowitz et al., 2003; Lichtenthal et al., 2004).

Criteria for identifying CG were proposed (Horowitz et al., 2003) and many have recognized the value of this new way of identifying patients at risk for serious complications after a loss. The CG criteria resonate with clinicians and give them a way of identifying persistent and atypical reactions to loss (Rando, 2013). Despite the movement to include CG as a unique mental health diagnosis, it was not specifically included in the *DSM-5* when it was released in 2013.

GRIEF AND THE *DSM-5*

Although CG was not included as a distinct diagnosis, the bereavement exclusion was removed from the newest edition of the *DSM*. The exclusion disallowed diagnosis of a mental health condition such as depression within the first 2 months of a loss because bereavement could include related symptoms, but would be expected to resolve over time (Doka, 2013) and would not be considered pathological in the aftermath of a loss. The American

Psychiatric Association (2013b), the publishers of the *DSM*, noted that many life stressors can precipitate mental health issues and current research no longer supports the specific exclusion of bereavement. The removal of this exclusion means that bereavement is now recognized as a possible trigger for several types of mental health issues, including major depression, adjustment disorder, persistent complex bereavement disorder, and separation anxiety (Parkes, 2014; Searight, 2014). Further, the American Psychiatric Association (2013a) noted that the removal of the bereavement exclusion indicates that bereavement normally lasts longer than 2 months, and can last 1 to 2 years.

CG, however, may last longer, and be more intense than typical grief reactions. Researchers continue to work toward delineating the scope, antecedents, and consequences of CG. Recent studies sought to identify how CG manifests in various circumstances, such as after a nondeath-related loss such as an earthquake (Li, Chow, Shi, & Chan, 2015), after the death of a family member in the intensive care unit (Ketish-Barnes et al., 2015), and after the loss of a child (Zetumer et al., 2015). Another type of loss that has attracted some attention in relation to CG is perinatal loss.

CG AND PERINATAL LOSS

Perinatal loss has been found to lead to feelings of grief (Barr & Cacciatore, 2008; Fenstermacher, 2014; St. John, Cooke, & Goopy, 2006), guilt (Wright, 2010), depression (Toffol, Koponen, & Partonen, 2013; van den Akker, 2011), altered relationships (Kagami et al., 2012; Sutan & Miskam, 2012; van den Akker, 2011), and lifelong occurrences of regrieving (Dyson & While, 1998; Wright, 2010). Outcomes of perinatal bereavement may include "negative long-term social, psychosocial, and biological outcomes such as anxiety, dysthymia, suicidality, loneliness, anhedonism, substance abuse, inorganic pain, and attachment, and relational problems" (Cacciatore, 2010, p. 691).

Perinatal loss has been viewed as a traumatic loss that can even lead to symptoms of PTSD (Christiansen et al., 2013; Hutti, Armstrong, Myers, & Hall, 2015; Murphy, Shevlin, & Elklit, 2014). PTSD and CG are distinct entities (Lichtenthal et al., 2004), but traumatic losses predispose individuals to CG (Rando, 1986). Another risk factor for CG is the perceived preventability of the loss (Rando, 1986). Bereaved mothers question whether they could have taken steps to protect their babies and thereby prevented the loss (Wojnar, Swanson, & Adolfsson, 2011; Wright, 2010). In fact, ruminations about the preventability of the loss and the reason for the loss are common features of perinatal loss (Black & Wright, 2012). Such ruminations often lead to self-blame (Wright, 2010). Intrusivity and rumination are also common features of CG (Horowitz et al., 2003; Shear, 2015).

Although not specifically identified as a risk factor for CG, previous loss experiences shape women's responses to perinatal loss (Boss & Clarke-Pounder, 2012). The perinatal loss literature indicates that certain key experiences can cause a deeper grief after perinatal loss (Kersting & Wagner, 2012). Women who have experienced infertility, repeated losses, or traumatic losses may be at greater risk for CG reactions (Kersting & Wagner, 2012; Price & McLeod, 2012). Lack of social support is also a risk factor for CG. This risk factor is especially noteworthy because women's perceptions regarding lack of emotional support from loved ones and from health care providers are well documented (Cacciatore, 2010; Lang et al., 2011; Wright, 2010). Often, perinatal loss is not socially recognized, which supports the notion that perinatal loss is a form of disenfranchised grief (Boss, 2007; Lang et al., 2011). When perinatal loss is not recognized, it can lead to feelings of isolation (Wright, 2010), which adds to the depth and complexity of the grief. Interestingly, while lack of social support can contribute to CG, impaired social relationships are also a symptom of CG (Kagami et al., 2012; Scheidt et al., 2012).

CG also involves "avoidance of situations that serve as reminders of the loss" (Shear, 2015, p. 156), which is quite common after perinatal loss. Some women avoid perceived triggers such as being around babies and pregnant women, and in subsequent pregnancies will often try to avoid going to the same hospital where the loss occurred (Wright, 2010). Interestingly, these responses from perinatally bereaved women are considered to be part of the normal trajectory of perinatal grief (Fenstermacher, 2014; Wright, 2010) and are generally not considered to be complicated within the context of perinatal loss.

Similarly, "the urge to hold onto the deceased person by constantly reminiscing or by viewing, touching, or smelling the deceased person's belongings" (Shear, 2015, p. 156) has been identified as a feature of CG. In contrast, dwelling with mementos of a baby who has died has been found to be healing after perinatal loss, possibly because the mementos serve to validate the loss (Blood & Cacciatore, 2014; Kavanaugh & Moro, 2006; McCreight, 2008). The line, then, between normal responses to perinatal loss and CG reactions after perinatal loss would seem to be, as in other cases, a matter of degree, based on self-report of how disruptive the grief is to the life of the bereaved.

The length of time that symptoms persist is at issue as well (Shear et al., 2011). In most cases, perinatal grief is expected to gradually decrease over the course of about 9 months to 1 year (Wright, 2010). Numerous studies have indicated that episodes of regrieving after perinatal loss can last for decades (Dyson & While, 1998; Lang et al., 2011; Wright, 2010) and can alter a woman's views of subsequent pregnancy (Côté-Arsenault, & Dombeck, 2001) and parenting of a subsequent child (Warland, O'Leary, McCutcheon, & Williamson, 2010). Thus, the ongoing nature of perinatal bereavement, in and of itself, may not indicate a CG response. However, distinguishing expected waves of grief from prolonged grief or CG is a matter of examining the intensity of the grief and the disruption of normal activities. When the grief is very intense, all-consuming, and disrupts the person's ability to engage in his or her normal daily activities, treatment should be considered and should include screening for suicidality.

TREATING CG

Although the concept of CG has been well documented and has been studied in depth, few studies have been conducted specifically related to the treatment of CG. The recommendations that have accrued thus far are reviewed in this section. Other insights regarding the support of perinatally bereaved parents, particularly those at risk for more CG responses, will also be discussed.

For perinatally bereaved parents, memories of getting the news of the loss coincide with their memories of how the health care provider delivered the news of the loss. The moment when a parent gets the news of the baby's death is a moment crystallized in time (Wright, 2010). The memories taken from that encounter by bereaved parents are lifelong and have bearing on the grief process (Lang et al., 2011). Thus, it is imperative that health care professionals have a well-rooted understanding of the communication skills needed to break bad news (Wright, 2016). A working understanding of grief theory is also necessary for all health care professionals because grief and loss are integral to the human experience and health care professionals regularly bear witness to human suffering.

This generalization is not to say that individual health care providers should be charged with providing comprehensive care for grieving patients alone. Rather, a case management approach is required to ensure proper coordination of services and continuity of care (Wool, 2013). Within the case management model, Wool (2013) recommended that pre-existing mental health issues be identified and addressed. Also, the case management team must work with grieving families to identify coping strategies and sources of support. In this way, a comprehensive program of care can be developed that addresses not only mental and physical manifestations of grief, but also religious, spiritual, and existential needs (Wool, 2013).

Programs of care must be structured enough to provide a framework for practitioners, but should be flexible enough to allow and promote patient-centered care. Cacciatore (2010) noted that when bereaved mothers received patient-centered care, psychological and somatic symptoms of grief decreased, particularly for those women who otherwise had poor support resources. Cacciatore and Flint (2012) recommended mindfulness-based bereavement care for perinatally bereaved parents (see also Chapter 6, this text).

Patient-centered care includes not only one-on-one support from a health care professional, but also provision for group support. Bereaved women benefit from a safe space to tell their stories of loss (Cacciatore, 2010). Such support venues allow for normalization of grief and provide the opportunity for bereaved mothers to both receive and give support (Cacciatore, 2010; Wright, Shea, & Gallagher, 2014).

In addition to face-to-face interventions, Internet-based interventions have also been found to alleviate distressing symptoms after perinatal loss. Kersting et al. (2013) found through a randomized controlled trial that a 5-week, Internet-based cognitive behavioral intervention significantly improved symptoms of PTSD, prolonged grief (measured using the Inventory of Complicated Grief), and anxiety. The intervention involved two 45-minute writing assignments each week designed to help participants process the most difficult aspects of their losses. The positive effects of the intervention were sustained at the 3-month and 12-month follow-up assessments.

Individualized psychotherapy has been found to effectively reduce symptoms of CG (Shear & Shair, 2005; Simon, 2013; see also Chapter 14, this text), but treatment with antidepressants or benzodiazepines has not been shown to decrease symptoms per se (Tol et al., 2014). Rather, antidepressant therapy seems to have the tangential benefit of improving adherence and response to individual psychotherapy. When used for this purpose, paroxetine and escitalopram have been found to be most beneficial (Simon, 2013). However, overuse of antidepressants for bereavement-related symptoms is an issue (Tol et al., 2014). In fact, Lacasse and Cacciatore (2014) found that when antidepressants are prescribed after loss, the treatment can lead to long-term use of the medications. Thus, the role of psychotropic medications in mediating grief symptoms is limited.

The World Health Organization (WHO) has begun preliminary work on the development of guidelines to treat those who have suffered traumatic stress, including bereavement (Tol et al., 2014). However, major challenges to this work include a paucity of evidence on results of clinical interventions. For bereavement care, there is strong evidence to recommend individual psychotherapy for adults without concomitant mental health illness (Tol et al., 2014), yet psychotherapy has been found to be less effective for CG (Shear & Shair, 2005; Shear et al., 2011).

CONCLUSION

CG has emerged as a potential negative consequence of loss. It involves severe and sometimes debilitating symptoms that prevent the griever from engaging in normal activities. This inability to re-engage in life carries on after acute grief was expected to resolve. Complicated reactions differ from expected bouts of regrieving in intensity, frequency, and duration. CG manifests differently in different groups.

Some features of CG that have been identified empirically have also been empirically identified as expected consequences of perinatal loss. In and of themselves, manifestations of grief such as avoiding reminders of the loss, the intense urge to hold the baby, and a constant desire to hold the baby's belongings are not atypical. Rather, when these feelings persist and intensify over time instead of gradually decreasing, evaluation of CG should be considered. Because several risk factors for CG are also inherent in the experience of perinatal loss, and an understanding of this type of loss is essential for those working with perinatally bereaved parents so that the distinction between typical and atypical grief responses can be accurately identified.

For example, perinatal grief is considered to be a form of disenfranchised grief that intrinsically involves a lack of social support and a lack of societal recognition of the loss. Because CG has been associated with a lack of support, it is important for clinicians to understand that perinatally bereaved families often report feeling ill-supported and isolated after their losses (Wright, 2010). Further, perinatal loss has been identified as a type of traumatic loss. Traumatic loss can precipitate very complex grief reactions, including PTSD. Health care professionals must be astute in distinguishing typical responses to perinatal loss from complicated reactions, and also complicated reactions from signs of PTSD.

Likewise, in working with bereaved individuals, preventability of the loss and self-blame and guilt are themes that emerge frequently. Ongoing self-blame and ruminations about how the bereft individual might have prevented the loss by acting differently can lead to CG reactions (Rando, 1986). After pregnancy loss, however, women are very likely to engage in these behaviors and, here again, the clinician must work to differentiate expected reactions from complicated reactions. This distinction should be based on the severity of the symptoms and the degree to which the symptoms interfere with the griever's ability to engage in normal daily activities (Shear, 2015).

On the surface, it would seem that some of the factors associated with CG cannot pinpoint CG among perinatally bereaved individuals because some perinatal grief reactions overlap with signs of CG. However, it is important to consider that most of the research conducted to date on perinatal loss has been qualitative. Thus, nuances of the experiences have been more easily identified and reported, which may lead to overreporting or underreporting of grief sequelae. Further, because qualitative research relies on self-selected participants who offer their own perceptions of a particular experience, it is possible that those women who chose to participate in the research were the most aggrieved with a complex story of loss to share. Research is ongoing into the variations and nuances of perinatal loss, and it is not yet known whether CG reactions after perinatal loss are the norm or the extreme. Research identifying atypical responses to perinatal loss, including CG, is badly needed.

At this point, what can be gleaned from the extant research is that CG reactions are now viewed as one potential outcome of a significant loss, including perinatal loss. Risk factors for CG include many of the features associated with responses to perinatal loss, and research is needed to clarify the parameters of CG in this particular population, its incidence, and effective support interventions. This information will move clinicians forward in terms of identifying families in need of focused support and in the development of patient-centered, effective interventions.

CASE STUDY

Concetta experienced the loss of a pregnancy 15 months ago. Concetta is 27 years old and has experienced the death of eight babies. She has no living children. She is concerned that her husband will want a divorce even though he assures her that he is concerned only about her well-being. Concetta keeps framed photos of her babies' ultrasounds in her living room. She often holds the blankets and clothing of those babies who had them. Concetta reports that she cries every day for long periods of time and sometimes uses sick time or vacation time because she feels that she cannot go to work. She is worried that she will lose her job. Concetta's family is very worried about her.

FOCUS QUESTIONS

1. Based on the information presented in the chapter, are you concerned about Concetta? Why or why not?
2. Symptoms of CG have been identified in the literature. Would Concetta's grief rise to the level of CG based on the criteria?
3. What supportive interventions would be most beneficial for Concetta?

REFERENCES

American Psychiatric Association. (2013a). *Highlights of changes from* DSM-IV-TR *to* DSM-5 [Adobe Digital Editions version]. Retrieved from http://www.dsm5.org/Documents/changes%20from%20dsm-iv-tr%20to%20dsm-5.pdf

American Psychiatric Association. (2013b). *Major depressive disorder and the "bereavement exclusion"* [Adobe Digital Editions version]. Retrieved from http://www.dsm5.org/Documents/Bereavement%20Exclusion%20Fact%20Sheet.pdf

Barr, P., & Cacciatore, J. (2008). Personal fear of death and grief in bereaved mothers. *Death Studies, 32,* 445–460. Retrieved from http://dx.doi.org/10.1080/07481180801974752

Black, B. P., & Wright, P. (2012). Posttraumatic growth and transformation as outcomes of perinatal loss. *Illness, Crisis, & Loss, 20,* 225–237. Retrieved from http://dx.doi.org/10.2190/IL.20.3.b

Blood, C., & Cacciatore, J. (2014). Parental grief and memento mori photography: Narrative, meaning, culture, and context. *Death Studies, 38,* 224–233. Retrieved from http://dx.doi.org/10.1080/07481187.2013.788584

Boss, P. (2007). Ambiguous loss theory: Challenges for scholars and practitioners. *Family Relations, 56,* 105–111. Retrieved from http://dx.doi.org/10.1111/j.1741-3729.2007.00444.x

Boss, R. D., & Clarke-Pounder, J. P. (2012). Perinatal and neonatal palliative care: Targeting the underserved. *Progress in Palliative Care, 20,* 343–348. Retrieved from http://dx.doi.org/10.1179/1743291X12Y.0000000039

Buckley, T., Sunari, D., Marshall, A., Bartrop, R., McKinley, S., & Tofler, G. (2012). Physiological correlates of bereavement and the impact of bereavement interventions. *Dialogues in Clinical Neuroscience, 14,* 129–139. Retrieved from http://www.dialogues-cns.org/

Cacciatore, J. (2010). Stillbirth: Patient-centered psychosocial care. *Clinical Obstetrics & Gynecology, 53,* 691–699. Retrieved from http://dx.doi.org/10.1097/GRF.0b013e3181eba1c6

Cacciatore, J., & Flint, M. (2012). ATTEND: Toward a mindfulness-based bereavement care model. *Death Studies, 36,* 61–82. Retrieved from http://dx.doi.org/10.1080/07481187.2011.591275

Christiansen, D. M., Elklit, A., & Olff, M. (2013). Parents bereaved by infant death: PTSD symptoms up to 18 years after the loss. *General Hospital Psychiatry, 35,* 605–611. Retrieved from http://dx.doi.org/10.1016/j.genhosppsych.2013.06.006

Côté-Arsenault, D., & Dombeck, M.-T. B. (2001). Maternal assignment of fetal personhood to a previous pregnancy loss: Relationship to anxiety in the current pregnancy. *Health Care for Women International, 22,* 649–665. Retrieved from http://dx.doi.org/10.1080/07399330127171

Doka, K. J. (2013, May 29). Grief and the *DSM*: A brief Q & A. *Huffington Post.* Retrieved from http://www.huffingtonpost.com/kenneth-j-doka/grief-and-the-dsm_b_3340216.html

Dyson, L., & While, A. (1998). The long shadow of perinatal bereavement. *British Journal of Community Nursing, 3,* 432–439. Retrieved from http://dx.doi.org/10.12968/bjcn.1998.3.9.7183

Fenstermacher, K. H. (2014). Enduring to gain perspective: A grounded theory study of the experience of perinatal bereavement in Black adolescents. *Research in Nursing & Health, 37,* 135–143. Retrieved from http://dx.doi.org/10.1002/nur.21583

Hogan, N. S., Worden, J. W., & Schmidt, L. A. (2004). An empirical study of the proposed complicated grief disorder criteria. *Omega—Journal of Death and Dying, 48,* 263–277. Retrieved from http://dx.doi.org/10.2190/GX7H-H05N-A4DN-RLU9

Horowitz, M. J., Siegel, B., Holen, A., Bonanno, G. A., Milbrath, C., & Stinson, C. H. (2003). Diagnostic criteria for complicated grief disorders. *PsychiatryOnline, 1,* 290–298. Retrieved from http://dx.doi.org/10.1176/foc.1.3.290

Hutti, M. H., Armstrong, D. S., Myers, J. A., & Hall, L. A. (2015). Grief intensity, psychological well-being, and the intimate partner relationship in the subsequent pregnancy after a perinatal loss. *Journal of Obstetric, Gynecologic, & Neonatal Nursing, 44,* 42–50. Retrieved from http://dx.doi.org/10.1111/1552-6909.12539

Kagami, M., Maruyama, T., Koizumi, T., Miyazaki, K., Nishikawa-Uchida, S., Oda, H., . . . Yoshimura, Y. (2012). Psychological adjustment and psychological stress among Japanese couples with a history of recurrent pregnancy loss. *Human Reproduction, 27,* 787–794. Retrieved from http://dx.doi.org/10.1093/humrep/der441

Kavanaugh, K., & Moro, T. (2006). Supporting parents after stillborn or newborn death: There is much that nurses can do. *American Journal of Nursing, 106*(9), 74–79. Retrieved from http://dx.doi.org/10.1097/00000446-200609000-00037

Kersting, A., Dölemeyer, R., Steinig, J., Walter, F., Kroker, K., Baust, K., & Wagner, B. (2013). Brief Internet-based intervention reduces posttraumatic stress and prolonged grief in parents after the loss of a child during pregnancy: A randomized controlled trial. *Psychotherapy and Psychosomatics, 82,* 372–381. Retrieved from http://dx.doi.org/10.1159/000348713

Kersting, A., & Wagner, B. (2012). Complicated grief after perinatal loss. *Dialogues in Clinical Neuroscience, 14,* 187–194. Retrieved from http://www.dialogues-cns.org/

Ketish-Barnes, N., Chaize, M., Seegers, V., Legriel, S., Cariou, A., Jaber, S., . . . Azoulay, É. (2015). Complicated grief after the death of a relative in the intensive care unit. *European Respiratory Journal.* Retrieved from http://dx.doi.org/10.1183/09031936.00160014

Lacasse, J. R., & Cacciatore, J. (2014). Prescribing of psychiatric medication to bereaved parents following perinatal/neonatal death: An observational study. *Death Studies, 38,* 589–596. Retrieved from http://dx.doi.org/10.1080/07481187.2013.820229

Lang, A., Fleiszer, A. R., Duhamel, F., Sword, W., Gilbert, K. R., & Corsini-Munt, S. (2011). Perinatal loss and parental grief: The challenge of ambiguity and disenfranchised grief. *OMEGA—Journal of Death and Dying, 63,* 183–196. Retrieved from http://dx.doi.org/10.2190/OM.63.2.e

Li, J., Chow, A. Y. M., Shi, Z., & Chan, C. L. W. (2015). Prevalence and risk factors of complicated grief among Sichuan earthquake survivors. *Journal of Affective Disorders, 175,* 218–223. Retrieved from http://dx.doi.org/10.1016/j.jad.2015.01.003

Lichtenthal, W. G., Cruess, D. G., & Prigerson, H. G. (2004). A case for establishing complicated grief as a distinct mental disorder in *DSM-V. Clinical Psychology Review, 24,* 637–662. Retrieved from http://dx.doi.org/10.1016/j.cpr.2004.07.002

McCreight, B. S. (2008). Perinatal loss: A qualitative study in northern Ireland. *Omega—Journal of Death and Dying, 57,* 1–19. Retrieved from http://dx.doi.org/10.2190/OM.57.1.a

Moore, J. (2011). Interconception care for couples after perinatal loss: A comprehensive review of the literature. *Journal of Perinatal and Neonatal Nursing, 25,* 44–51. Retrieved from http://dx.doi.org/10.1097/JPN.0b013e3182071a08

Murphy, S., Shevlin, M., & Elklit, A. (2014). Psychological consequences of pregnancy loss and infant death in a sample of bereaved parents. *Journal of Loss & Trauma, 19,* 56–69. Retrieved from http://dx.doi.org/10.1080/15325024.2012.735531

Parkes, C. M. (2014). Diagnostic criteria for complications of bereavement in the *DSM-5. Bereavement Care, 33,* 113–117. Retrieved from http://dx.doi.org/10.1080/02682621.2014.980987

Price, S. K., & McLeod, D. A. (2012). Definitional distinctions in response to perinatal loss and fertility barriers. *Illness, Crisis, and Loss, 20*(3), 255–273. doi: 10.2190/IL.20.3.d

Prigerson, H. G., Bierhals, A. J., Kasl, S. V., Reynolds, C. F., III, Shear, M. K., Day, N., . . . Jacobs S. (1997). Traumatic grief as a risk factor for mental and physical morbidity. *American Journal of Psychiatry, 154,* 616–623. Retrieved from http://dx.doi.org/10.1176/ajp.154.5.616

Prigerson, H. G., Bierhals, A. J., Kasl, S. V., Reynolds, C. F., III, Shear, M. K., Newsom, J. T., & Jacobs, S. (1996). Complicated grief as a disorder distinct from bereavement-related depression and anxiety: A replication study. *American Journal of Psychiatry, 153*, 1484–1486. Retrieved from http://dx.doi.org/10.1176/ajp.153.11.1484

Prigerson, H. G., Frank, E., Kasl, S. V., Reynolds, C. F., III, Anderson, B., Zubenko, G. S., . . . Kupfer, D. J. (1995). Complicated grief and bereavement-related depression as distinct disorders: Preliminary empirical validation in elderly bereaved spouses. *American Journal of Psychiatry, 152*, 22–30. Retrieved from http://dx.doi.org/10.1176/ajp.152.1.22

Rando, T. A. (Ed.). (1986). *Parental loss of a child.* Champaign, IL: Research Press.

Rando, T. A. (2013). On achieving clarity regarding complicated grief: Lessons from clinical practice. In M. Stroebe, H. Schut, & J. van den Bout (Eds.), *Complicated grief: Scientific foundations for health care professionals* (pp. 40–54). New York, NY: Routledge.

Scheidt, C. E., Hasenburg, A., Kunze, M., Waller, E., Pfeifer, R., Zimmermann, P., . . . Waller, N. (2012). Are individual differences of attachment predicting bereavement outcome after perinatal loss? A prospective cohort study. *Journal of Psychosomatic Research, 73*, 375–382. Retrieved from http://dx.doi.org/10.1016/j.jpsychores.2012.08.017

Searight, H. R. (2014). Expanding the boundaries of major depressive disorder in *DSM-5*: The removal of the bereavement exclusion. *Open Journal of Depression, 3*, 9–12. Retrieved from http://dx.doi.org/10.4236/ojd.2014.31004

Shear, M. K. (2015). Complicated grief. *New England Journal of Medicine, 372*, 153–160. Retrieved from http://dx.doi.org/10.1056/NEJMcp1315618

Shear, M. K., & Shair, H. (2005). Attachment, loss, and complicated grief. *Developmental Psychobiology, 47*, 253–267. Retrieved from http://dx.doi.org/10.1002/dev.20091

Shear, M. K., Simon, N., Wall, M., Zisook, S., Neimeyer, R., Duan, N., . . . Keshaviah, A. (2011). Complicated grief and related bereavement issues for *DSM-5. Depression and Anxiety, 28*, 103–117. Retrieved from http://dx.doi.org/10.1002/da.20780

Simon, N. M. (2013). Treating complicated grief. *Journal of the American Medical Association, 310*, 416–423. Retrieved from http://dx.doi.org/10.1001/jama.2013.8614

St. John, A., Cooke, M., & Goopy, S. (2006). Shrouds of silence: Three women's stories of prenatal loss. *Australian Journal of Advanced Nursing, 23*(3), 8–12. Retrieved from http://www.ajan.com.au

Stroebe, M., Schut, H., & van den Bout, J. (2013). Introduction. In M. Stroebe, H. Schut, & J. van den Bout (Eds.), *Complicated grief: Scientific foundations for health care professionals* (pp. 1–10). New York, NY: Routledge.

Stroebe, M., van Son, M., Stroebe, W., Kleber, R., Schut, H., & van den Bout, J. (2000). On the classification and diagnosis of pathological grief. *Clinical Psychology Review, 20*, 57–75. Retrieved from http://dx.doi.org/10.1016/S0272-7358(98)00089-0

Sutan, R., & Miskam, H. M. (2012). Psychological impact of perinatal loss among Muslim women. *BMC Women's Health, 12*, Art. No. 15. Retrieved from http://dx.doi.org/10.1186/1472-6874-12-15

Thieleman, K., & Cacciatore, J. (2013). The DSM-5 and the bereavement exclusion: A call for critical evaluation. *Social Work, 58*, 277–280. Retrieved from http://dx.doi.org/10.1093/sw/swt021

Toffol, E., Koponen, P., & Partonen, T. (2013). Miscarriage and mental health: Results of two population-based studies. *Psychiatry Research, 205*, 151–158. Retrieved from http://dx.doi.org/10.1016/j.psychres.2012.08.029

Tol, W. A., Barbui, C., Bisson, J., Cohen, J., Hijazi, Z., Jones, L., . . . van Ommeren, M. (2014). World Health Organization guidelines for management of acute stress, PTSD, and bereavement: Key challenges on the road ahead. *PLoS Medicine, 11*(12), Art. No. e1001769. Retrieved from http://dx.doi.org/10.1371/journal.pmed.1001769

van den Akker, O. B. A. (2011). The psychological and social consequences of miscarriage. *Expert Review of Obstetrics & Gynecology, 6*, 295–304. Retrieved from http://dx.doi.org/10.1586/eog.11.14

Warland, J., O'Leary, J., McCutcheon, H., & Williamson, V. (2010). Parenting paradox: Parenting after infant loss. *Midwifery, 27*, e163–e169. Retrieved from http://dx.doi.org/10.1016/j.midw.2010.02.004

Wojnar, D. M., Swanson, K. M., & Adolfsson, A.-S. (2011). Confronting the inevitable: A conceptual model of miscarriage for use in clinical practice and research. *Death Studies, 35*, 536–558. Retrieved from http://dx.doi.org/10.1080/07481187.2010.536886

Wool, C. (2013). State of the science on perinatal palliative care. *Journal of Obstetric, Gynecologic, & Neonatal Nursing, 42*, 372–382. Retrieved from http://dx.doi.org/10.1111/1552-6909.12034

Worden, J. W. (1991). *Grief counselling and grief therapy: A handbook for the mental health practitioner* (2nd ed.). New York, NY: Routledge.

Wright, P. M. (2010). *Pushing On: A grounded theory study of maternal perinatal bereavement* (Doctoral dissertation). Retrieved from ProQuest Dissertations and Theses database. (AAT No. 3404182).

Wright, P. M. (2016). The Pushing On theory of maternal perinatal bereavement. In B. P. Black, P. M. Wright, & R. Limbo. *Perinatal and pediatric bereavement in nursing and other health professionals.* New York, NY: Springer.

Wright, P. M., Shea, D. M., & Gallagher, R. (2014). From seed to tree: Developing community support for perinatally bereaved mothers. *Journal of Perinatal Education, 23*(3), 151–154.

Zetumer, S., Young, I., Shear, M. K., Skritskaya, N., Lebowitz, B., Simon, N., . . . Zisook, S. (2015). The impact of losing a child on the clinical presentation of complicated grief. *Journal of Affective Disorders, 170*, 15–21. Retrieved from http://dx.doi.org/10.1016/j.jad.2014.08.021

CHAPTER 8

Lesbians, Parenthood, and Reproductive Loss

Danuta M. Wojnar

*F*or many people, the desire to have children is vital to achieve life fulfillment regardless of sexual orientation (Boivin & Pennings, 2005). The availability of statistics, however, regarding the prevalence of homosexual identity and the desire to have children varies greatly across the world. This is due in part to the diverse religious and political views on homosexuality and the delicate nature of questions regarding sexuality and the people's desire to have children (Borneskog, Skoog Svanberg, Lampic, & Sydsjo, 2012).

Historically, women and men who were attracted to same-sex individuals faced strong societal pressure to enter heterosexual relationships and have children (Renaud, 2007). Because of heterosexist societal attitudes, many individuals repressed same-sex feelings or expressed them in highly secretive ways (Borneskog et al., 2012). The gay liberation movement in the 1970s brought radical changes to what was considered the "normal" family constellation and "normal" human reproduction. As a result, increasing numbers of people came out as lesbian or gay and formed same-sex households (Wojnar & Swanson, 2006). When not precluded by legal action, children from previous heterosexual relationships were often raised in the same-sex households (Borneskog et al., 2012).

Since the 1970s, a series of societal changes has afforded all people in the United States the same rights with regard to children and family formation (Gates, 2013). In 1986, the last relic of homosexuality as a psychiatric illness was removed from the *Diagnostic and Statistical Manual of Mental Disorders Third Edition* (*DSM-III*). Subsequently, same-sex couples were given rights to legally enter civil unions and, most recently, to receive marriage licenses in many regions of the United States (Gonzales, 2014). Concurrently, child adoption, assisted reproduction and, when necessary, fertility treatments became available to persons across all sexual orientations (Ross, Steele, & Epstein, 2006).

LGBTQ FAMILIES IN THE UNITED STATES

Recent national statistics indicate that nearly 8.5 million Americans self-identify as lesbian, gay, bisexual, transgender, or queer (LGBTQ; Gates, 2011; U.S. Census Bureau, 2011). Approximately 3 million LGBTQ people have had a biological child and as many as 6 million American children under 18 years of age have had a parent who self-identifies as a member of the LGBTQ community (Gates, 2013). The majority of LGBTQ parents are lesbians who became mothers through donor insemination, adoption, or short-lived heterosexual relationships (Gates, 2013). It is therefore imperative to consider the unique challenges associated with seeking and achieving motherhood by this sizeable population of women. Although a growing body of research has addressed the issues associated with lesbian family formation, parenting, and the well-being of children born to lesbian mothers, less is known about their experiences of unexpected pregnancy loss and even less about culturally appropriate therapeutic interventions subsequent to loss. While the biological uniqueness of women in itself creates grounds for universal research on women's health, life experiences that shape the mental, spiritual, and social well-being of lesbians and other members of the LGBTQ community deserve special consideration (McDonald, McIntyre, & Anderson, 2003). In this chapter, an overview of research findings regarding lesbian couples' journeys toward biological parenthood and their experiences of early, unexpected pregnancy loss is provided, and recommendations for clinical practice and research are offered.

HUMAN DESIRE TO BECOME A PARENT

The desire to become parents is considered to be central to life fulfillment of women and men in most cultures (Boivin & Pennings, 2005). In the Western world, there have been various interpretations of the meaning of parenthood and what drives people's desire to become parents. In the past, scientists interpreted people's desire to have children primarily as a biological drive (Benedeck, 1970). Others saw it as an essential component of developing a female identity (Boss, Van Balen, & Van Den Boom, 2003). From the feminist perspective, the desire to have children has often been viewed as a social enforcement of gender roles and a potential barrier to one's personal development and achievement of life goals (Thompson, 2002). Recent research on the motivation to have children in persons across sexual orientation showed that most individuals share the desire to experience stable family life, happiness, and love (Boss et al., 2003; Erickson Zink, 2012). Interestingly, research findings suggest that happiness from being able to parent was ranked highest by lesbian couples (Boss et al., 2003) and heterosexual couples with a history of infertility (Dyer, Mokoena, Maritz, & Van Der Spuy, 2008).

PREGNANCY LAUNCHING BY LESBIAN COUPLES

A planned lesbian family is when two women have chosen biological motherhood within the context of their couple relationship (Wojnar & Katzenmeyer, 2014). Contrary to the popular belief that roles in same-sex families are similar to those in heterosexual families, variation is a distinctive feature in lesbian family narratives (Dahl, Fylkesnes, Sorlie, & Malterud, 2013). Planned lesbian families differ from other family constellations because of the complexity of issues and decisions they face as the future parents (Black & Fields, 2014). These issues are often intertwined in complex ways and the decisions are often not easy to make (Black & Fields, 2014; Wojnar, 2007).

One of the first decisions lesbian couples must consider prior to achieving pregnancy is to decide on the source of the donor. The decision is typically made based on the partners' personal beliefs about the importance of knowing the biological origins of the child (Wojnar & Swanson, 2006). This decision results in two possible consequences: the first one is to decide on the route and the location of conception; the second is to decide what role if any the donor will have in parenting the child. The second consequence may have important emotional implications that can affect the parents and their children in profound ways (Nordqvist, 2012; Wojnar & Swanson, 2006). For example, the literature suggests that many lesbian couples select an anonymous donor in a sperm bank to ensure donor anonymity to the couple and child throughout the lifetime. The risk of such a decision is the psychological impact on the child who may one day wish to identify his or her biological origins (Renaud, 2007). Hence, some couples select an identifiable donor, that is, a donor who is anonymous to the couple but can be identifiable to the child upon request. Still, others negotiate with a trusted male acquaintance or a friend to become a donor or seek a "stranger donor" through newspaper or Internet advertising (Borneskog, Sydsjo, Lampic, Bladh, & Skoog Svanberg, 2013; Wojnar & Swanson, 2006). A lot of these options allow the child to uncover his or her biological origins upon request. Additionally, a "dedicated donor" concept has emerged as an increasingly popular choice among lesbian families (Wojnar & Katzenmeyer, 2014). According to this arrangement, the donor or the donor and his partner have no parental rights but are introduced to the child and are actively engaged in the child's life (Borneskog et al., 2012).

Regardless of the donor decision, each of the choices made by lesbian couples carries considerable risk and stress. For example, when a "known" or a "stranger" donor is selected and nonclinical insemination is performed in the privacy of the couple's home, the threat of potential custody battles and battles over parenting rights may emerge. These stressors can be perceived as especially threatening to the position of the lesbian comother, who lacks biological substantiation to the child (Nordqvist, 2011).

An equally important decision is which lesbian partner will take on the role of the biological parent. This decision is typically made based on the partners' age and physical health, income, access to health insurance, and the desire to become pregnant (Wojnar & Swanson, 2006). Regardless, in spite of the social and legal progress made to acknowledge the rights of the comother, taking on the role carries unique challenges that are not a typical part of the heterosexual parenting experience. For example, it has been reported that the attachment process to the child is longer and less uniform among lesbian comothers than biological mothers (Wojnar & Katzenmeyer, 2014). There are also reports that despite the legal threats faced by comothers, their psychosocial experience of living through a partner's pregnancy is similar to that of expectant fathers in terms of emotional investment, empathy, and attachment process (Sandelowski & Black, 1994).

However, some comothers have questioned their right to think of themselves as the future parents, especially when insensitive comments were made by well-meaning but ill-informed health care providers, family, and friends (Dahl et al., 2013). Such legitimate concerns frequently lead lesbian couples considering biological parenthood to delay pregnancy plans until they come to a conclusion that they can face any unanticipated challenges related to pregnancy and parenthood (Wojnar & Katzenmeyer, 2014).

MISCARRIAGE EXPERIENCES OF LESBIAN COUPLES

Achieving pregnancy is a joyful and happy time for the vast majority of lesbian couples, because their pregnancies are typically carefully planned and wanted (Peel, 2010; Wojnar, 2007). However, similar to heterosexual couples, the joy of lesbian pregnancy may be interrupted by miscarriage, an early, unexpected pregnancy loss prior to the point of fetal viability (Peel, 2010). Conservative estimates suggest that approximately 12% to 30% of confirmed pregnancies and up to 50% of all pregnancies (Cramer & Wise, 2000) end in miscarriage, making it one of the most common losses experienced by people of reproductive age. Epidemiological research suggests that risk of pregnancy loss is higher for non-White women, teens, women older than 35 years of age, unmarried women, and women with multiple deliveries (MacDorman & Kirmeyer, 2009). There is no epidemiological research that refers specifically to lesbian pregnancy loss.

Regardless of sexual orientation, most women experience miscarriage as a traumatic, unforeseen, and unwelcome event (Beutel, Deckardt, von Rad, & Weiner, 1995) and respond with distress that may include grief, anger, depression, anxiety, self-blame, or guilt (Adolfsson, Larsson, Wijma, & Bertero, 2004; Swanson, 2000; Swanson, Connor, Jolley, Pettinato, & Wang, 2007; Peel, 2010; Wojnar, 2007). Partner and social support has been consistently linked to women's ability to effectively cope with pregnancy loss (Swanson, Karmali, Powell, & Pulvermakher, 2003). Lack of social support and the failure of practitioners to offer compassionate counseling have been associated with prolonged emotional distress (Wojnar, 2007).

The majority of studies exploring heterosexual women's emotional responses to miscarriage have been interpretive or descriptive in nature. A few intervention studies (Swanson, 1999a, 1999b; Swanson, Chen, Graham, Wojnar, & Petras, 2009) suggest that women benefit from counseling sessions with an empathetic practitioner.

Only a few published studies have addressed the experiences of lesbian miscarriage. Wojnar (2007) investigated the experience of miscarriage from the perspective of 20 lesbian women (10 couples) who were in a committed couple relationship, and miscarried within 2 years of enrollment. The women experienced anywhere from one to four miscarriages. They had been in a committed couple relationship from 2 to 15 years. All participants received some form of emotional support from practitioners after the loss, but the majority claimed it was insufficient.

Wojnar (2007) discovered that before one can appreciate the magnitude of grief after lesbian miscarriage, the unique circumstances that surround pregnancy launching must be understood. The challenges encountered by lesbian couples in Wojnar's (2007) study included (a) confronting internalized homophobic attitudes about having a family with children; (b) negotiating which partner will become the biological parent; (c) deciding on the right source of donor, method, and place of conception; (d) confronting societal judgments about their desire to parent; and (e) dealing with the lack of biological connection to the child by the comother and anxiety related to the adoption process. Clearly, findings of this study suggest that when supporting lesbians who miscarry one must also consider the complexity of becoming pregnant, the joy of pregnancy, and the loss of control and sadness subsequent to miscarriage. The overarching theme of the phenomenological model proposed by Wojnar (2007) was "we are not in control." The overarching theme encapsulated two subthemes: "we work so hard to get a baby" and "it hurts so bad: the sorrow of miscarriage," which suggest that the experience of lesbian miscarriage is compounded by the complexities of planning and achieving pregnancy as a same-sex couple.

In a subsequent study that explored lesbian miscarriage, Peel (2010) found three themes: *processes and practices for conception; amplification of loss;* and *heterosexism in health care*. Of the 60 respondents who completed the survey, 84% conceived using donor sperm, the majority used various available resources to plan the pregnancy, and most engaged in preconception care. The experience of loss was potentiated by the contextual factors and the emotional investment of study participants in becoming mothers. Most women felt that their loss(es) had made a significant negative impact on their lives. Although many respondents in Peel's study were satisfied with their care, some reported experiencing heterosexism from health professionals.

Most recently, Wojnar, Swanson, and Adolfsson (2011), using data from 42 lesbian and heterosexual women, developed the theoretical model Miscarriage: Confronting the Inevitable for use in clinical practice and research. The model depicts the common experiences and events encountered by lesbian and heterosexual women. The experience of miscarriage depicted in the model consists of these processes: coming to know, losing and gaining, sharing the loss, going public, getting through it, and trying again. When miscarriage occurred, study participants experienced a series of challenging events that were beyond their control. The overarching theme, "we are not in control," illustrates what it is like for most women to miscarry. It points to the feelings of helplessness, hopelessness, powerlessness, and lack of control over keeping the pregnancy and living through the unexpected loss.

In order to truly understand the magnitude of this invisible loss, one has to recognize the meaning most women attribute to pregnancy as a journey toward motherhood. In this study, regardless of women's sexual orientation or the geographical location where the miscarriage took place (United States, Canada, and Sweden), the meaning of loss was framed by women's developing maternal identity. In Wojnar and colleagues' theoretical model, "getting pregnant" refers to the events surrounding conception and early pregnancy.

How women come to recognize that the miscarriage has taken place is captured in the model by the event of "Coming to Know." It refers to the woman's realization that "something is wrong" and involves contrasting the evidence of impending loss, such as bleeding, abdominal cramping, and lower back pain against hopes of sustaining the pregnancy. "Coming to Know" is characterized by moving through a series of hope/no-hope cycles described by some women as a rollercoaster that ends with confirmation that the pregnancy is no longer viable.

Bleeding and cramping are the physical symptoms that accompany "Coming to Know." While the severity of physical symptoms can vary from woman to woman, study participants described it as a frightening and painful experience that provided physical evidence that miscarriage was taking place.

The next theme, "Losing and Gaining," captures the highly emotional process of the study participants' ability to identify what was lost and gained through miscarriage. In this study, the vast majority of women equated their miscarriage with the loss of a baby that negatively impacted their intimate partner relationship. While some women felt that the miscarriage challenged their couple relationship, others felt that miscarriage brought them closer to their partner.

The physical events of miscarriage were frequently experienced as intensely private, unforgettable moments. Some of the women shared stories captured by the event of scooping it up as they remembered examining the fetal tissue for membranes, or recognizable body parts.

After the physical part of miscarriage was over, study participants encountered mixed responses from others when they felt ready to embark on "Sharing the Loss" journey. Women in this study consistently revealed that they wanted their loss to be acknowledged by their partner or family members, health care providers, and friends and considered compassionate responses as therapeutic.

Feeling empty refers to the women's understanding that their womb is no longer carrying a baby. It refers to the physical void and emotional emptiness many women in the study felt for weeks or even months after their loss.

Ultimately, regardless of the immediate emotional response, women who experience miscarriage have to learn about "Going Public"; that is, learn to live with the loss, encounter other pregnant mothers and babies, and deal with people's comments, be they empathetic and compassionate or not.

A step in the process of going public includes making memories, which refers to organizing events, creating rituals, or keeping objects that helped to memorialize the pregnancy and significance of their loss. Memories included simple gestures such as lighting a candle, planting a rose bush, burying the remains in special places, or hosting a small memorial gathering.

The next process, "Getting Through It," refers to moving from preoccupation with the miscarriage to an emotional place where the positive events appear to outweigh the negative and the women feel they returned to "their old selves." Hearing from their health care provider that miscarriages often occur for reasons beyond anybody's control and that pregnancies end because the fetus might not have been healthy may help some women alleviate their guilt and self-blame. "Resuming Menses" is an important event in the model. For some it may be perceived as a flashback to the experience of miscarriage, for others it can be seen as a symbol of returning to fertility.

"Trying Again" is the experience of considering the next pregnancy while dealing with fears of another pregnancy loss. Women in the study worried about miscarrying again, not conceiving, or making an inappropriate choice to forego another pregnancy.

CONCLUSION

The model of Miscarriage: Confronting the Inevitable describes several common processes women experience when they go through miscarriage. Women shared their experiences of feeling *Not in Control* with regard to keeping their pregnancy. Feeling *Not in Control* coexists with the experiences of Coming to Know, Losing and Gaining, Sharing the Loss, Going Public, Getting Through It, Resuming Menses, and Trying Again. While the physical events of miscarriage are common cross-culturally, the expression of each woman's grief after miscarriage may be as unique as the expression of other feelings in everyday life. For example, in some cultures women must overcome folk beliefs that they somehow contributed to their miscarriage (Schaffir, 2007; Van, 2001). In some instances, such as having a history of infertility, women may feel particularly guilty after miscarriage (Freda, Devine, & Semelsberger, 2003). Interestingly, lesbian mothers in Wojnar's (2007) sample did not include guilt as a central issue in their narratives about miscarriage, while Swedish women in the study by Adolfsson et al. (2004) experienced a great deal of guilt.

Societal awareness of the impact of miscarriage on women and their partners and expectations for grief after early pregnancy loss continue to lag in Western cultures and beyond (Callister, 2006; Schaffir, 2007). Over the past few decades, many heterosexual women reported dissatisfaction with indifference or mixed reactions in terms of empathy and support from their spouse, providers, family members, and close friends. Likewise, recent research conducted with lesbians who miscarried provides evidence that interventions could and should be improved. It is particularly important that health care providers at the time of miscarriage and in subsequent pregnancy treat women with compassion, respect, and in a culturally informed manner. One promising model to guide clinical practice in obstetrical care or counseling for lesbian and heterosexual women after pregnancy loss is Wojnar, Swanson, and Adolfsson's (2011) model of miscarriage that considers pregnancy loss experiences of lesbian and heterosexual women. Although it may take decades to change societal attitudes toward the legitimacy of grieving after miscarriage, research with women from diverse cultural backgrounds that tests the effectiveness of the revised miscarriage model in clinical practice may be an important next step. Health care providers may want to start with evaluating their own beliefs and communication styles when caring for women who have miscarried before offering help.

CASE STUDY

Nancy and Taryn have been in a committed relationship for 8 years. After planning a pregnancy for the past 2 years, they learned that Nancy was pregnant through in vitro fertilization. At their 12-week prenatal visit, the couple stated they were looking forward to hearing the baby's heartbeat and were beginning to share the news with their families and friends. When the nurse could not hear fetal heart sounds, an ultrasonogram confirmed that a miscarriage was inevitable.

FOCUS QUESTIONS

1. Based on the information presented in the chapter, what aspects of family planning need to be considered when providing support for lesbian couples who are experiencing perinatal loss?
2. What specific issues may lesbian couples face when their baby dies?
3. What societal changes have influenced the experiences of family planning among lesbian couples?
4. What clinical interventions would be most helpful in supporting Nancy and Taryn?

REFERENCES

Adolfsson, A., Larsson, P. G., Wijma, B., & Bertero, C. (2004). Guilt and emptiness: Women's experiences of miscarriage. *Health Care for Women International, 25*(6), 543–560.

Benedeck, T. (1970). The family as a psychological field. In E. J. Anthony & T. Benedeck (Eds.), *Parenthood, its psychology and psychopathology* (pp. 109–136). Boston, MA: Little, Brown, & Co.

Beutel, M., Deckardt, R., von Rad, M., & Weiner, H. (1995). Grief and depression after miscarriage: Their separation, antecedents, and course. *Psychosomatic Medicine, 57*(6), 517–526.

Black, B. P., & Fields, W. S. (2014). Contexts of reproductive loss in lesbian couples. *MCN, The American Journal of Maternal Child Nursing, 39*(3), 157–162.

Boivin, J., Griffiths, E., & Venetis, C. A. (2011). Emotional distress in infertile women and failure of assisted reproductive technologies: Analysis of prospective psychological studies. *British Medical Journal, 342*, d223.

Borneskog, C., Skoog Svanberg, A., Lampic, C., & Sydsjo, G. (2012). Relationship quality in lesbian and heterosexual couples undergoing treatment with assisted reproduction. *Human Reproduction, 27*, 779–786.

Borneskog, C., Sydsjö, G., Lampic, C., Bladh, M., & Skoog Svanberg, A. S. (2013). Symptoms of anxiety and depression in lesbian couples treated with donated sperm: A descriptive study. *British Journal of Obstetrics and Gynecology, 120*(7), 839–846. doi: 10.1111/1471-0528.12214.

Boss, H. M., Van Balen, F., & Van Dem Boom, D. C. (2003). Planned lesbian families: Their desire and motivation to have children. *Human Reproduction, 18*(10), 2216–2224.

Callister, L. C. (2006). Perinatal loss: A family perspective. *Journal of Perinatal and Neonatal Nursing, 20*(3), 227–234.

Cramer, D. W., & Wise, L. A. (2000). The epidemiology of recurrent pregnancy loss. *Seminars in Reproductive Medicine, 18*(4), 331–339.

Dahl, B., Fylkesnes, A. M., Sorlie, V., & Malterud, K. (2013). Lesbian women's experiences with healthcare providers in the birthing context: A meta ethnography. *Midwifery, 25*(6), 682–690.

Dyer, S., Mokoena, N., Maritz, J., & Van Der Spuy, Z. (2008). Motives for parenthood among couples attending a level 3 infertility clinic in the public sector in South Africa. *Human Reproduction, 23*(2), 352–357.

Erickson Zink, A. (2012). Adoptive homes and the meaning of family: Implications for gay and lesbian prospective parents. *Columbia Social Work Review, 3,* 52–60.

Freda, M. C., Devine, K. S., & Semelsberger, C. (2003). The lived experience of miscarriage after infertility. *Journal of Maternal Child Nursing, 28,* 16–23.

Gates, G. J. (2011). *How many people in the United States are Lesbian, Gay, Bisexual, and Transgender?* Los Angeles, CA: The Williams Institute, UCLA School of Law. Retrieved from http://williamsinstitute.law.ucla.edu/research/census-lgbt-demographics

Gates, G. J. (2013). *LGBT parenting in the United States.* Los Angeles, CA: The Williams Institute, UCLA School of Law. Retrieved from http://williamsinstitute.law.ucla .edu/wp-content/uploads/LGBT-Parenting.pdf

Gonzales, G. (2014). Same-sex marriage—prescription for better health. *New England Journal of Medicine, 370*(15), 1373–1376. doi: 10.1056/NEJMp1400254.

MacDorman, M. F., & Kirmeyer, S. (2009). Fetal and perinatal mortality, United States, 2005. (2009). *National Vital Statistics Report, 57,* 1–19.

McDonald, C., McIntyre, M., & Anderson, B. (2003). The view from somewhere: Locating lesbian experience in women's health. *Health Care for Women International, 24,* 697–711.

Nordqvist, P. (2011). Dealing with sperm: Comparing lesbians' clinical and non-clinical donor conception process. *Sociology of Health and Illness, 33*(1), 114–119.

Nordqvist, P. (2012). Origins and originators: Lesbian couples negotiating parental identities and sperm conception. *Culture, Health, and Sexuality, 14*(3), 297–311.

Peel, E. (2010). Pregnancy loss in lesbian and bisexual women: An online survey of experiences. *Human Reproduction, 25*(3), 721–727.

Renaud, M. T. (2007). We are mothers too: Childbearing experiences of lesbian families. *Journal of Obstetrical, Gynecologic and Neonatal Nursing, 36*(2), 190–199.

Ross, L. E., Steele, L. S., & Epstein, R. (2006). Lesbian and bisexual women's recommendations for the provision of assisted reproductive technology services. *Fertility and Sterility, 86*(3), 735–738.

Sandelowski, M., & Black, B. P. (1994). The epistemology of expectant parenthood. *Western Journal of Nursing Research, 16*(6), 601–614.

Schaffir, J. (2007). Do patients associate adverse pregnancy outcomes with folkloric beliefs? *Archives of Women's Mental Health, 10*(6), 301–304.

Swanson, K. M. (1999a). Research-based practice with women who have had miscarriages. *Image. Journal of Nursing Scholarship, 31,* 339–345.

Swanson, K. M. (1999b). The effects of caring, measurement, and time on miscarriage impact and women's well-being in the first year after loss. *Nursing Research, 48,* 288–298.

Swanson, K. M. (2000). Predicting depressive symptoms after miscarriage: A path analysis based on the Lazarus Paradigm. *Journal of Women's Health and Gender-Based Medicine, 65,* 902–910.

Swanson, K. M., Chen, H., Graham, C., Wojnar, D., & Petras, A. (2009). Resolution of depression and grief during the first year after miscarriage: A randomized controlled clinical trial of couples-focused interventions. *Journal of Women's Health, 18*(8), 1245–1257.

Swanson, K. M., Connor, S., Jolley, S. N., Pettinato, M., & Wang, T. J. (2007). Contexts and evolution of women's responses to miscarriage during the first year after loss. *Research in Nursing and Health, 30*(1), 2–16.

Swanson, K. M., Karmali, Z. A., Powell, S. H., & Pulvermakher, F. (2003). Miscarriage effects on couples' interpersonal and sexual relationships during the first year after loss: Women's perceptions. *Psychosomatic Medicine, 65*, 902–910.

Thompson, C. M. (2002). Fertile ground: Feminists theorize infertility. In M. C. Inhorn & F. Van Balen (Eds), *Infertility around the globe. New thinking on childlessness, gender and reproductive technologies* (pp. 52–78). Berkeley, CA: University of California Press.

U.S. Census Bureau. (2011). *General Social Survey, 2008/2010. The epidemiology of recurrent pregnancy loss.* Los Angeles, CA: The Williams Institute, UCLA School of Law. Retrieved from http://williamsinstitute.law.ucla.edu/wp-content/uploads/Census2010Snapshot-US-v2.pdf

Van, P. (2001). Breaking the silence of African-American women: Healing after pregnancy loss. *Health Care for Women International, 22*(3), 229–243.

Wojnar, D., & Swanson, K. M. (2006). Why shouldn't lesbian women who miscarry receive equal consideration? A viewpoint. *Journal of GLBT Family Studies, 2*(1), 1–12.

Wojnar, D. M. (2007). Miscarriage experiences of lesbian couples. *Journal of Midwifery and Women's Health, 52*(5), 479–485.

Wojnar, D. M., & Katzenmeyer, A. (2014). Experiences of preconception, pregnancy, and new motherhood for lesbian non-biological mothers. *Journal of Obstetrical, Gynecologic, and Neonatal Nursing, 43*(1), 50–60. doi: 10.1111/1552-6909.12270

Wojnar, D. M., Swanson, K. M., & Adolfsson, A. (2011). Confronting the inevitable: A conceptual model of miscarriage for use in clinical practice and research, *Death Studies, 35*, 536–558.

CHAPTER 9

Early Pregnancy Loss During Adolescence

Sara Rich Wheeler and Marlene G. S. Sefton

*A*dolescence, generally defined as beginning between ages 11 and 12 years and ending between ages 18 and 23 years (Sass & Kaplan, 2012), is a time of rapid physical, emotional, and cognitive growth and development coupled with changes in relationships with parents, siblings, and peers. For adolescents, pregnancy is often unplanned and may represent developmental and situational crises for everyone involved. Approximately 6% of U.S. adolescents became pregnant in 2010, the most recent statistic available. This represents 625,310 pregnancies in women younger than age 20 years or 57.4 per 1,000 adolescent women. Of these pregnancies, the rates per 1,000 women for abortions, births, and loss (miscarriage or stillbirth) were 14.7, 34.4, and 8.3, respectively, or 372,177 live births, 162,450 abortions, and 90,600 miscarriages or stillbirths (Krost & Henshaw, 2014). The purpose of this chapter is to highlight key elements of adolescent growth and development, provide a summary of research findings on the adolescent female bereavement response to an early pregnancy loss prior to 20 weeks gestation (miscarriage, ectopic pregnancy, or elective termination), and outline communication strategies to serve as a guide for health care clinicians. The chapter is built upon theoretical frameworks as a way to conceptualize and organize the material.

When a pregnancy ends too soon the experience may include a sense of loss, grief, and changes in relationships. These can occur whether the pregnancy is planned, wanted, or not wanted. Adolescent pregnancy loss research reveals that adolescents who have experienced an early pregnancy loss have significant physical, emotional, social, and cognitive responses and are at risk for depression and a rapid repeat pregnancy (Barglow, Istiphan, Bedger, & Welbourne, 1973; Horowitz, 1978; Sefton, 2002, 2007; Smith, 1999; Wheeler, 1997a, 1997b; Wheeler & Austin, 2000, 2001).

ADOLESCENT GROWTH AND DEVELOPMENT

To gain a greater understanding of the adolescent response to pregnancy loss, it is helpful to review normal adolescent emotional and psychological development. Erik Erikson's (1968) classic developmental theory offers an outline of the psychosocial tasks of adolescents. During this developmental stage, adolescents work through identity versus identity diffusion. The tasks associated with this stage illustrate a transition from childhood to adulthood. In the adolescent's search for ego identity, the initial identity formation may take place within the peer group. The adolescent is most concerned with how he or she is perceived by other members of his or her peer group. Both boys and girls are concerned about their appearance and fitting in with their peer group. Erikson maintains adolescents usually fall in love to help define their ego identity, not for the satisfaction of a sexual drive. The ego image is clarified and strengthened as it is reflected on a like-minded and loved friend. For some adolescents, trying to integrate their ego identity and/or sexual maturity may produce a crisis. An adolescent in crisis must learn to trust his or her own self and then to trust others. Trust is placed in those peers and adults who the adolescent perceives can help him or her. Anyone who might suggest limits or disagree with the adolescent's aspirations might be met with accusations of a lack of caring (American Psychological Association, 2002).

Piaget (1950) studied cognitive development from infancy to adulthood. His observations of adolescents revealed a transition from concrete operations to formal operations and the ability to think abstractly. Some adolescents are focused on logic and others are able to combine logical and abstract thinking. New thinking skills are practiced on parents, teachers, and peers through arguing, sarcasm, and humor. Higher level thinking allows adolescents to become introspective, think about the future, and to set personal goals (Keating, 1990).

Blos (1979) described three separate phases of adolescence (early, middle, and late), which evolve throughout the transition from childhood to adulthood. The age ranges are arbitrarily set and mirror educational milestones. The middle school stage represents the early adolescence period, ages 10 to 14 years. Entrance to and completion of high school, ages 15 to 17 years, connote middle adolescence, and graduation from high school and entrance into college, ages 18 to 23 years, represent later adolescence (Balk, 2014).

Early Adolescence

The onset of puberty heralds early adolescence. The variations in the age of the adolescent at the time of puberty and growth spurts can cause adolescents of the same age to physically look very different (Kipke, 1999). This wide range in physical development creates stress and anxiety in some adolescents as they worry about their physical appearance and how they look to others. Body image can affect self-image as social comparisons are made (Steinberg, 1993). There are frequent mood swings and a desire for privacy. Early adolescents are well aware of their weaknesses, even when they appear self-confident (Erikson, 1968). An increase in cognitive abilities leads the adolescent to want to make his or her own decisions. Some early adolescents have difficulty in understanding the potential consequences of their decisions. Problems arise when the decision made by the adolescent is in direct conflict with a parent(s) or guardian. Socially, early adolescents begin to spend more time with their friends, as peers begin to be more important than their family (Balk, 2014). They want to feel a part of the group and conform to group norms. This can put the early adolescent in conflict with his or her family, with the mother frequently the primary target (Pipher, 1999).

Middle Adolescence

Most adolescents have entered or completed puberty during this phase (Kipke, 1999). Middle adolescence physical growth is near adult size. Emotions are unpredictable and swing widely from euphoria to depression (Steinberg, 1999). A middle adolescent girl is hungry for recognition, with drama and creativity as basic ingredients for her behavior. The process of identity formation is intense with experimentation of different roles, looks, sexuality, values, friendships, ethnicity, and occupations (Erikson, 1968). Some middle adolescents demonstrate an increased ability to empathize with others, a greater vulnerability to worrying, and depression. Many middle adolescents are able to think abstractly and can apply lessons learned in one situation to another; think about the future; and see many potential possibilities (Keating, 1990). This can lead to an increase in responsible behaviors and willingness to confer with trusted adults in important life decisions (Cole & Cole, 1996; Eccles et al., 1993). Peers become an essential replacement for parents, with the adolescent pushing for more autonomy and independence (Balk, 2014).

Late Adolescence

Late adolescents are typically fully developed (Kipke, 1999). They are more emotionally stable and have a stronger sense of themselves (Steinberg, 1993). Cognitive skills and logical thought are at a peak (Keating, 1990). Socially, late adolescents begin to enjoy more secure and intimate love relationships and are comfortable with loosened family ties (Cole & Cole, 1996; Steinberg,

1993). Peer relationships remain important. Late adolescents are able to sustain intimate and love relationships. They show a greater maturity in their capacity to become their own person, to determine a direction in life that meshes with their self-concept (Balk, 2014).

INTEGRATED THEORY OF BEREAVEMENT

Sanders's (1989) Integrated Bereavement Theory has been used to organize grief responses and the bereavement process. The theory identifies antecedents, processes, and possible outcomes of grief. The bereaved are conceptualized as moving in and out of the phases toward renewal. At times, phases may overlap when a setback occurs that slows the forward motion of the grief process. Sanders's five phases of bereavement that constitute mourning are (a) shock, (b) awareness of the loss, (c) conservation/withdrawal, (d) healing, and (e) renewal. The first three phases are predominantly physiological in nature. These phases are more stressful to the bereaved from a physiological, emotional, social, and cognitive standpoint. The final two phases are predominantly psychological in nature and focus more on the outcome of bereavement.

External mediators from the environment can influence the bereaved and include social support systems (i.e., family, friends, church, school), socioeconomic status, relationship with the deceased, type of death, and cultural background. Internal mediators are inherent within the person and include age, gender, personality, ego strength, cognitive ability, physical health, dependency needs, and perception of the loss. The internal and external mediators interact and effect grief responses in either positive or negative ways at the time of the loss and throughout the grief. Interactions over time eventually affect the bereaved adolescent's ability to cope with and adapt to his or her loss. Ultimately, the adolescent's physical/mental health, support systems, and perception of self are affected.

According to Sanders (1989), there are three general possibilities for the outcome of grief: (a) a new way to go on with life with feelings of increased psychosocial functioning, (b) maintenance of life as if the situation never occurred, and (c) complications after the loss that are directly related to the loss (i.e., lowered self-esteem, depression, negative changes in social or family functioning, hypochondriasis, alcohol use, and suicide).

Adolescent Pregnancy Loss Overview

To our knowledge, there have been only six research studies on adolescent girls' responses to pregnancy loss, some of which have resulted in more than one publication (Barglow, Istiphan, Bedger, & Welbourne, 1973;

Hatcher, 1973; Horowitz, 1978; Sefton, 2002, 2007; Smith, 1999; Wheeler, 1997a, 1997b; Wheeler & Austin, 2000, 2001). Barglow et al.'s (1973) study of 31 adolescent girls experiencing a miscarriage, stillbirth, or newborn death found that they moved through a mourning process with stages similar to Sanders's stages of bereavement. Initial feelings of shock were followed by a yearning characterized by daydreaming about the infant and a desire to become pregnant again. These adolescents also experienced guilt, anger, and many somatic symptoms. Apathy was typically expressed by neglect in caring about themselves or an inability to visualize their future. This was perceived by the researchers as a way for the adolescents to cover their pain and despair. Recovery occurred when adolescents became more purposeful in their behavior and began to think about their future.

Barglow and colleagues (1973) further identified criteria for assessing complicated mourning as a persistent or abnormal emotional state, an acute psychosis or hypochondriasis, self-destructive behavior, and/or long-term denial of the loss. Based on their criteria for complicated mourning, they found that more than three fourths of the adolescents experienced a complicated mourning process related to a pregnancy loss.

Six adolescents were interviewed by Hatcher (1973) 6 weeks after a therapeutic abortion. Hatcher categorized the participants' developmental stages and noted reaction differences between the stages. Stage classifications were early, middle, and late adolescence, which were determined by evaluation of developmental status and not chronological age. In general, all six girls expressed minimal consequences following their abortion. The early adolescents were relieved to no longer be pregnant but also wanted to avoid thinking about it or discussing it, as if denying that the pregnancy and abortion ever occurred. Sexual activity was not resumed due to fear. For a short time, the middle adolescent participants experienced more guilt, lower self-esteem, sense of loss, and depressive symptoms than the participants in the other stages. Although participants in late adolescence also felt guilt, they felt the experience matured them. They continued to have thoughts about the fetus and worked through their grief. Hatcher concluded that denial was the prevalent response for the early adolescents, unexpected sadness occurred for the middle adolescents, and late adolescents understood their sadness and anticipated it.

Horowitz (1978) interviewed 40 adolescent girls whose abortion, miscarriage, or infant loss was followed by a subsequent pregnancy. Interviews took place within 3 months after they had given birth. Although these adolescents demonstrated few grief responses, some found it difficult to talk about their previous pregnancy loss. Horowitz hypothesized these young women had received little social support for their loss and were afraid of feeling overwhelmed by their emotional reactions.

A dissertation study (Smith, 1999) and subsequent publications (Sefton, 2002, 2007) examined the long-term effects of miscarriage for 14 Latina adolescent girls 2 to 5 years after they had experienced a miscarriage. All of the young women experienced grief responses to their miscarriage and a period of bereavement after their loss. Support from their families and boyfriends were identified as key in helping them to work through their grief, reach resolution, and to feel better about themselves. These young women did not feel a need to conceive after their loss, with many expressing concerns of experiencing a second miscarriage. The participants were found to experience the stages of bereavement as outlined by Sanders (shock, awareness of the loss, conservation/withdrawal, healing, renewal), but some reported still feeling grieved even years after the loss.

Wheeler (1997a) conducted a pilot study of 34 adolescents who had experienced a miscarriage/ectopic pregnancy (38%), elective termination (53%), newborn death (2%), or a loss attributed to sudden infant death syndrome (5%). This study focused on the physical, emotional, social, and cognitive responses to pregnancy loss. When asked to rate their perception of loss, 85% of the adolescents reported a perception of loss. Older gestational age at the time of loss was also positively associated with a perceived relationship with the unborn child. Those adolescents who had made preparations for the pregnancy or baby had higher grief responses than those who had not made preparations. Younger adolescents and those who had wanted the baby had higher physical responses (i.e., sleep disturbances and appetite), emotional responses (i.e., crying, guilt, mood changes), and social response scores (feeling different, alone, and socially isolated). At the time of the study, 59% ($n = 20$) of the adolescents were pregnant again.

Wheeler's (1997b) dissertation study of 164 low socioeconomic status, never married, adolescent girls aged 13 to 19 years ($m = 16.9$) compared the results for 52 adolescents who had experienced a miscarriage (62%) or elective termination of a pregnancy (35%) with those of adolescents who had never been pregnant ($n = 62$) and those currently pregnant ($n = 50$). All of the miscarriages or elective terminations occurred between 4 and 18 weeks gestation. Approximately two thirds of all participants in the never-pregnant group indicated they had experienced a significant loss in the past 2 years. In comparing the grief responses of the adolescents who had experienced an early pregnancy loss with those of adolescents who had experienced other types of significant loss, the early pregnancy loss group reported more intense physical, emotional, and cognitive responses than their never-pregnant counterparts. Furthermore, 25% of these pregnancy loss women responded "own child" in response to the type of significant loss they had experienced in the past 2 years. The early pregnancy loss group had higher overall depression, physical, emotional, and social grief scores than the other groups. The group that experienced an early pregnancy loss and were subsequently pregnant had lower overall depression and higher self-esteem scores than the other three groups in the study. These studies suggest that miscarriage, elective termination, stillbirth, or newborn death are significant life events for most adolescents with grief responses and bereavement processes.

Adolescent Grief Responses

When adolescents have experienced an early pregnancy loss they will experience grief responses that are physical, emotional, social, and cognitive in nature (Barglow et al., 1973; Sefton, 2007; Wheeler & Austin, 2001). These grief responses can last for years, but for most adolescents, reactions to the pregnancy loss will decrease after 6 months and be resolved by 12 months (Horowitz, 1978; Smith, 1999). Limited research has been conducted on the grief response of adolescents who have experienced an early pregnancy loss, but from this research insights can be gained and applied to the care of adolescents during bereavement. To gain a greater understanding of the bereavement response of adolescents to pregnancy loss, evidence regarding bereavement responses of adolescents experiencing any type of loss and women older than 19 years who have lost a pregnancy are compared and contrasted.

Physical Responses

Adolescents who had experienced a pregnancy loss reported more physical responses than adolescents who were currently pregnant or had never been pregnant (Wheeler, 1997a, 1997b; Wheeler & Austin, 2001). Crying, staying in bed, and loss of appetite with subsequent weight loss were physical responses identified soon after the loss (Smith, 1999; Wheeler, 1997b). As one adolescent recalled, "I miscarried in November and it took me a while. I didn't eat and I got real sick cause I was not eating and I was losing weight. I was like that for a good five months" (Smith, 1999). It is important to note that many did not cry at the time of the loss but cried at a later time. Sleep disturbances can also occur, including insomnia, waking during the middle of the night, dreaming about the baby, and nightmares. This can be illustrated by the comments from two young women. One expressed, "I just can't seem to relax enough to go to sleep." Another had a stronger reaction, "I have really bad dreams, sometimes nightmares. . .the other night I dreamed about babies and blood all over my bed" (Wheeler, 1997a). Some adolescents reported dry mouth and throat, while others felt a lump-in-the-throat sensation and feelings of emptiness. The feelings of emptiness may be related to the physical changes that begin to occur in early pregnancy (i.e., breast, blood volume, uterine, growing embryo) and the subsequent changes that occur after a miscarriage or elective termination. Muscle aches and pains in the neck and shoulders were also identified. Some adolescents indicated they felt restless. Younger adolescents had more physical symptoms such as sleep disturbances and changes in appetite. A positive association existed between adolescents wanting the baby and increased physical responses. The intensity of the grief responses did not appear to be influenced either by knowledge of the pregnancy at the time of the miscarriage or by elective termination (Wheeler, 1997a, 1997b).

In comparison, adolescents who experienced other losses and women older than 19 years who experienced a pregnancy loss also had physical responses to the loss. Adolescents who experienced the death of a sibling or parent had similar somatic complaints when compared with adolescents who experienced a pregnancy loss. Grief responses among adolescents who experienced a sibling or parent loss included trouble eating (e.g., loss of appetite and stomach pains), sleep disturbances, and being ill more often. Sleeping problems often were the result of dreams that were nightmarish in quality. The dreams were very frightening and repetitive (Balk, 1991; Boelen & Spuij, 2013; Fanos & Nickerson, 1991; Hogan & Greenfield, 1991; Opie, Goodwin, Finke, Beattey, Lee, & van Epps, 1991; Torbic, 2011). Somatic expressions in the study by Fanos and Nickerson (1991) included severe headaches, ulcers, and chronically tensed, painful muscles and joints. Opie and colleagues (1991) found that bereaved adolescents missed school because they did not feel well and had general somatic complaints and affective distress. As with adolescents who experience any type of loss, women older than 19 years also experienced physical sensations after their pregnancy loss such as crying, insomnia, and aching arms (Beutel, Deckardt, von Rad, & Weiner, 1995; Janssen, Cuisinier, deGraauw, & Hoogduin, 1996; Madden, 1994). Wheeler (1997b) reported that adolescents who experienced an early pregnancy loss had more intense grief responses than those who had experienced other types of losses (i.e., peer, parent, grandparent, pet).

Emotional Responses

The emotional response to a loss is probably the best known and studied response. The emotional response examines the feelings about the loss. Merriam-Webster's defines emotion as "a conscious mental reaction (as anger or fear) subjectively experienced as strong feeling usually directed toward a specific object and typically accompanied by physiological and behavioral changes in the body" (Emotion, n.d.). Adolescents who experienced an early pregnancy loss had a wide range of emotional responses.

Some adolescents reported crying at the time of the loss, while others were unable to cry at the time of the loss. Guilt, anger, and frequent mood swings were reported. Anger at a mother, boyfriend, God, and one's self was expressed, with some adolescents indicating they had a strong desire to scream. Various teens reported feeling like "less of a woman" or "a nobody" (Sefton, 2007; Wheeler, 1997a). These comments highlight the emotional reaction to an early pregnancy loss. "I was happy to know something was living inside me. . . .I cried. . . .Oh, how I cried. I was really mad. I wanted that baby" and "Sometimes I feel like I'm just going through the motions, I'm so tired of being sad and depressed" (Wheeler, 1997b).

Responses to pregnancy loss and to other losses can be compared to gain a better understanding of this phenomenon during the adolescent period. Initially, after the death of a family member, adolescents report feeling dazed, shocked, confused, numb, lonely, fearful of death, afraid, vulnerable, angry at God, and sometimes responsible for the death. They also feel frustrated, depressed, sad, uncomfortable when happy, guilty, anxious, powerless/helpless, and more irritable. These responses are intense at the time of the death and diminish over time (Balk, 1991; Boelen & Spuij, 2013; Fanos & Nickerson, 1991; Hogan & Greenfield, 1991; Kaplow, Layne, Pynoos, Cohen, & Lieberman, 2012; McNeil, Stilliman, & Swilhart, 1991; Rosenberg et al., 2014; Torbic, 2011). These emotional responses to the loss of a family member highlight the similarities to the emotional responses of adolescents who have experienced a pregnancy loss.

Adolescent emotional responses are similar to those of women who have experienced an early miscarriage. Psychological and emotional symptoms reported in the literature include yearning to see their loved one, sensing the presence of their baby, crying, anger, guilt, frustration, shame, oversensitivity, denial, and fear of another loved one's death. Emotional responses identified include crying, anxiety, despair, disappointment, irritability, anger, difficulty in coping, helplessness, avoidance of reminders of the pregnancy, emotional distancing of self, depression, guilt, low self-esteem, feelings of inadequacy or failure, and self-blame for causing the early pregnancy loss (Abboud & Liamputtong, 2003; Limbo & Wheeler, 1986; Robinson, 2014; Schaper, Hellwig, Murphy, & Gensch, 1996). For the majority of women, bereavement decreased over time, often resolving by 12 months after miscarriage (Beutel et al., 1995; Robinson, 2014; Stirtzinger, Robinson, & Stewart, 1999).

Social Responses

The dynamics of interpersonal relationships are affected by many factors, with a loss possibly having the greatest impact. When an adolescent experiences an early pregnancy loss, the grief response can affect her social relationships and how she interacts with family and friends. Many adolescents who have experienced a pregnancy loss have reported feeling different from their peers. The loss experience changed them, and they felt that friends did not understand what they were going through due to their friends' lack of maturity and exposure to similar experiences. Some felt that their peers were intolerant of their grief and so withdrew from their peers, exacerbating feelings of isolation and of being all alone with their loss (Smith, 1999; Wheeler, 1997a, 1997b). Some adolescents intentionally separated themselves from their friends and needed to be alone to grieve: "I was always in my room, just locked in. I would let nobody come in. I was always crying because of what happened" (Smith, 1999).

Others felt a strong need to act as if nothing had happened: "I try to laugh along with people, but it sometimes doesn't help. If I can't handle it and it makes me really upset, I go to my special spot and just sit and think" (Wheeler, 1997a, 1997b). Feeling different, alone, and isolated from friends has been shown to be positively associated with the length of pregnancy. The longer the gestational age, the more these feelings were experienced (Wheeler, 1997a, 1997b). When considering relationship influences and emotional healing, a perceived lack of positive interpersonal relationships or support has been found to have a negative impact on the emotional health of some adolescents who experience an early pregnancy loss. Conversely, feeling supported by the boyfriend, parents, and/or friends positively affected the healing process for the teen (Sefton, 2002; Smith, 1999). Two positive outcomes for some adolescents experiencing this type of loss were feeling closer to their family, particularly their mother, and feeling more mature than their friends (Sefton, 2002; Smith, 1999; Wheeler, 1997a, 1997b). This positive change was expressed by one girl when she stated, "My parents are very important to me. I am finding out that I can trust my parents enough to tell them things about me no matter how bad it is" (Wheeler, 1997b).

In a review of the literature of adolescents who had experienced the death of a loved one, social grief reactions were found to be similar to those of adolescents who had experienced pregnancy loss (Balk, 1990; Boelen & Spuij, 2013; Kaplow et al. 2012, Rosenberg et al., 2014; Torbic, 2011). Some adolescents reported feeling different from their peers after the death of a loved one. These adolescents perceived their peers to be intolerant of their grief, thus leading them to socially isolate themselves from their peers (Davies, 1991; Martinson & Campos, 1991, Torbic, 2011). Adolescents also expected their parents and other friends to recognize their feelings and to offer them support (McNeil et al., 1991; O'Brien, Goodenaw, & Espin, 1991). Still others established deep, serious relationships early and felt they were more mature than their peers (Oltjenbruns, 1991).

When considering how grief for an early pregnancy loss affected social reactions of adult women, research also showed that these women experienced reactions similar to those of their adolescent counterparts. Some experience grief, guilt, self-doubt, and anxiety; some experience reactions severe enough to be considered symptoms of posttraumatic stress disorder (Engelhard, van den Hout, & Arntz, 2001; Robinson, 2014). Relationship quality affected a woman's reaction also. Increased anxiety and decreased coping strategies were present when women felt a lack of support from the father of the baby (Beutel et al., 1995; Janssen et al., 1997; Rajan, 1994). Relationships with a spouse often suffered, with women having a greater difficulty with communication and a higher incidence of dissolution of marital or cohabitation relationships (Gold, Sen, & Hayward, 2010; Robinson, 2014; Serrano & Lima, 2006). On the other hand, women who felt supported during their grieving had a more positive grief resolution. For example, being allowed to talk about the experience and having their loss acknowledged was helpful to women experiencing a miscarriage (Madden, 1994; Rajan, 1994).

Cognitive Responses

The cognitive response to a pregnancy loss is another aspect that provides insight into the loss experience for young women. *Cognition* reflects the awareness, perception, knowing, or reasoning of an event. It is the intellectual response to the loss (Cognition, n.d.). It has been found that adolescents who have experienced an early pregnancy loss conceptualize or give meaning to the loss in several different ways that include (a) thinking their miscarriage or elective termination was just a life experience and not a significant loss, (b) thinking of it as a nondescript pregnancy loss, or (c) thinking the loss was the loss of an actual baby (Sefton, 2002; Wheeler, 1997a).

As with conceptualizing the loss, the significance of the loss varied among adolescents ranging from not significant to moderately significant or very significant. How significant the loss was perceived to be was highly individualized for most adolescents, with research not finding specific correlates that predicted significance. Although some did not feel the event was significant to them, others considered the event very significant and were still affected by the loss even months or years later (Barglow et al., 1973; Horowitz, 1978; Sefton, 2002; Wheeler, 1997a, 1997b). In reflecting upon her miscarriage, one girl said, "It was real important to me, to tell you the truth, cause that was supposed to be my first child. That's something I'm never going to forget. It was a real big deal to me cause whether or not the child was there or not I really did care about it" (Smith, 1999).

Some contemplated the meaning or purpose of the loss. For many, having a pregnancy loss as an adolescent, though a significant and difficult experience, did allow them to pursue other interests and goals, including continuing with their education. Some philosophized, thinking that "It was for the best" or "It was God's will." Meaning and significance has also been shown to be related to the emotional response to the loss. As the meaning and significance increased, the emotional response increased (Smith, 1999).

Although responses varied, several thoughts were common among adolescents and again did not depend on the type of loss—either miscarriage or elective abortion. For some adolescents, a pregnancy loss precipitated a time of reflection about what their life would have been like if the baby had lived. They expressed having hopes and dreams for their child. Others reflected on how difficult it would have been to have the baby and be a teenaged mother (Smith, 1999; Wheeler, 1997a). They also thought about why the loss happened to them and became more thoughtful about the meaning of life and how short life can be. Some reflected on what they might have done to cause their miscarriage and if more could have been done at the time of the loss. Others had a more severe reaction to the loss, wishing they were dead or could die (Wheeler, 1997a).

School performance was found to be influenced by the pregnancy loss. After a loss, the adolescent girls expressed experiencing concentration difficulties and feeling distracted by thoughts of the baby: "It's like I can't shut my brain off" (Wheeler, 1997a). A lack of interest in school ensued for some, leading to dropping out of or prolonging high school (Smith, 1999; Wheeler, 1997a).

In a comparison to adolescents who have experienced pregnancy loss, those who have experienced other types of loss have shown similar cognitive responses (Balk & Corr, 2009; Boelen & Spuij, 2013; Fanos & Nickerson, 1991; Hogan & DeSantis, 1994; Kaplow et al., 2012; Rosenberg et al., 2014; Torbic, 2011). Many adolescents experienced a decline in school performance after the death of a parent or sibling. These adolescents found concentration difficult, were preoccupied, had intrusive thoughts, and felt distracted. All of these responses might have contributed to poor school performance and attendance (Balk & Corr, 2009; Hogan & DeSantis, 1994; McNeil et al., 1991; O'Brien et al., 1991; Torbic, 2011). Hogan and DeSantis (1994) identified the intrusive thoughts as painful, uninvited, spontaneous, and related to the circumstances and events surrounding the death. The intrusive thoughts and feelings fell into three subcategories: guilt and shame, sense of loneliness, and a realization of the permanency of death. Fanos and Nickerson (1991) found that many adolescents struggled with why the death occurred, why it happened to someone close to them, and why God let it happen. See Table 9.1 for a summary of emotional, physical, cognitive, and social responses to early pregnancy loss during adolescence.

TABLE 9.1 Adolescent Responses to Early Pregnancy Loss

EMOTIONAL	PHYSICAL	COGNITIVE	SOCIAL
Depression	Sleep disturbances	Low self-esteem	Isolation
Grief	Exhaustion	Shock	Relationship
Guilt	Appetite changes	Denial	changes (+/−)
Anger	Aches and pains	Difficulty concentrating	
Mood changes	Dry mouth	Fantasizing about the	
Apathy	Crying	infant	
Emptiness	Quickly become	"For the best"	
Fear of failure	pregnant to replace		
Desire to die	loss		
Difficulty speaking			
about loss			
Healing			

Adolescent Pregnancy Loss Bereavement Outcomes

In summary, several points can be made about adolescent bereavement following an early pregnancy loss. Grieving adolescents are at risk for developing clinical depression and suicidal ideation, and moreover are vulnerable to becoming pregnant again within the next 2 years (Barglow et al., 1973; Horowitz, 1978; Sefton, 2007; Stevens-Simon, Dolgan, Kelly, & Singer, 1997; Wheeler, 1997a, 1997b; Wheeler & Austin, 2001). Adolescents can have various grief responses and at various intensities that can be manifested as physical, emotional, social, and cognitive responses. When an adolescent exhibits more grief responses, she is more likely to have lower self-esteem, less satisfaction with family relationships, and feelings that her life will not change (Smith, 1999; Wheeler & Austin, 2001). Adolescents who experience a pregnancy loss may suppress their feelings to live their lives as they did before the loss. This may be based on a lack of acknowledgment, support, and understanding from family, friends, and professionals who cared for them at the time of the loss. Doka (1989) calls this "disenfranchised grief." This means that support from family and friends may be limited or even absent.

Along with lack of support, other circumstances can contribute to disenfranchised grief. A prominent circumstance is when a sense of shame surrounds the death. Negative stigma associated with adolescent pregnancy may create stress for the adolescent, and a loss then adds additional stress. The negative stigma against adolescent pregnancy may inhibit the mourner's ability to publicly grieve a subsequent loss because society may see it as "for the best" or even as a punishment for becoming pregnant as an adolescent, resulting in even more stress for the girl. Another context can be when the mourner is not thought to have the ability to grieve. Some may assume that the very young, the very old, or the mentally handicapped may not have the capability to grieve. Again, if that assumption is made, support and understanding may not be given to the adolescent, contributing to a disenfranchised grief response. Sanders (1989) also identified an additional circumstance that could contribute to disenfranchised grief: sudden, unexpected death. This type of death has been found to have a more long-term debilitating effect on the survivors than anticipated death. The vast majority of miscarriages are unanticipated and sudden, which result in a more intense or prolonged grief. Some of the signs and symptoms of prolonged grief and complicated bereavement in adolescents include:

• Depression
• Suicidal ideation
• Prolonged crying/sadness (>1 year)
• Daily thoughts of the loss
• Unemployment
• Incomplete schooling
• Hypochondriasis
• Denial of loss
• Self-destructive behavior

Implications for Care

There are many challenges in working with adolescents who have experienced an early pregnancy loss. Based on current statistics, many of the adolescents who experience a pregnancy loss are younger, with complicated life situations. Health care professionals need to determine who the adolescent considers to be her support and to include them in her care. Health care professionals need to know the state laws that pertain in the situation of an adolescent pregnancy, pregnancy loss, and adoption. For example, when the adolescent becomes pregnant, does she become emancipated from her parents/guardian? Can she make health care decisions for herself, her pregnancy, and her baby? Or are her parent(s) responsible for making health care decisions for the adolescent and the adolescent responsible for making health care decisions for her baby? What rights does the father of the baby have? Who is financially responsible for the adolescent and her baby's health care, autopsy, and burial? The socioeconomic status of the adolescent and/or her family may make it difficult to make final arrangements for the baby. Knowing who to contact, what paperwork needs to be completed, and the costs involved to ensure that the baby's final disposition is complete and respectful are important considerations. Do the services that existed for the adolescent and the father of her baby during the pregnancy end after the death of the baby? (See Appendix 9.1 for lay and professional bereavement resources.)

Most adolescents do not spontaneously "open up" and talk with adults. Furthermore, the presence of a parent, foster parent, and/or guardian may foster complicated interpersonal dynamics, which have the potential for keeping the adolescent from expressing herself. Adolescents need to perceive they are in a safe, nonjudgmental environment where they feel listened to and understood. Health care professionals working with adolescents need to establish a connection with the adolescent, regardless of how brief the encounter may be. Reflective listening can be helpful in working with adolescents, because the basic goal of such listening is to give a person the chance to express, explore, and understand his or her own feelings (Parlakian, 2001; see Appendix 9.2 for communication tips). The desire for some adolescents to want as many family and friends to be present at the time of the loss and/or to want to use social media to share their feelings and emotions may be difficult for some health care professionals to understand and support. It is important to remember that supporting the adolescent also means supporting her support system, in the hopes her social support system will be understanding and supportive of her after discharge.

When possible, offering adolescents and their loved ones the opportunity to see, hold, and have special time with the remains can be important in actualizing the loss and creating support at the time of the loss and after. Creating memories (e.g., pictures, footprints, handprints, blessing or baptism, special mementos) for adolescents who describe their loss in terms of the loss of a baby can be comforting (Alexander, 2001; Limbo & Kobler, 2013). It is important to remember that some adolescents have limitations on their living space. Being sensitive to adolescents in this situation is important so as to not overburden them with mementos that may have to be discarded in the future, thus creating another sense of loss.

Hospital discharge planning should include anticipatory guidance with regard to the physical, emotional, social, and cognitive grief responses and potential responses from family and friends (Soto, 2011). Further physical responses should also include written and verbal information on afterpains, caring for the perineum, changes in lochia, inhibiting lactation, identifying postpartum infection, and when to notify health care providers of problems. Adolescents should also be given information on birth control. Follow-up care should focus on assessment of grief responses (e.g., physical complaints, eating and sleep habits, signs and symptoms of depression, school attendance/performance, family functioning, boyfriend/peer relationships). Referrals may be in the form of information about local pregnancy support groups, bereavement programs for adolescents who have experienced a pregnancy loss, or counseling. Referral is necessary for those adolescents struggling with clinical depression, suicidal thoughts with intention, homelessness, and/or not attending school.

CONCLUSION

This chapter has focused on the grief responses of female adolescents who have experienced an early pregnancy loss. Theoretical frameworks for understanding adolescent growth and development, grief responses, and the bereavement process were offered to help the health care provider better understand the impact of loss. Information on assessing adolescents for developing negative outcomes/complicated bereavement was offered, as were strategies for care and tips for communicating with adolescents at the time of the loss and after.

CASE STUDY

Samira is a 15-year-old patient who experienced a miscarriage at 12 weeks gestation. Samira's parents are relieved that the pregnancy ended "before anyone could see [she] was pregnant." Two weeks after the loss, Samira reported that she cries a lot but feels that she needs to keep it to herself. When asked about her loss, she shares that it was probably for the best, she feels very sad, and no one seems to understand her sadness. She also expresses concern that her boyfriend will break up with her because she is hesitant to engage in sexual activity again.

FOCUS QUESTIONS

1. What aspects of Samira's loss experience are expected for a patient of her age? What aspects are unexpected?
2. What supportive interventions would be most helpful for Samira?
3. What interventions would help Samira express her feelings to others, particularly her parents?
4. How could Samira's concerns about her boyfriend be addressed?

REFERENCES

Abboud, L., & Liamputtong, P. (2003). Pregnancy loss: What it means to women who miscarry and their partners. *Social Work Health Care, 36*(3), 37–62. doi: 10.1300/J010v36n03_03

American Psychological Association. (2002). *Developing adolescents: A reference for professionals.* Washington, DC: Author. Retrieved from http://www.apa.org/pi/families/resources/develop.pdf

Anderson, K. V. (2001). "The one thing you can never take away": Perinatal bereavement photographs. *MCN, The American Journal of Maternal/Child Nursing, 26*(3), 123–127.

Balk, D. E. (1990). The self-concepts of bereaved adolescents: Sibling death and its aftermath. *Journal of Adolescent Research, 5,* 112–132.

Balk, D. E. (1991). Sibling death, adolescent bereavement, and religion. *Death Studies, 15*(1), 1–20. doi:10.1080/07481189108252406

Balk, D. E. (2014). Adolescence and emerging adulthood: A developmental perspective. In K. J. Doka & A. S. Tucci (Eds.), *Helping adolescents cope with loss.* Washington, DC: Hospice Foundation of America.

Balk, D. E., & Corr, C. A. (2009). *Adolescent encounters with death, bereavement and coping.* New York, NY: Springer.

Barglow, P., Istiphan, I., Bedger, J., & Welbourne, C. (1973). Response of unmarried adolescent mothers to infant or fetal death. *Adolescent Psychiatry, 2,* 285–300.

Beutel, M., Deckardt, R., von Rad, M., & Weiner, H. (1995). Grief and depression after miscarriage: Their separation, antecedents, and course. *Psychosomatic Medicine, 57*(6), 517–526.

Blos, P. (1979). *The adolescent passage: Developmental issues.* Madison, CT: International Universities Press, Inc.

Boelen, P., & Spuij, M. (2013). Symptoms of post-traumatic stress disorder in bereaved children and adolescents: Factor structure and correlates. *Journal of Abnormal Child Psychology, 41,* 1097–1108. doi:10.1007/s10802-013-9748-6

Cognition. (n.d.). *Merriam-Webster.com.* Retrieved from http://www.merriam-webster .com/dictionary/cognition

Cole, M., & Cole, S. R. (1996). *The development of children.* New York, NY: W. H. Freeman and Company.

Davies, B. (1991). Long-term outcomes of adolescent sibling bereavement. *Journal of Adolescent Research, 6*(1), 83–96. doi:10.1177/074355489161007

Doka, K. J. (1989). *Disenfranchised grief: Recognizing hidden sorrow.* Lexington, MA: Lexington Books.

Eccles, J., Midgley, C., Wigfield, A., Buchanan, C. M., Reuman, D., Flanangan, C., & MacIver, D. (1993). Development during adolescence: The impact of stage-environment fit on young adolescents' experience in schools and in families. *American Psychologist, 48,* 90–101.

Emotion. (n.d.). *Merriam-Webster.com.* Retrieved from http://www.merriam-webster .com/dictionary/emotion

Engelhard, I., van den Hout, M., & Arntz, A. (2001). Posttraumatic stress disorder after pregnancy loss. *General Hospital Psychiatry, 23,* 62–66. doi:10.101 61S0163-8343(01)00124-4

Erikson, E. H. (1968). *Identity, youth, and crisis.* New York, NY: W. W. Norton and Company.

Fanos, J. H., & Nickerson, B. G. (1991). Long-term effects of sibling death during adolescence. *Journal of Adolescent Research, 5*(1), 70–82. doi:10.1177/074355489161006

Gold, K., Sen, A., & Hayward, R. (2010). Marriage and cohabitation outcomes after pregnancy loss. *Pediatrics, 125,* e1202–e1207. doi:10.1542/peds.2009-3081

Hatcher, S. (1973). The adolescent experience of pregnancy and abortion. *Journal of Youth and Adolescence, 2*(1), 28–61.

Hogan, N. S. & DeSantis, L. (1994). Things that help and hinder adolescent sibling bereavement. *Western Journal of Nursing Research, 16*(2), 132–153. doi:10.1177 /019394599401600202

Hogan, N. S., & Greenfield, D. B. (1991). Adolescent sibling bereavement symptomatology in a large community sample. *Journal of Adolescent Research, 6*(1), 97–112. doi:10.1177/074355489161008

Horowitz, N. (1978). Adolescent mourning reactions to infant and fetal loss. *Social Casework, 59,* 551–559.

Janssen, H., Cuisinier, M., deGraauw, K., & Hoogduin, K. (1996). Controlled prospective study on the mental health of women following pregnancy loss. *American Journal of Psychiatry, 153,* 226–230.

Janssen, H., Cuisinier, M., deGraauw, K., & Hoogduin, K. (1997). A prospective study of risk factors predicting grief intensity following pregnancy loss. *Archives of General Psychiatry, 54,* 54–61. doi:10.1001/archpsyc.1997.01830130062013

Kaplow, J., Layne, C., Pynoos, R., Cohen, J., & Lieberman, A. (2012). DSM-5 diagnostic criteria for bereavement related disorders in children and adolescents: Developmental considerations. *Psychiatry: Interpersonal Biological Processes, 75*(3), 243–266. doi:10.1521/psyc.2012.75.3.243

Keating, D. P. (1990). Adolescent thinking. In S. S. Feldman & G. R. Elliot (Eds.), *At the threshold: The developing adolescen*t. Cambridge, MA: Harvard University Press.

Kipke, M. (Ed.). (1999). *Adolescent development and the biology of puberty: Summary of a workshop on new research.* Washington, DC: National Academy Press.

Krost, K., & Henshaw, S. (2014). *U.S. teenage pregnancies, births and abortions 2010: National and state trends by age, race, and ethnicity.* New York, NY: Guttmacher Institute. Retrieved from http://www.guttmacher.org/pubs/USTPtrends10.pdf

Limbo, R. K., & Kobler, K. (2013). *Meaningful moments: Rituals and reflections when a child dies.* LaCrosse, WI: Gundersen Medical Foundation.

Limbo, R. K., & Wheeler, S. R. (1986). Women's response to the loss of their pregnancy through miscarriage: A longitudinal study. *The Forum Newsletter: Newsletter of the Association for Death Education and Counseling, 10*(4), 1–2.

Madden, M. (1994). The variety of emotional reactions to miscarriage. *Women and Health, 21*(2/3), 85–104. doi:10.1300/J013v21n02_06

Martinson, I. M., & Campos, R. G. (1991). Adolescent bereavement: Long-term responses to a sibling's death from cancer. *Journal of Adolescent Research, 6*(1), 54–69. doi:10.1177/074355489161005

McNeil, J. N., Stilliman, G., & Swilhart, J. J. (1991). Helping adolescents cope with the death of a peer: A high school case study. *Journal of Adolescent Research, 6*(1), 132–145. doi:10.1177/074355489161010

O'Brien, J. M., Goodenow, C., & Espin, O. (1991). Adolescent reactions to the death of a peer. *Adolescence, 26*(102), 431–440. Retrieved from http://web.a.ebscohost.com/ehost/detail?sid=b1fb6ff2-ad8b-48ef-8ba0-106f75b17276%40sessionmgr4004&vid=1&hid=4101&bdata=JnNpdGU9ZWhvc3QtbGl2ZQ%3d%3d#db=rzh&AN=2009455354

Oltjenbruns, K. A. (1991). Positive outcomes of adolescents, experiences with grief. *Journal of Adolescent Research, 6*(1), 43–53. doi:10.1177/074355489161004

Opie, N. D., Goodwin, T., Finke, L. M., Beattey, J. M., Lee, B., & Van Epps, J. (1991). The effect of a bereavement group experience on bereaved children's and adolescents' affective and somatic distress. *Journal of Child Psychiatric Nursing, 5*(1), 20–26. doi:10.1111/j.1744-6171.1992.tb00108.x

Parlakian, R. (2001). *Look, listen and learn: Reflective supervision and relationship-based work.* Washington, DC: Zero to Three Center for Program Excellence.

Piaget, J. (1950). *The psychology of intelligence.* New York, NY: International Universities Press.

Pipher, M. (1999). *Reviving ophelia: Saving the selves of adolescent girls.* Westminister, MD: Ballantine Publishing Group.

Rajan, L. (1994). Social isolation and support in pregnancy loss. *Health Visit, 67*(3), 97–101.

Robinson, G. (2014). Pregnancy loss. *Best Practices & Research Clinical Obstetrics and Gynaecology, 28,* 169–178. doi:10.1016/j.bpobgyn.2013.08.012

Rosenberg, A., Postier, A., Osenga, K., Kreicbergs, U., Neville, B., Dussel, V., & Wolfe, J. (2014). Long-term psychosocial outcomes among bereaved siblings of children with cancer. *Journal of Pain and Symptom Management, 49*(1), 55–65. doi:10.1016/j.jpainsymman.2014.05.006

Sanders, C. M. (1989). *Grief: The mourning after—dealing with adult bereavement.* New York, NY: Wiley InterScience.

Sass, A., & Kaplan, D. (2012). Adolescence. In W. Hay, Jr., M. Levin, R. Deterding, M. Abzug, & J. Sondheimer (Eds.), *Current diagnosis and treatment: Pediatrics* (21st ed.). New York, NY: McGraw-Hill Companies.

Schaper, A. M., Hellwig, M. S., Murphy, P., & Gensch, B. K. (1996). Ectopic pregnancy loss during fertility management. *Western Journal of Nursing Research, 18*(5), 503–517. doi:10.1177/019394599601800503

Sefton, M. (2002). The long-term effects of an early miscarriage for Latina adolescents. *Hispanic Health Care International, 1*(2), 71–78.

Sefton, M. (2007). Grief analysis of adolescents experiencing an early miscarriage. *Hispanic Health Care International, 5*(1), 13–20.

Serrano, F., & Lima, M. L. (2006). Recurrent miscarriage: Psychological and relational consequences for couples. *Psychological Psychotherapy, 79*(4), 585–594. doi:10.1348/147608306X96992

Smith, M. (1999). *The long-term effects of a miscarriage for adolescent Latinas* (Unpublished doctoral dissertation). University of Illinois at Chicago, Chicago, IL.

Soto, M. (2011). Anticipatory guidance: A hospital-based intervention for adolescents with perinatal loss. *Journal of Child Adolescent Social Work, 28,* 49–62. doi:10.1007/s10560-010-0219-4

Steinberg, L. (1993). *Adolescence.* New York, NY: McGraw-Hill.

Stevens-Simon, C., Dolgan, J., Kelly, L., & Singer, D. (1997). The effect of monetary incentives and peer support groups on repeat adolescent pregnancies. *JAMA, 277,* 977–982. doi:10.1001/jama.1997.03540360045029

Stirtzinger, R., Robinson, G., & Stewart, D. (1999). Parameters of grieving in spontaneous abortion. *International Journal of Psychiatry in Medicine, 29*(2), 235–249. doi:10.2190/UDW4-2EAG-1RTY-D1Y4

Torbic, H. (2011). Children and grief: But what about the children? *Home Health Nurse, 29*(2), 67–77. doi:10.1097/NHH.0b013e31820861dd

Wheeler, S. R. (1997a). Adolescent pregnancy loss. In J. R. Woods & J. L. Woods (Eds.), *Loss during or in the newborn period: Principles of care with clinical cases and analyses.* Pitman, NJ: Jannetti Publications, Inc.

Wheeler, S. R. (1997b). The i*mpact of early pregnancy loss on adolescent women age 13-19: A comparison study* (Unpublished doctoral dissertation). Indiana University-Purdue University, Indianapolis, IN.

Wheeler, S. R., & Austin, J. K. (2000). The Loss Response List (LRL): A tool for measuring adolescent grief responses. *Death Studies, 24,* 21–34. doi:10.1080/074811800200676

Wheeler, S. R., & Austin, J. K. (2001). The impact of early pregnancy loss on adolescents. *The American Journal of Maternal/Child Nursing, 26*(3), 154–159.

APPENDIX 9.1: BEREAVEMENT RESOURCES

- American Psychological Association
  - http://www.apa.org/pi/families/resources/develop.pdf
- *A teenager's grief: When a baby dies.* A Place to Remember. Item #: AT0501
  - www.aplacetoremember.com/pdshop/shop/item.aspx?itemid=579
- Guttmacher Institute: Provides a summary of state laws regarding minor's consent, abortion, and access to prenatal care and contraceptive services
  - www.guttmacher.org/sections/adolescents.php
- Nykiel, C. (2004, Revised Edition). After the loss of your baby: For teen mothers. Centering Corporation. ISBN-13: 978-1561231560
- Resolve Through Sharing Bereavement Services: Online bereavement education courses for health care providers
  - www.bereavementservicesonline.org
- American College of Obstetricians and Gynecologists (ACOG): Webtreats are lists of links to additional Internet resources.
  - Webtreats: Adolescent Health
  - www.acog.org/About_ACOG/ACOG_Departments/ Resource_Center/WEBTREATS_Adol_Ped_Health
  - Webtreats: Pregnancy
  - www.acog.org/About_ACOG/ACOG_Departments/ Resource_Center/WEBTREATS_Pregnancy
  - Webtreats: High-risk pregnancy and pregnancy loss
  - www.acog.org/About_ACOG/ACOG_Departments/ Resource_Center/WEBTREATS_High_Risk_Preg_Preg_Loss_Infertility
  - Webtreats: List of all
  - www.acog.org/About_ACOG/ACOG_Departments/ Resource_Center/WEBTREATS
  - Adolescent Health Care
  - www.acog.org/About_ACOG/ACOG_Departments/ Adolescent_Health_Care
  - Ordering information for the Guidelines for Adolescent Health Care
  - sales.acog.org/Guidelines-for-Adolescent-Health-Care-P698C54.aspx

APPENDIX 9.2: TIPS FOR TALKING WITH ADOLESCENTS WHO EXPERIENCED A PREGNANCY LOSS

- Whenever possible, try to position yourself at the same eye level as the adolescent.
- Listen more than talk; keep the focus on the adolescent.

- Attend to support system dynamics. When asked a question, if the teen looks to someone to help her answer, consider this person's thoughts and feelings when providing care.
- To help frame conversation and support, be aware and knowledgeable of cultural, religious, family, and peer influences, as well as individual coping skills.
- Listen nonjudgmentally; let the adolescent know her thoughts and opinions are valued.
- Help the adolescent actualize the loss by asking when she learned she was pregnant. Who did she tell she was pregnant? What plans had she made? How did she learn she was going to experience a loss? What was that experience like? Note the term she uses for the loss, which may give some indication of the meaning and significance of the loss.
- If needed, provide further information regarding the pregnancy and baby to aid comprehension of the loss event. It may be helpful to show a graphic or model of an embryo or fetus representing the weeks of gestation at the time of the loss, an ultrasound picture of an embryonic gestational sac (missed pregnancy), and/or a drawing of a uterus with fallopian tubes. Base approach on the adolescent's cognitive development stage.
- Use empathetic facial expressions and touch to convey caring.
- Sharing others' experience could be helpful for the adolescent in working through problems, finding solutions, and making decisions.
- When discussing or inquiring about family planning, be sensitive that the discussion could evoke a grief response regarding past pregnancy loss, even years later.
- Support feelings of grief, reminding the adolescent that these feelings are normal, valid, and will diminish over time.

CHAPTER 10

Understanding the Experience of Pregnancy Subsequent to a Perinatal Loss

Denise Côté-Arsenault and Joann O'Leary

*B*ecoming pregnant again when a prior pregnancy ended in death requires courage because subsequent pregnancies tend to be fraught with fear and anxiety (Côté-Arsenault, 2007; Côté-Arsenault, Donato, & Earl, 2006; O'Leary, 2004; O'Leary & Thorwick, 1997). There is also an equal dose of optimism and hope that this subsequent pregnancy will result in a live baby at the end of 9 months (Côté-Arsenault et al., 2006). This chapter discusses the challenge for parents, then, to find a balance between anxiety and hope on a daily, weekly, and monthly basis while holding the prize carefully in one's mind's eye throughout the 9 months of pregnancy.

Pregnancy is a unique state that is simultaneously biophysical, psychological, developmental, and social (Rubin, 1984). All experiences of pregnancy, both positive and negative, remain with a woman. She is in a different "life space" with each pregnancy, as life goes on and as relationships evolve. Rubin (1984) stated that a woman develops a maternal identity for each baby, a distinct emotional binding-in of mother to a particular child that remains even if the child does not survive. Pregnancy experiences become cumulative; past experiences inform current ones (Armstrong, Hutti, & Myers, 2009; Chez, 1995; Côté-Arsenault & Morrison-Beedy, 2001; Rubin, 1984), especially unresolved emotional issues (Raphael-Leff, 2004). Regardless of the cause of the death, it is impossible to have another experience of pregnancy without stimulating memories of the painful past loss (Chez, 1995). Women report comparing their signs and symptoms of pregnancy with those they had in the past to reassure themselves that this pregnancy is okay, at least for today (Côté-Arsenault & Mahlangu, 1999).

Perinatal losses can occur at any time from conception to the neonatal period, with the most common time frame in the first trimester. Preterm births are the most common cause of infant death (Martin & Osterman, 2013). Intense feelings of grief and loss are experienced by most mothers, but definitely not by all, and mothers attribute greater meaning to the loss than do fathers (Côté-Arsenault, 2003; Swanson, 2000). In a subsequent pregnancy, the timing of past losses become periods of high anxiety prior to the antici-pated milestone, but some women feel some relief after successfully passing those dates, while others continue to have high anxiety. Some parents report posttraumatic stress symptoms in a new pregnancy where trauma had been previously experienced, especially during an ultrasound where the previous loss was confirmed (O'Leary, 2005). Therefore, it is important to get a history from the parents' perspective of the previous loss, as the parents' definition of what they viewed as trauma can be very different from what may be reported in the medical records (Creedy, Shochet, & Horsfall, 2000). Women with a prior miscarriage or termination were found to be more fearful of childbirth and had an increased risk of depression postpartum (Räisänen et al., 2013). The majority of women who suffer a perinatal loss become preg-nant again (estimates are 50%–85%) with an awareness that not all preg-nancies end with a live birth (Cordle & Prettyman, 1994; Cuisinier, Kuijper, Hoogduin, de Graauw, & Janssen, 1996). This realism greatly influences their expectations. Worries and concerns about the current pregnancy and its potential outcomes are the hallmarks of pregnancy after perinatal loss (Armstrong & Hutti, 1998; Côté-Arsenault, 2003; Côté-Arsenault, Bidlack, & Humm, 2001).

THEORETICAL PERSPECTIVES OF PREGNANCY

Pregnancy is much more than the physical condition of growing a baby. Pregnancy is an anticipated route to motherhood that impacts a woman's psyche, partner and family relationships, and status in society (Côté-Arsenault, Brody, & Dombeck, 2009). We describe three theoretical per-spectives to facilitate one's understanding of the impact of pregnancy and perinatal loss on parents: (a) pregnancy as a developmental process, (b) pregnancy as a liminal phase within a rite of passage, and (c) prenatal attachment.

Pregnancy as a Developmental Process

Theoretical perspectives of human development focus on anticipated change and growth across the life span and seek to describe, understand, and explain how and why people change throughout their lives. Erikson (1963) identified eight stages in the psychosocial life cycle of humans as "ages of man" (pp. 247–274). The majority of young girls imagine being a mother in the future, and they often play out this fantasy with their dolls and strollers. A similar fantasy is true for boys. Erikson described that young adults face a developmental dualism between intimacy (which includes bearing offspring) and social isolation. The ideal outcome is intimacy, a commitment to others such as a life partner, and children (Erikson, 1963). Pregnancy and parenthood are thus commonly expected parts of adulthood; when these milestones are desired but not achieved, a developmental crisis can ensue. This can be the case of perinatal loss of a wanted pregnancy.

Several theorists have identified normative phases or tasks of pregnancy that are part of an anticipated developmental process. Rubin (1984) described four tasks that pregnant women strive to ensure: (a) safe passage for self and baby, (b) social acceptance of self as mother to *this* baby, (c) binding-in to baby, and (d) giving of self. With previous unsuccessful pregnancies, women learn that they cannot always ensure safe passage of a healthy baby, nor can they make sure that all of their deceased babies, who are often forgotten, are accepted into the family. Their experience likely includes babies who died and are often forgotten by others. Therefore, in a new pregnancy after a loss, women's anxiety is due in part to knowing that some of their desired successful tasks, as outlined by Rubin, are not entirely in their control (Côté-Arsenault, 1995).

Pregnancy has also been seen as a transition to parenthood. Galinsky (1987) calls it the first stage of parenthood: "the image-making stage." Reviewing images of parenthood provides parents-to-be with the opportunity of taking on some images and rejecting others, based on one's own past experiences. As images are reviewed, parents become bonded to their unborn child, wonder what that child will be like, and wonder what it will be like to be a parent to that child (Galinsky, 1987). Similarly, Bergum (1989) found being "with child" to be a transformative process; the child's presence transforms a woman into a mother. Simultaneously, relationships evolve with one's partner, one's parents, and oneself. One's view of self is inextricably tied to images of being a parent to this anticipated child. Mercer (2005) contends that a woman's "progress through the stages in becoming a mother is influenced by her life experiences, creativity, and her and her infant's unique characteristics" (p. 650).

The transitions and transformations described by developmental theorists such as Rubin, Galinsky, Bergum, and Mercer imply that a parent never goes back to the way she was prior to her first pregnancy. It follows then that when a pregnancy has not ended with a live baby, the mother is transformed during her time with that wished-for child and subsequent pregnancies will be altered processes. This transformation has also been seen in fathers (O'Leary & Thorwick, 2006a). They have embarked on an imagined developmental process that did not result in a healthy baby and are therefore skeptical and scared when trying again.

Pregnancy as a Liminal Phase in a Social Process

Anthropologist van Gennep (1908/1960) analyzed life crisis ceremonies in global cultures, called *rites of passage*, that accompany social events such as birth, death, puberty, and marriage. The rites of passage enable individuals to move to a new social status (e.g., single to married) with new rules, roles, and relationships. The transition period of time between the old and the new status is referred to as a liminal phase, a time of adjustment and support (Turner, 1967/1987). Pregnancy in American culture includes several rituals such as regularly scheduled prenatal care visits, changing to maternity clothes, baby showers, and childbirth classes. Accordingly, pregnancy changes how a woman views herself and how others view her (Côté-Arsenault et al., 2009).

Rites of passage cushion the transition. Turner described that liminal phase as being "betwixt and between" (Turner, 1967/1987, p. 3) and described liminality as dangerous and unsettling. Pregnancy can be viewed as a rite of passage between "woman-not-mother" and "woman-mother" (Côté-Arsenault et al., 2009). He argued that a person must be successful in traversing the liminal state in order to achieve the new social status. This easily applies to pregnancy after perinatal loss.

When a woman announces her pregnancy, she may be seen as different from simply a "woman," but not yet identified as a "woman-mother," culturally. Thus, she is betwixt and between the two statuses. When the pregnancy ends with a fetal or infant death, she is caught in liminality, not socially seen as mother to the dead baby even though she feels that she *is* a mother. When she enters another pregnancy, she knows the risks and is traversing a liminality that is difficult and uncertain. Thus, she is anxious and concerned about the outcome.

Prenatal Attachment

The relationship of a mother and her fetus has been the focus of scholars such as Cranley (1981) and Rubin (1984) as well as more recent literature systematic reviews (Alhusen, 2008; Cannella, 2005). Condon (1985, 2006) recognized that fathers too have an emotional bond with their unborn child. Recognizing the unique emotional connection parents have to babies who have died and to those in utero in a new pregnancy is particularly important when talking about pregnancy after loss (PAL). The idea that pregnancy is the beginning stage of parenting is particularly understood by families who have experienced a perinatal death (O'Leary, Warland, & Parker, 2011).

Bowlby (1988) defined attachment as a behavioral system in which the child seeks security and protection from the caretaker (mother/father) in order to have a secure base. The attachment relationship a child develops with his parents is crucial for long-term emotional development (Karen, 1998; Stroufe, 2005). Bowlby (1988) believed that without attachment there would be no bereavement. It follows therefore, that parental bereavement implies the existence of a parental attachment relationship (Condon, 1987; O'Leary & Thorwick, 2008).

Prenatal motherhood involves an embodied relationship with the unborn child that provides the mother's awareness of her unborn baby that no one knows or understands (O'Leary, Warland, & Parker, 2011). There is significant research today to support that the mother and unborn baby are connected intimately, both biologically and psychologically (Côté-Arsenault & Dombeck, 2001; DiPietro et al., 2013; Dirix, Nijhuis, Jongsma, & Hornsta, 2009; Glover, 2011; O'Leary & Thorwick, 1997; Sandman, Davis, Buss, & Glynn, 2011; Thomson, 2007).

For the purposes of this chapter, the definition of prenatal attachment is defined as the emotional bond between the parents and the unborn baby (Condon, 1993). Using Condon's (1993) definition, it is clear that many bereaved parents can develop a strong attachment to a baby lost during pregnancy, and this emotional connection continues into a subsequent pregnancy (Armstrong, 2002; O'Leary, 2004). Emotional cushioning, holding back attachment, can be strong in families experiencing PAL due to their fear of another loss (Côté-Arsenault & Donato, 2011) and their loyalty to the deceased baby (O'Leary & Thorwick, 2008). The ability to keep the unborn baby in mind to form an emotional connection makes PAL a complex developmental process (Côté-Arsenault, Bidlack, & Humm, 2001; O'Leary, Gaziano, & Thorwick, 2006; O'Leary et al., 1997; O'Leary & Thorwick, 2006b). In a study of adults who were born after a perinatal loss, researchers found attachment issues with their parents to be a common theme (O'Leary, Gaziano, & Thorwick, 2006).

CHARACTERISTICS OF PREGNANCY AFTER LOSS

Parents who experience a stillbirth or miscarriage are often advised to become pregnant again and to try to forget about the past loss. However, research on perinatal loss indicates that parents do not want to forget their babies and that the pregnancy loss is an experience that stays with them for many years (Côté-Arsenault & Morrison-Beedy, 2001; O'Leary & Warland, 2013). The decision to become pregnant again after loss is not a carefree undertaking. In fact, anxiety, depression, and fear of attachment are prime characteristics of pregnancy after perinatal loss (Côté-Arsenault, 2011; Wood & Quenby, 2010). After discussing each in turn, we then share fathers' experience of PAL and describe milestones that serve as key markers during pregnancy.

Anxiety is the hallmark of pregnancy subsequent to perinatal loss. Pregnancy-specific anxiety (PSA), defined as worries and concerns about this pregnancy and its outcome (Côté-Arsenault & Dombeck, 2001), dominates women's anxiety due to the fear of having another loss. However, previous anxiety disorders can be exacerbated in PAL (Austin & Priest, 2005). PSA is higher in women with a history of perinatal loss as compared with women with no such history (Côté-Arsenault, 2003; Theut, Pedersen, Zaslow, & Rabinovich, 1988; Woods-Giscombe, Lobel, & Crandell, 2010). PSA has been reported as highest in the first trimester, with significant decrease throughout the pregnancy for women with miscarriage (Côté-Arsenault, 2007).

Pregnancy anxiety generally decreases throughout the pregnancy for most, but it often fluctuates throughout the day and from one day to another. In her pregnancy diary from an unpublished study (Côté-Arsenault & Moore, in press), one mother wrote at 21 weeks about how worried she had been about the lack of fetal movement all day at work, and then "I came right home, got in comfortable clothes, and went to bed to lie on my left side and poked around. Sure enough, I got about four kicks. It was such a relief, I cried." High anxiety is common leading up to prenatal appointments, due to the fear that something bad will be found (which had occurred in the past pregnancy). Once they hear or see the baby, the anxiety plummets with a huge sigh of relief, only to start creeping upward over the coming days (Côté-Arsenault, Donato, & Earl, 2006). Those with a history of stillbirth have reported elevation of their PSA as they approach the time of their past loss (Côté-Arsenault, 2007). This increased anxiety can be true for parents, regardless of the gestation of their previous loss, thinking, "Get the baby out while it is still alive" (O'Leary & Thorwick, 2006b).

Depression and anxiety often go hand in hand, and this is true after perinatal loss and in PAL (Adeyemi et al., 2008; Armstrong, 2002). Women with prior pregnancy loss have been found to have higher levels of depression during pregnancy and for up to 33 months after the birth of a healthy child (Blackmore et al., 2011). Bergner and associates (Bergner, Beyer, Klapp, & Rauchfuss, 2008) suggest that women who responded to their miscarriage with more depressive coping and anxiety in their grieving were more likely to have higher anxiety and depression in their subsequent pregnancies. So, even though anxiety is often the most obvious negative emotion in PAL, depression warrants careful attention. It often accompanies anxiety but is a frequent component of grief. Depression and death-related grief are often treated as the same phenomenon (Corless, Cartier, & Guarino, 2011). Grief for the deceased baby does not go away just because there is a new pregnancy, but parents often feel that they must choose between their babies. Therefore, it is important to assess whether what is seen as depression in parents experiencing PAL can be their struggle to redefine grief as their ongoing continued bond and attachment to their previous baby (O'Leary, Thorwick, & Parker, 2012). The ability to differentiate between grief and depression is important (Corless, Cartier, & Guarino, 2011). Perinatal depression is of concern in PAL because it is a risk factor for postpartum depression and has negative effects on parenting (Räisänen et al., 2013). Clinical screenings and interventions to support women who are experiencing symptoms of depression and anxiety are essential. It is important to keep in mind that not understanding that a new layer of grief surfaces in the new pregnancy for both a mother and her partner can undermine a normal experience that often lacks social support from others, sometimes causing more anxiety in these families (O'Leary, 2004).

Fathers

Fathers have been described as the "forgotten bereaved" both at the time of loss and in the pregnancy that follows (Armstrong, 2001; McCreight, 2004; Murphy, 1998; O'Leary, 2005). After perinatal loss, men's perception of their role of fathering changes drastically as described by one father, "Why did I have to lose a baby before I realized I was already a father?" (O'Leary & Thorwick, 2006a). Assessment of how fathers are coping during a pregnancy after loss is important as some can blame themselves for the previous loss and not support the mother's concerns (O'Leary, Warland, & Parker, 2011). O'Leary (2002) reported that some fathers downplayed their partner's worry that something was wrong with the baby and did not encourage the mother to seek medical care.

In an earlier study investigating mothers' and fathers' relationship with their unborn, Condon (1985) found fathers to be strikingly more similar to than different from mothers in how they related to the unborn baby, but first-time fathers reported less time spent and less frequent engagement in palpating and thinking about the fetus. Condon speculated this was due to the biological immediacy of the women's connection with the fetus and of men spending less time in inner preoccupation with the fetus. This finding changes drastically for fathers after perinatal loss. Fathers paid more attention to the behavior and presence of their unborn babies, sought reassurance from the mother by asking frequently about fetal movement, and acknowledged this was different from previous pregnancies where they took the baby's wellness for granted (Armstrong, 2002; O'Leary & Thorwick, 2006a). This behavior is consistent with other studies suggesting that fathers need the mothers, because they have less opportunity than their pregnant spouses to palpate or inspect the outline of the fetus (Condon, 2000; O'Leary et al., 2006).

Milestones

Given that 9 months is a very long period of time filled with many developmental and social tasks, it is not surprising that women and their partners identify upcoming markers as goals they hope to reach. Early pregnancy is a time of high vigilance not only because the risk of loss is the highest but also because the indicators of a healthy pregnancy are subtle and subjective. Miscarriage is watched for at each trip to the bathroom, when the toilet tissue is checked for blood. Nausea, vomiting, and tender full breasts are viewed as positive signs of high pregnancy hormones and thus the reassurance that everything is fine. Key milestones include hearing or seeing a heartbeat, gestational age of prior complications or loss(es), time of highest risk of loss (first trimester), detection of fetal movements, the time of fetal viability and, most importantly, birthing a healthy baby (Côté-Arsenault & Mahlangu, 1999; Côté-Arsenault et al., 2006).

Many women who have experienced PAL anxiously await hearing the fetal heartbeat because they believe that the risk of miscarriage drops after it is heard. It is common for some parents to ask for more heartbeat checks in the office to make sure the baby is still alive (Côté-Arsenault et al., 2006; Hutti, Armstrong, & Myers, 2011). Prior events where critical incidents occurred, such as the 20-week fetal anatomic ultrasound, may also hold special significance. Remembering that an ultrasound scan confirmed their previous loss, health care providers need to be aware that this exam can elicit increased anxiety and fear that this baby may also be dead and, for some, may cause flashbacks to the previous loss (O'Leary, 2005). Confirming that there is a heartbeat first is very helpful in helping parents with these anxieties (Côté-Arsenault, 2011). The experience of quickening, when mothers begin to feel the flutter of their baby, can be very comforting and a sign that can be experienced at home on their own.

INTERVENTIONS FOR SUPPORTING PARENTS

Prenatal Care

Parents need additional and ongoing support from their health care provider for reassurance that their baby is safe (Côté-Arsenault et al., 2006; Côté-Arsenault & Donato, 2007). Care providers need to recognize that parental anxiety is normal and not to take this as lack of trust in them as providers. Both mothers and fathers often display heightened anxiety and vigilance of fetal movement (Armstrong & Hutti, 1998; Côté-Arsenault & Marshall, 2000; Grout & Romanoff, 2000; O'Leary & Thorwick, 1997; O'Leary et al., 1997; O'Leary, 2005; O'Leary et al., 2006). A good time to "check in" to gauge how both parents are doing emotionally is during prenatal visits or antenatal testing. Before an examination or placing the belt on the mother's abdomen, it is sensible to ask "Tell me about your baby." This simple statement can reframe paying attention to fetal movements by understanding the patterns of sleep–awake cycles of her baby. This can help a mother who may be avoiding paying attention to fetal movement begin to trust that the baby will let her know if he or she is in trouble if the movements change. This approach shifts the focus of care from the health care provider telling the parent how the baby is doing to the mother reporting what she knows about her baby (O'Leary et al., 2012). Alternatively, when mothers call with anxiety about the baby's movements, it is important to ask more questions and offer for them to come in for confirmation that all is well through objective data. This is especially important for mothers who intuitively felt something was wrong with their baby in their previous pregnancy but were dismissed by the health care providers and their babies died (O'Leary, Warland & Parker, 2011; Warland, 2014).

That said, parents do need to know that the new unborn baby is separate from the deceased baby, and some parents will need guidance in this work. Interventions to reinforce this can more easily be introduced once fetal movement becomes more consistent. Then, care providers can ask parents about the deceased baby, call the baby by name, and stress this baby is still an important member of the family as they embark on a new pregnancy with a new baby. Continuing to acknowledge their parenting role to the deceased baby has been found to help the parents make way for emotional energy to embrace a new baby (O'Leary et al., 2012; O'Leary & Thorwick, 1997; Prigerson et al., 2009; Romanoff, 2001). Educating parents on the developmental competencies of their new unborn child at each gestational age, such as hearing at 16 weeks and recognizing the mother's voice by term (Hepper & Shahidullah, 1994; Voegtline, Costigan, Pater, & DiPietro, 2013), helps parents know the unborn baby has an awareness of the world outside the uterus. This may also help parents understand that the unborn baby may sense their grief (O'Leary et al., 2006) and also their love and desire to protect him from harm (O'Leary et al., 2012). Using mindfulness care such as journaling to the baby can help parents put their grief into words.

Experience tells us that there are several things that help many parents experiencing PAL prepare for labor and birth. Encourage parents to seek birthing support after they reach 32 weeks gestation (Midland-Gensvh & Rybarik, 2004). If a separate class is not available, it is important for the childbirth educator to ask parents to share their story (Wright & Black, 2013), noting statements that may be triggers for symptoms of trauma from the last experience. At a minimum, a tour of the birthing area prior to active labor is beneficial for parents who birthed a visible baby in their last experience, no matter how small (O'Leary et al., 2012). While some parents will not want to "go there" before they actually have to present for active labor, it is helpful to explain that a tour now will help them focus on this labor and this baby. Touring often can bring up potential triggers for posttraumatic stress disorder (PTSD), such as the same visual surroundings, smells, blanket the deceased baby may have been wrapped in, equipment in the room, and others. Processing this can help parents identify their anticipated needs and serve as a way to communicate past history and concerns to care providers (O'Leary, Warland, & Parker, 2012). The birth plan also can include their preference for continuous or intermittent fetal monitoring and their choice of additional support persons or a doula for either the mother or the partner (O'Leary, Throwick, & Parker, 2012).

Those providing prenatal care for mothers with a history of pregnancy loss should acknowledge and address the prior losses in the following ways.

Guidance for Prenatal Care in Pregnancy After Loss

- Learn the stories of unsuccessful pregnancies and babies who are missed
- Ask the names of all other children and request to use the names of deceased babies as well as of the unborn baby
- Note significant dates or gestational ages from past experience that might be anxiety triggers in the current pregnancy
- Acknowledge that anxiety about this pregnancy is normal in PAL
- Recognize that fetal surveillance may be stressful for the parents, including fetal movements
- Provide suggestions for ways to cope with their anxiety
- Encourage attachment to this unborn baby
- Recognize the significance of all babies while noting that they are separate (Côté-Arsenault, 2011; Midland-Gensvh & Rybarik, 2004)

Support Groups for Pregnancy After Loss

Support groups are often the only available source of intervention for couples experiencing PAL. While it has been difficult to draw confident conclusions on the effectiveness of support groups for people seeking help with grief-related issues (Jordan & Neimeyer, 2003; Neimeyer, 2000), support groups can serve as a rite of passage and cushioning during the liminality of PAL. Meeting with others who experienced similar losses has been found to be extremely important to restore the feeling of normality (Dyregrov et al., 2014) and to understand that parental grief is lifelong because of one's continued bond with a deceased baby (Arnold & Gemma, 2008).

Parents have the ability to find meaning through narrative telling (Keesee, Currier, & Neimeyer, 2008; Neimeyer, 2006), and support groups provide a space where experiences can be shared (Carlson, Lammert, &

O'Leary, 2012). A PAL group that focuses on helping parents reconstruct meaning in their continued bond and attachment to a deceased baby and the narrative sharing of their fear to attach to a new unborn baby have been found to be helpful for women and some men in processing their new identity (O'Leary et al., 2012). This is different from an infant loss group where the focus is on bereavement; rather, it is about being a parent to two babies and the attention the new unborn baby needs now. Educating parents on the unborn baby's competencies will help them attach to a baby already present.

Support groups such as these exist sparsely across the United States, but one focused ethnographic study of two pregnancy-after-loss support groups (Côté-Arsenault & Freije, 2004) revealed that pregnancy was viewed differently by those with a history of prior perinatal loss compared to the dominant culture where pregnancy was viewed as essentially failsafe. Five paradoxes within the two views of pregnancy emerged from the data: (a) while, to most people, pregnancy is assumed to end in *birth*, in PAL pregnancy involves *birth and death*; (b) in the dominant culture, pregnancy means that there will be a new *baby*, but in PAL pregnancy is a biological fact but it *does not equal baby*; (c) pregnancy is seen as *a positive, hopeful* time by many, but for those experiencing PAL pregnancy is *a time of hope and fear*; (d) pregnancy touches the hearts of many in our culture with strong, positive emotions, but in PAL women often avoid the emotional (heart) aspects of pregnancy by focusing on the intellectual, factual (head) experience to protect themselves from future grief; and, finally; (e) those in PAL prefer to keep pregnancy private, share with a select few, rather than the often public display of pregnancy in the dominant culture. Within such a group, parents learned how to cope with these paradoxes in a supportive environment where loss was the common thread, worry was normal, all babies were honored, new skills were gained for advocating for self and baby with providers, and personal growth was achieved. Support groups were found to serve as safe places for those experiencing PAL, where feelings did not need to be explained, references to all children (those alive, deceased, and in utero) were welcome, and PAL experiences were viewed as normal (Côté-Arsenault & Freije, 2004).

An anonymous, open-question follow-up survey mailed to former participants of the second author's PAL support group yielded 75 returned surveys. When asked what was helpful about the support group, all of the respondents said that participation in the group reduced their anxiety, but it never completely went away until the birth of their babies. This unpublished finding indicates that, even with intervention, PSA remains until the birth of a healthy baby. The parents also reported that the group helped them learn to advocate for themselves and their baby, suggesting that the model of relationship-based prenatal parenting can be useful (O'Leary, Thorwick,

& Parker, 2012). Providing psychosocial support to families experiencing PAL has been described as at least as important as medical management of the pregnancy, warranting the same degree of consideration (Aho, Tarkka, Astedt-Kurki, & Kaunonen, 2006; Condon, 2006; O'Leary & Thorwick, 2006a, 2006b; Turton et al., 2006).

Nurse Home Visit Intervention

Although support groups are not an option for many women, a nurse home visitation intervention was developed and pilot tested based on the theory of caring (Swanson, 1991). The overall goal was to provide a supportive environment similar to that found in support groups but delivered through a caring relationship with an experienced nurse throughout the pregnancy. The aim was to normalize the PAL experience, reduce pregnancy anxiety and depression by teaching anxiety-reducing skills, and facilitate prenatal attachment (Côté-Arsenault, Schwartz, Krowchuk, & McCoy, 2014). The skills were relaxation techniques including guided imagery, problem solving, "I" messages, and daily fetal movement records. Those women who received the intervention reported a significant increase in social support compared to those in the control condition, and each woman utilized at least one of the new skills. Women felt that their anxiety was lessened; however, the differences were not statistically significant. Home visits were the highest rated aspect of the intervention.

Each mother in the intervention received a pregnancy diary to encourage journaling as a way to relieve stress and anxiety (Côté-Arsenault et al., 2014). Some wrote in it every day, while others wrote weekly. These women found the diary very helpful. A minority of women stated that they either did not like to write or did not have time to do so.

Another journaling suggestion is to encourage parents to share their feelings for the deceased baby with the new baby coming. This approach can help parents who believe they cannot express their feelings in writing because they do not want their unborn baby to know the loyalty they have to the previous baby or their fear of attachment to this pregnancy. As the pregnancy progresses, they then are more able to focus on the present baby, telling him or her about the deceased sibling. This gives words to the emotions parents are carrying rather than keeping the feelings inside (O'Leary et al., 2012) and integrates their parenting of both babies. A cognitive behavioral Internet-based therapy for parents after the loss of a child during pregnancy that included 10 writing assignments of their experience found that overall mental health and depression significantly improved after treatment (Kersting, Kroker, Schlicht, Baust, & Wagner, 2011). Acknowledging these feelings as their reality sometimes helps them understand that feelings are just feelings, which also opens the conversation to ways of working with their anxiety. Research suggesting that an unborn baby is affected by the emotions of its mother (Dirix et al., 2009; Glover, 2011, 2012; O'Leary & Thorwick, 1997; Sandman et al., 2011; Thomson, 2007) underscores the importance of helping parents learn ways to cope with their anxiety.

The theories, principles, and interventions presented thus far are illustrated in the following two clinical examples.

CLINICAL EXAMPLE: PREGNANCY LOSS AT 18 WEEK

After the loss of her baby at 18 weeks gestation the previous year, Julia learned she was 6 weeks pregnant. She and her husband, Drew, hoping this would happen, were very excited, but fear quickly followed that something would go wrong again. Their first pregnancy had been going along very well until it all ended with no warning signs and no fetal heartbeat at 18 weeks.

Like most families who have not experienced a pregnancy loss, Julia and Drew had immediately shared the news of their first pregnancy with family and good friends. Then, just 10 weeks later, they painfully had to tell them the pregnancy was over. This time they agreed not to share the news until they were sure everything was fine. Julia soon realized she needed to have at least one person to talk to, so they decided to tell a couple they were both close to who did not have any children. They were relieved to be able to share but swore their friends to secrecy.

Drew went to early prenatal visits with Julia and were thrilled to hear their new baby's heartbeat at 11 weeks. Fetal growth and all lab values were textbook perfect, so they relaxed a little. Julia was experiencing morning sickness and her breasts were tender, which she saw as a good sign; she felt pregnant, so she reasoned her hormones must be high. Before her next prenatal visit, Julia felt well but realized she was anxious, fearing she could not know for sure that everything was okay with her baby because during the previous pregnancy she had no clue that something was wrong. When everything checked out as normal at the next appointment she began to relax again. In the next visit would an ultrasound be done and they were very excited. But the confidence slowly faded as Julia and Drew realized that they were approaching 18 weeks, (the time of loss of their first baby). Julia thought that she might be feeling the baby move, but the flutters were so light and unpredictable, she could not be sure. She did not want to get her hopes up just to have them dashed.

The night before their 19-week prenatal check Julia had trouble sleeping. She tried to relax but kept waiting to feel the baby's flutters, which did not happen. Eager to have their ultrasound, they were also afraid of the unknown. Thankfully, there was only good news. Their baby girl looked perfectly normal and healthy. They hugged and cried with relief and happiness. Although they had tried not to get attached to their baby, fearing another loss, it was clear they had been in love with the idea of her and now had a visual image of her posted on their refrigerator and on their cellphones.

Relationships with friends during this pregnancy were challenging for Julia. She had several good friends from medical school who were all having babies and was surprised and hurt by their lack of understanding her reluctance to go to their baby showers or hold their newborns. Some of those babies were the same age as the child she never had a chance to hold, so she could not push through her fear. One friend tried to be understanding, and eventually they talked through their relationship; she was able to support Julia and waited until she was more confident to come for a visit. The other friends never reached out, and Julia went through a difficult grieving process about relationships that she had assumed would be there to support her through tough times.

Knowing that they had passed some major milestones, fetal movement became more frequent. As they approached viability, and Drew could feel a little movement through Julia's belly, there were still waves of anxiety but also more time feeling confident that everything was going to be okay. Sharing their news with everyone, Julia proudly began wearing maternity clothes, and they named their daughter Emma. However, when Julia's sister brought up planning a baby shower, Julia became nervous, not sure she was ready for that. Fetal movements were comforting, but it was nerve-wracking when the baby did not move for several hours. Prenatal visits brought her anxiety down until she was diagnosed with gestational diabetes.

At 30 weeks gestation, Julia and Drew felt comfortable and ready for planning. They signed up for birthing classes, chose nursery furniture, and Julia gave her sister the okay to plan a shower. Fears of labor and birth were part of their thinking, especially when Julia's blood pressure started rising. They were very anxious to hold their baby in their arms. Although the baby was born very healthy, Julia found herself checking Emma as she slept, to make sure that she was breathing.

Analysis

Julia and Drew's responses to a new pregnancy were normal responses for anyone who has suffered the death of a baby, no matter the gestation. The death of their first baby in the second trimester made them skeptical about this pregnancy and afraid to bond with this baby. The "selective telling" to a few people is very common in pregnancy after loss, as parents try to avoid the "un-telling" if something were to happen. However, many parents do choose to tell someone so that if there is another loss, they have support.

This couple's anxiety about this pregnancy went up and down like a see-saw as they awaited each week, for each milestone to be successfully achieved (Côté-Arsenault et al., 2006). This is a common experience. The anxiety never fully goes away, but confidence that the baby will be fine generally increases throughout the pregnancy (Côté-Arsenault, 2007).

It would be very appropriate and helpful for nurses, physicians, and sonographers to note Julia's OB history and ask her and her husband about their feelings. This would give Julia and Drew an opening to express their concerns, share their past experience about the loss, and talk about the missing sibling. Providers should ask if they named the deceased baby and begin to talk about this new baby as a sibling. Asking about their anxieties will also normalize them as part of PAL. Attachment can be encouraged during these early weeks with descriptions of fetal development and capabilities, while reminding them that the deceased baby also knew them as parents, which can support their continued bond with that baby.

Hopefully, the birthing class nurse educator recognizes the OB histories of all the parents in the class and includes comments about fears and worries. If they are seen as normal, then parents will feel comfortable asking questions about how to cope with them.

Julia and Drew's continued concern for their daughter, even though she is healthy, is to be expected. Parents often feel that their child is vulnerable in the world, although they should be able to reduce their hypervigilance when they realize that the baby is fine and through positive self-talk. Several studies have found that parenting after prior perinatal loss differs from parenting of those who have not had similar experiences (O'Leary & Warland, 2012; Warland, O'Leary, McCutcheon, & Williamson, 2011). It is helpful to warn parents about the risk of being overly protective and for pediatricians to be aware of the family history of loss.

CLINICAL EXAMPLE: FATHER AFTER STILLBORN SON

Fathers/partners during pregnancy after loss are often overlooked and yet can carry just as much fear and anxiety as the mother. Often, two themes are seen in their behaviors; withdrawing emotionally or excessively monitoring the progress of the pregnancy (Armstrong, 2001; O'Leary et al., 1997; O'Leary et al., 2006; Samuelsson, Radestad, & Segesten, 2001). David fell into the first category.

David and his wife Sarah suffered the stillbirth of a son at 36 weeks gestation for unknown reason. At the time of their son Noah's death, they also had a healthy 2-year-old daughter. David and Sarah had been very close during Sarah's pregnacy with Noah, building memories as they had done with their daughter. David attended all the prenatal visits with Sarah and actively helped in preparing the nursery for the upcoming birth. Although when Noah died David seemed to shut down all emotions. When Sarah became pregnant again he withdrew emotionally from her. He did not want to talk about the pregnancy and would not attend any prenatal appointments. The staff encouraged Sarah to have David come to her weekly nonstress tests, where

(continued)

he might get some reassurance this baby was being watched closely. He refused. Sarah attended the weekly support group throughout the pregnancy and shared her own fears and her loneliness in this pregnancy. David was also not open to participating in the special birth class. Sarah felt much to her pain, he had simply emotionally withdrawn, they were not close through the pregnancy, building no memories, and both fearing another loss.

In the last 2 weeks of the pregnancy Sarah was encouraged to ask him to at least come back for a tour of the birthing area as they were birthing in a different hospital. He agreed, and went with one of the facilitators of the group on the tour. It was while in the birthing room that the educator saw him tearing up. Rather than being a father with no feelings, it was apparent he was just as frightened as Sarah that death would strike again. The educator arranged to meet with them for Sarah's last nonstress test 3 days before she was to be induced. While Sarah sat with the baby being monitored, she and David were given a guided imagery/relaxation, which they were both open to. They closed their eyes and the educator began to talk with them about this new unborn baby they would soon meet. The conversation focused on acknowledging how difficult the pregnancy had been for them and that this new little baby was a sibling to their son Noah. She talked about their deceased baby boy, validating how much they both missed him and wished he was here to meet the new baby, that he would always be a part of their family and this baby would not replace him. During this relaxation, both parents cried and, interestingly, the fetal monitor stayed at a steady, comfortable pace with no variability until they were done, almost as if the baby was "listening too." When they left, the nurse asked the educator, "Are they going to be alright?" The simple reply was, "They are both scared to death."

The birth occurred 3 days later, and both facilitators of the support group were in attendance. There was a brief period where they lost the baby's heartbeat on the monitor, which freaked out both parents and the nurse caring for them because they became so alarmed. They all quickly calmed when the nurse found the heartbeat again. When their healthy daughter was born, everyone in the room celebrated. It was not until the next day that David came up to the educator and shared what really was going on with him after the birth, behavior no one else in the room realized had occurred. He shared: "During the birth I was crying tears of joy but after she was born I began to get angry at the people in the room. They were calling her a "she" and I thought it was a boy. I thought it was my son." He was still in deep grief over the loss of his son and continued to struggle into the postpartum period. The story does not have a happy ending. This couple divorced 10 years later, Sarah believing one cause was due to David never really having resolved the loss of their first son and withdrawing into himself.

Analysis

This case illustrates many issues: how difficult it can be for men to reach out for help and how important it is for health care providers to encourage their involvement. When this is difficult, the mother will need more support herself. It is not uncommon for some couples to cope in a pregnancy following loss by not talking with each other. Finding out how each person is coping emotionally is helpful, and in this case, the older sibling too. The consequence of the loss of a baby is uniquely different for every family. One can never really know what lies behind a partner's withdrawal (in this case, extreme fear of another loss to the point that he possibly did not even want to think there was a baby inside, resulting in the loneliness of Sarah throughout the pregnancy).

CONCLUSION

Experiences of pregnancy and childbearing have a profound impact on parents and their children and no less so when those experiences are ones of perinatal loss. Theoretical perspectives provide a variety of lenses through which to understand why PAL can be challenging but also aid to direct interventions for these families to support them through pregnancy and parenting. Interventions can be undertaken by parents themselves, such as journaling or support group attendance, or provided by health care providers throughout the pregnancy. The goals of all interventions are recognizing the characteristics of PAL, empowering parents to believe in themselves and their baby, integrating all of their experiences and children into their evolving development, and supporting parents.

This chapter addressed the complexity of a pregnancy following perinatal loss for both mothers and their partners and offer supportive interventions to help families manage their journey. While the behaviors of families experiencing PAL have been well documented for the past 20 years, there continues to be a need for further research on the kinds of intervention that will be most helpful in decreasing fears and anxieties and facilitating attachment to the baby being carried.

CASE STUDY

Rita and Tariq have arrived at the clinic for their prenatal appointment. They experienced the loss of their previous pregnancy at 30 weeks. The couple learns that the baby is a boy, and Tariq leaves the exam room. Rita appears bewildered by her husband's reaction and shares that she is glad that they will have "another boy." Tariq tells the provider that he is concerned that Rita will want to give the baby the same name as their first baby. He states that he does not want to share his feelings with Rita because "she was so sad when we lost our son. I don't want to do or say anything that would upset her."

FOCUS QUESTIONS

1. What theoretical perspectives would be most helpful in determining the best approach to developing a plan of care for Rita and Tariq?
2. What interventions would be most useful for facilitating communication between Rita and Tariq?
3. What interventions would be most helpful to support Rita and Tariq as they parent their expected baby while still coping with their previous loss?

REFERENCES

Adeyemi, A. A., Mosaku, K., Ajenifuja, O., Fatoye, F., Makinde, N., & Ola, B. (2008). Depressive symptoms in a sample of women following perinatal loss. *Journal of the National Medical Association, 100*(12), 1463–1468.

Aho, A., Tarkka, M., Astedt-Kurki, P., & Kaunonen, M. (2006). Fathers' grief after the death of a child. *Mental Health Nursing, 26*(8), 647–663.

Alhusen, J. L. (2008). A literature update on maternal-fetal attachment. *JOGNN: Journal of Obstetric, Gynecologic & Neonatal Nursing, 37*(3), 315–328. doi:10.1111/j.1552-6909.2008.00241.x

Armstrong, D. (2001). Exploring fathers' experiences of pregnancy after a prior perinatal loss. *Maternal Child Nursing, 26*(3), 147–153.

Armstrong, D. S. (2002). Emotional distress and prenatal attachment in pregnancy after perinatal loss. *Journal of Nursing Scholarship, 34*(4), 339–345. doi: http://dx.doi.org.libproxy.uncg.edu/10.1111/j.1547-5069.2002.00339.x

Armstrong, D., & Hutti, M. (1998). Pregnancy after perinatal loss: The relationship between anxiety and prenatal attachment. *Journal of Obstetric, Gynecologic, and Neonatal Nursing, 27*(2), 183–189.

Armstrong, D. S., Hutti, M. H., & Myers, J. (2009). The influence of prior perinatal loss on parents' psychological distress after the birth of a subsequent healthy infant. *Journal of Obstetric, Gynecologic, and Neonatal Nursing JOGNN / NAACOG, 38*(6), 654–666. doi:10.1111/j.1552-6909.2009.01069.x

Arnold, J., & Gemma, P. (2008). The continuing process of parental grief. *Death Studies, 32*(3), 658–673.

Austin, M., & Priest, S. R. (2005). Clinical issues in perinatal mental health: New developments in the detection and treatment of perinatal mood and anxiety disorders. *Acta Psychiatric Scandinavia, 112,* 97–104. doi: 10.1111/j.1600-0447.2005.00549.x

Bergner, A., Beyer, R., Klapp, B. F., & Rauchfuss, M. (2008). Pregnancy after early pregnancy loss: A prospective study of anxiety, depressive symptomatology and coping. *Journal of Psychosomatic Obstetrics and Gynaecology, 29*(2), 105–113. doi:10.1080/01674820701687521

Bergum, V. (1989). *Woman to mother: A transformation.* Granby, MA: Bergin & Garvey Publishers.

Blackmore, E. R., Côté-Arsenault, D., Tang, W., Glover, V., Evans, J., Golding, J., . . . ALSPAC Research team. (2011). Previous prenatal loss as a predictor of perinatal depression and anxiety. *British Journal of Psychiatry, 198*, 373–378. doi:10.1192/bjp .bp.110.083105

Bowlby, J. (1988). *A secure base*. New York, NY: Basic Books.

Cannella, B. L. (2005). Maternal-fetal attachment: An integrative review. *Journal of Advanced Nursing, 50*(1), 60–68. doi:10.1111/j.1365-2648.2004.03349.x

Carlson, R., Lammert, C., & O'Leary, J. (2012). The evolution of group and online support for families who have experienced perinatal or neonatal loss. *Illness, Crisis and Loss*, 20(3), 275–293.

Chez, R. (1995). After hours. *Obstetrics & Gynecology, 85*(6), 1059–1061.

Condon, J. (1985). The parental-fetal relationship: A comparison of male and female expectant parents. *Journal of Psychosomatic Obstetrics and Gynaecology, 4*(4), 271–284.

Condon, J. (1987). Prevention of emotional disability following stillbirth: The role of the obstetric team. *Australian New Zealand Journal of Obstetrics and Gynecology, 27*(4), 323–329.

Condon, J. (1993). The assessment of antenatal emotional attachment: Development of a questionnaire instrument. *British Journal of Medical Psychology, 66*(2), 167–183.

Condon, J. (2000). Pregnancy loss. In M. Steiner, P. Yonkers, & P. P. Eriksson (Eds.), *Mood disorders in women* (pp. 353–369). London: Martin Dunitz.

Condon, J. (2006). What about dad? Psychosocial and mental health issues for new fathers. *Australian Family Physician, 35*(9), 690–692.

Cordle, C., & Prettyman, R. (1994). A two year follow-up of women who have experienced early miscarriage. *Journal of Reproductive and Infant Psychology, 12*(1), 37–43.

Corless, I. B., Cartier, J. M., & Guarino, A. J. (2011). Depression and grief—overlapping phenomena or lack of individuation. *Crisis, Illness & Loss, 19*(2), 125–141. doi:10.2190/IL.19.2.c

Côté-Arsenault, D. (2003). The influence of perinatal loss on anxiety in multigravidas. *Journal of Obstetric, Gynecologic, and Neonatal Nursing, 32*(5), 623–629. doi: http:// dx.doi.org.libproxy.uncg.edu/10.1177/0884217503257140

Côté-Arsenault, D. (2007). Threat appraisal, coping, and emotions across pregnancy subsequent to perinatal loss. *Nursing Research, 56*(2), 108–116. doi:10.1097/01 .NNR.0000263970.08878.87

Côté-Arsenault, D. (2011). *Loss and grief in the childbearing period*. White Plains, NY: March of Dimes.

Côté-Arsenault, D., Bidlack, D., & Humm, A. (2001). Women's emotions and concerns during pregnancy following perinatal loss. *MCN, The American Journal of Maternal Child Nursing, 26*(3), 128–134.

Côté-Arsenault, D., Brody, D., & Dombeck, M. T. (2009). Pregnancy as a rite of passage: Liminality, rituals and communitas. *Journal of Prenatal & Perinatal Psychology & Health, 24*(2), 69–87.

Côté-Arsenault, D., & Dombeck, M. T. (2001). Maternal assignment of fetal personhood to a previous pregnancy loss: Relationship to anxiety in the current pregnancy. *Health Care for Women International, 22*(7), 649–665.

Côté-Arsenault, D., & Donato, K., (2007). Restrained expectations in late pregnancy following loss. *Journal of Obstetric, Gynecologic, and Neonatal Nursing, 36*, 550–557. doi: 10.1111/J.1552-6909.2007.00185.x

Côté-Arsenault, D., & Donato, K. (2011). Emotional cushioning in pregnancy after perinatal loss. *Journal of Reproductive and Infant Psychology, 29*(1), 81–92. doi: 10.1080/02646838.2010.513115

Côté-Arsenault, D., Donato, K. L., & Earl, S. S. (2006). Watching & worrying: Early pregnancy after loss experiences. *MCN, The American Journal of Maternal Child Nursing, 31*(6), 356–363.

Côté-Arsenault, D., & Freije, M. M. (2004). Support groups helping women through pregnancies after loss. *Western Journal of Nursing Research, 26*(6), 650–670. doi: 10.1177/0193945904265817

Côté-Arsenault, D., & Mahlangu, N. (1999). Impact of perinatal loss on the subsequent pregnancy and self: Women's experiences. *Journal of Obstetric, Gynecologic, and Neonatal Nursing, 28*(3), 274–282. doi: http://dx.doi.org.libproxy.uncg .edu/10.1111/j.1552-6909.1999.tb01992.x

Côté-Arsenault, D., & Marshall, R. (2000). One foot in-one foot out: Weathering the storm of pregnancy after perinatal loss. *Research in Nursing & Health, 23*, 473–485.

Côté-Arsenault, D., & Moore, S. (in press). *Exploring women's experiences of pregnancy after loss through diary entries.* Unpublished manuscript.

Côté-Arsenault, D., & Morrison-Beedy, D. (2001). Women's voices reflecting changed expectations for pregnancy after perinatal loss. *Journal of Nursing Scholarship, 33*(3), 239–244.

Côté-Arsenault, D., Schwartz, K., Krowchuk, H., & McCoy, T. M. (2014). Evidence-based intervention for women pregnant after perinatal loss. *MCN, The American Journal of Maternal Child Nursing, 39*(3), 177–186.

Côté-Arsenault, D. Y. (1995). Tasks of pregnancy and anxiety in pregnancy after perinatal loss. *Dissertation Abstracts International, 56–12*, 66–69.

Cranley, M. (1981). Development of a tool for the measurement of maternal attachment during pregnancy. *Nursing Research, 30*, 281–284.

Creedy, D., Shochet, I., & Horsfall, J. (2000). Childbirth and the development of acute trauma symptoms: Incidence and contributing factors. *Birth, 27*(2), 104–111.

Cuisinier, M., Kuijper, J., Hoogduin, C., de Graauw, C., & Janssen, H. (1996). Miscarriage and stillbirth: Time since the loss, grief intensity and satisfaction with care. *European Journal of Obstetrics and Gynecology, 52*(2), 163–168.

DiPietro, J. A., Voegtline, K. M., Costigan, K. A., Aguirre, F., Kivlighan, K., & Chen, P. (2013). Physiological reactivity of pregnant women to evoked fetal startle. *Journal of Psychosomatic Research, 75*, 321–326. doi: http://dx.doi.org/10.1016/j .jpsychores.2013.07.008

Dirix, C., Nijhuis, J., Jongsma, H., & Hornsta, G. (2009). Aspects of fetal learning and memory. *Child Development, 80*(4), 1251–1258. doi:10.1111/j.1467-8624.2009.01329.x

Dyregrov, K., Dryregrov, A., & Johnsen, I. (2014). Positive and negative experiences from grief group participation: A qualitative study. *Omega, 68*(1), 45–62.

Erikson, E. H. (1963). *Childhood and society.* New York, NY: Norton & Company.

Galinsky, E. (1987). *The six stages of parenthood.* Reading, MA: Addison-Wesley.

Glover, V. (2011). Annual research review: Prenatal stress and the origins of psychopathology: An evolutionary perspective. *Journal of Child Psychology and Psychiatry, 52*(4), 356–367. doi:10.111/j.1469-7610/2011.02371.x

Glover, V. (2012, October). *Effects of prenatal anxiety, depression and stress on fetal and child development. Mechanisms and questions.* Presentation at the Marce International Conference, Paris, France.

Grout, L., & Romanoff, B. (2000). The myth of the replacement child: Parents' stories and practices after perinatal death. *Death Studies, 24*(2), 93–113.

Hepper, P., & Shahidullah, S. (1994). The beginnings of mind: Evidence from the behavior of the fetus. *Journal of Reproductive and Infant Psychology, 12*(3), 143–154.

Hutti, M. H., Armstrong, D. S., & Myers, J. (2011). Healthcare utilization in the pregnancy following a perinatal loss. *MCN, The American Journal of Maternal Child Nursing, 36*(2), 104–111. doi:10.1097/NMC.0b013e3182057335

Jordan, J., & Neimeyer, R. (2003). Does grief counseling work? *Death Studies, 27*(9), 765–786.

Karen, R. (1998). *Becoming attached: First relationships and how they shape our capacity to love.* New York, NY: Oxford Press.

Keesee, N., Currier, J., & Neimeyer, R. (2008). Predictors of grief following the death of one's child: The contribution of finding meaning. *Journal of Clinical Psychology, 64*(10), 1145–1163.

Kersting, A., Kroker, K., Schlicht, S., Baust, K., & Wagner, B. (2011). Efficacy of cognitive behavioral Internet-based therapy in parents after the loss of a child during pregnancy: Pilot data from a randomized controlled trial. *Archives of Women's Mental Health, 14*, 465–477.

Martin, J. A., & Osterman, M. (2013). Preterm births—United States 2006 & 2010. National Center for Health Statistics. *CDC Supplements, 62*(03), 136–138.

McCreight, B. S. (2004). A grief ignored: Narratives of pregnancy loss from a male perspective. *Sociology of Health and Illness, 26*(3), 326–350.

Mercer, R. T. (2005). Nursing support of the process of becoming a mother. *JOGNN: Journal of Obstetric, Gynecologic, and Neonatal Nursing, 35*(5), 649–651. doi: 10.1111/J.1552-6909.2006.00086.x

Midland-Gensvh, D., & Rybarik, F. (Eds.). (2004). Subsequent pregnancy. *RTS bereavement and training in pregnancy loss and newborn death.* Gundersen Lutheran Medical Foundation, LaCrosse, WI.

Murphy, F. (1998). The experience of early miscarriage from a male perspective. *Journal of Clinical Nursing, 7*(4), 325–332.

Neimeyer, R. A. (2000). Searching for meaning of meaning: Grief therapy and the process of reconstruction. *Death Studies, 24*(6), 541–558.

Neimeyer, R. (2006). Complicated grief and the reconstruction of meaning: Conceptual and empirical contributions to a cognitive-constructivist model. *Clinical Psychology: Science and Practice, 13*(2), 141–145.

O'Leary, J. (2002). *The meaning of parenting during pregnancy after the loss of a previous baby* (Doctoral Dissertation). University of Minnesota, Minneapolis, MN.

O'Leary, J. (2004). Grief and its impact on prenatal attachment in the subsequent pregnancy. *Archives of Women's Mental Health, 7*(1), 7–18. doi:10.1007/s00737-003-0037-1

O'Leary, J. (2005). The trauma of ultrasound during a pregnancy following perinatal loss. *Journal of Loss and Trauma, 10*, 183–204.

O'Leary, J., Gaziano, C., & Thorwick, C. (2006). Born after loss: The invisible child in adulthood. *Journal of Pre and Perinatal Psychology and Health, 21*(1), 3–23.

O'Leary, J., & Thorwick, C. (2006b). *When pregnancy follows a loss: Preparing for the birth of your new baby.* Minneapolis, MN: Author.

O'Leary, J., Thorwick, C., & Parker, L. (2012). In K. Ragland (Ed.), *The baby leads the way: Supporting the emotional needs of families' pregnant following perinatal loss* (2nd ed., pp. 32–36). Minneapolis, MN: Author. Retrieved from aplacetoremember.com

O'Leary, J., & Warland, J. (2012). Intentional parenting of children born after a perinatal loss. *Journal of Loss and Trauma, 17*(2), 137–157. doi 10.1080/15325024.2011.595297

O'Leary, J., & Warland, J. (2013). Untold stories of infant loss: The importance of contact with the baby for bereaved parents. *Journal of Family Nursing, 19*(3), 1–24. doi:10.1177/1074840713495972

O'Leary, J., Warland, J., & Parker, L. (2011). Prenatal parenthood. *Journal of Prenatal Educators, 20*(4), 218–220.

O'Leary, J., Warland, J., & Parker, L. (2012). Childbirth preparation for families pregnant after loss. *International Journal of Childbirth Education, 27*(2), 44–50.

O'Leary, J. M., & Thorwick, C. (1997). Impact of pregnancy loss on the subsequent pregnancy. In J. R. Woods & J. Esposito-Woods (Eds.), *Loss during pregnancy or in the newborn period* (pp. 431–463). Pitman, NJ: Jannetti.

O'Leary, J. M., & Thorwick, C. (2006a). "It affects me too." Fathers' experience in a pregnancy after loss. *Journal of Obstetrics, Gynecologic, and Neonatal Nursing, 35*(1), 78–86.

O'Leary, J. M., & Thorwick, C. (2008). Attachment to the unborn child and parental representations of pregnancy following perinatal loss. *Attachment: New Directions in Psychotherapy & Relational Psychoanalysis, 2*, 292–320.

Prigerson, H. G., Horowitz, M. J., Jacobs, S. C., Parkes, C. M., Aslan, M., Goodkin, K., & Maciejewski, P. K. (2009). Prolonged grief disorder: Psychometric validation of criteria proposed for *DSM-5* and ICD-11. *PLOS Medicine, 6*(8), 1–12. doi: 10.1371/journal.pmed.1000121

Räisänen, S., Lehto, S. M., Nielsen, H. S., Gissler, M., Kramer, M., & Heinonen, S. (2013). Fear of childbirth predicts postpartum depression: A population-based analysis of 511,422 singleton births in Finland. *BMJ Open, 3*(11), e004047. doi:10.1136/bmjopen-2013-004047

Raphael-Leff, J. (2004). Transitions to parenthood in societies in transition. Mental health priorities in perinatal disturbances. *The Signal, 12*(3,4), 6–13.

Romanoff, B. (2001). Research as therapy: The power of narrative to effect change. In R. Neimeyer (Ed.), *Meaning reconstruction and the experience of loss* (pp. 245–257). Washington, DC: American Psychological Association.

Rubin, R. (1984). *Maternal identity and the maternal experience.* New York, NY: Springer.

Samuelsson, M., Radestad, I., & Segesten, K. (2001). A waste of a life: Fathers' experience of losing a child before birth. *Birth, 28*(2), 124–130.

Sandman, C. A., Davis, E. P., Buss, C., & Glynn, L. M. (2011). Exposure to prenatal psychobiological stress exerts programming influences on the mother and fetus. *Neuroendocrinology, 95*(1), 7–21. doi: 10.1159/00032701715

Stroufe, A. (2005). Attachment and development: A prospective, longitudinal study from birth to adulthood. *Attachment & Human Development, 7*(4), 349–367. doi:10.1080/14616730500365928

Swanson, K. M. (1991). Empirical development of a middle range theory of caring. *Nursing Research, 40*(3), 161–166.

Swanson, K. M. (2000). Predicting depressive symptoms after miscarriage: A path analysis based on the Lazarus paradigm. *Journal of Women's Health & Gender-Based Medicine, 9*(2), 191–206. doi:10.1089/152460900318696

Theut, S. K., Pedersen, F. A., Zaslow, M. J., & Rabinovich, B. A. (1988). Pregnancy subsequent to perinatal loss: Parental anxiety and depression. *Journal of the American Academy of Child and Adolescent Psychiatry, 27*(3), 289–292.

Thomson, P. (2007). "Down will come baby": Prenatal stress, primitive defenses and gestational dysregulation. *Journal of Trauma & Dissociation, 8*(3), 85–113.

Turton, P., Badenhorst, W., Hughes, P., Ward, J., Riches, S., & White, S. (2006). Psychological impact of stillbirth on fathers in the subsequent pregnancy and puerperium. *British Journal of Psychiatry, 188*, 165–172.

Turner, V. (1967/1987). Betwixt and between: The liminal period in rites of pasage. In L. C. Mahdi, S. Foster, & M. Little (Eds.), *Betwixt & between: Patterns of masculine and feminine initiation* (2nd ed., pp. 3–19). La Salle, IL: Open Court.

van Gennep, A. (1908/1960). *The rites of passage* (M. B. Vizedome, G. L. Caffee Trans.). Chicago, IL: The University of Chicago Press.

Voegtline, K., Costigan, K., Pater, H., & DiPietro, J. (2013). Near-term fetal response to maternal spoken voice. *Infant Behavior and Development, 36*(4), 526–533.

Warland, J. (2014). *The star program.* Presented at the stillbirth summit. Minneapolis, MN.

Warland, J., O'Leary, J., McCutcheon, H., & Williamson, V. (2011). Parenting paradox: Parenting after infant loss. *Midwifery, 27*(5), 163–169. doi:10.1016/ j.midw.2010.02.004

Wood, L., & Quenby, S. (2010). Exploring pregnancy following a preterm birth or pregnancy loss. *British Journal of Midwifery, 18*(6), 350–356.

Woods-Giscombe, C. L., Lobel, M., & Crandell, J. L. (2010). The impact of miscarriage and parity on patterns of maternal distress in pregnancy. *Research in Nursing & Health, 33,* 316–328. doi:10.1002/nur.20389

Wright, P., & Black, B. (2013). Perinatal loss. *International Journal of Childbirth Education, 28*(1), 15–19.

Pediatric Bereavement

Mary Muscari

*M*y acute care pediatric years are long behind me, but memories of children lost remain: Chris worrying more about the family he was leaving behind than the inevitable loss of his own life; Nancy asking if it was okay to die as her body lay ravaged by the effects of terminal illness; Mrs. S. wanting to hold her son one last time after all medical intrusions were removed from his lifeless body. These recollections also merge with images of these very same children on better days, when, even though hospitalized and quite ill, they still exuded the amazing personalities that made them so unforgettable.

Children should not die, and they certainly should not be murdered. But life does not work that way. Thousands of children die in the United States every year, most taken unexpectedly by accidents and many from families whose lives intersect with health care providers at what may be the most difficult moment of their lives.

Health care providers can make a difference in those moments. They can hold empty hands, say soothing words, and just be there with their presence. However, to do so effectively and professionally, they need the know-how. This book provides the necessary knowledge to empower health care providers to assure that their clients not face bereavement alone. This section provides foundations that include theoretical perspectives on pediatric palliative care, the concept of hope in end-of-life care, and the effects of a child's death on other young children. It also addresses the affected family members, including those who lose a child through trauma, and how to help children cope with death. Each chapter takes the reader to a higher level of awareness. For example, the chapter "Supporting Grieving Children" addresses grieving children's needs: the truth, healthy relationships with the adults in their lives, acknowledgment, respect, boundaries, routine, predictability, and choices. The authors then move on to discuss how to talk to children about death and their involvement in rites and funerals.

This section adds a critical element to the libraries of all those who work with children as it supplements the ever-shrinking undergraduate and graduate pediatric curricula through discussions of evidence-based practices and ideas for future research. It is a breath of fresh air that tackles a taboo topic of pediatric palliative care and transforms it into the everyday knowledge necessary for the science of evidence-based practice and the art of caring.

CHAPTER 11

Conceptual Approaches to Understanding Parental Grief After the Death of a Child

Margaret Shandor Miles

*T*he grief of parents following the death of an infant or child involves many painful and complex emotional, behavioral, cognitive, and physical responses. Unique to the grief of parents is the close relationship between parent and child, the central importance of a child in the parental identity, the responsibility and role of parents in caring for their children, and society's perception of the death of an infant or child as a rare occurrence. In the case of perinatal loss, parental grief is complicated by the loss of a fetus or infant for whom one's attachment is developing but not fully actualized; thus, it involves grieving for the inability to live into the relationship and the many plans and dreams revolving around the planned-for child. Losses during early pregnancy such as miscarriage, abortion, or fetal death are often a private experience, leaving parents to grieve alone. Stillbirth and neonatal death related to prematurity or a serious health problem at birth is devastating for parents who generally have, over time, become acquainted with the fetus via ultrasonography, fetal movement, and their own fantasies about their baby. Generally, parents have high expectations of becoming parents of a healthy child; however, some parents also anticipate with hope and fear the birth of an infant diagnosed with a defect prenatally. All of these parents experience a complicated period of emotional pain as they grieve the loss of their anticipated child.

The purpose of this chapter is to place our understanding of parental grief within the literature of grief across history to provide a perspective on the universality of grief over the ages. Of particular importance is a summary of various theoretical perspectives and conceptual models of grief and the context and time in which they were written, as well as conceptual models focused specifically on parental grief. The final goal of the paper is to synthesize the literature in conceptualizing the grief of parents to guide clinicians and researchers.

DEFINITIONS OF GRIEF

The concept *grief* is defined in a variety of ways by different authors and disciplines (Howarth, 2011; Weiss, 2008). As noted by Scheff (2015), "anarchy rules" in the literature in defining grief, the emotion generally associated with loss. Some authors define grief as an emotion along with joy, anger, and guilt or link grief with the emotion of sadness. Grief is often interchanged with bereavement or mourning (Neimeyer, Harris, Winokuer, & Thornton, 2011). Bereavement refers to the state of having lost a significant other through death, and mourning is generally considered the social, religious, and other practices of a cultural group (Stroebe, Hansson, Schut, & Stroebe, 2008). The *Diagnostic and Statistical Manual of Mental Disorders* (5th ed.; *DSM–5*; American Psychiatric Association, 2013) describes the dysphoric mood or sadness of grief, differentiating grief from a major depressive disorder. In most publications, grief is not defined because the author assumes that the definition is clear. When it is described, grief is often defined by its manifestations or, more commonly, in conjunction with modifiers such as normal, typical, complicated, pathological, or dysfunctional (Cowles & Rodgers, 1991; Shear, 2011). Most conceptualizations of grief define it inclusively, encompassing many differing states of emotional distress as well as other responses (Scheff, 2015; Weiss, 2008). This inclusive view of grief is used in the North American Nursing Diagnosis Association's (NANDA's) definition of grieving: "A normal complex process that includes emotional, physical, spiritual, social, and intellectual responses and behaviors by which individuals, families, and communities incorporate an actual, anticipated, or perceived loss into their daily lives" (Herdman, 2012, p. 363).

HISTORICAL LITERATURE ABOUT PARENTAL GRIEF

Although we think of the grief of parents from our own perspective of time and culture, literature, poetry, and art are replete with evidence that parents across cultures and over centuries have faced the devastating loss of an infant or child, and often more than one child. Many ancient Chinese poets and philosophers wrote poignant poems about the death of an infant or child (Rexroth, 1971). Mei Yao Ch'en (1002–1060), a scholar of the Sung dynasty, wrote this poem, *On the Death of a New Born Child*, about his infant daughter and son:

> The flowers in bud on the trees
> Are pure like this dead child
> The East wind will not let them last.

It will blow them into blossom,
And at last into the earth.
It is the same with this beautiful life
Which was so dear to me.
While his mother is weeping tears of blood,
Her breasts are still filling with milk.

Shakespeare (1606/1623) in *Macbeth* recognized the need to openly confront the intense feelings of a man following the slaughter of his wife and children: "Give sorrow words; the grief that does not speak whispers the oe'r-fraught heart and bids it break." Charles Lamb (1827) wrote a long and touching poem about the death of his daughter at birth, *On an Infant Dying as Soon as Born*. Chekhov (1886) in a short story, "Misery" (subtitled "To Whom Shall I Tell My Grief?"), poignantly illuminated the need of a bereaved father to share his story of loss, to which no one would listen. John Gunther's memoir, *Death Be Not Proud* (1949), is a classic account of the death of his own beloved son. Although he generally avoided sharing his own grief, his wife described her intense grief each time she missed her son. This brief overview of accounts of grief in literature provides us with an awareness of the universality and profound pain of the grief of parents across centuries and across cultures. For additional literary and artistic perspectives on grief, see *A Child Dies: A Portrait of Family Grief* (Arnold & Gemma, 1983) and *In the Midst of Winter* (Moffat, 1982).

CONCEPTUALIZATION MODELS OF GRIEF

Psychoanalytic and Psychobiological Models

The modern Western views about grief as a psychological concept emerged in the 20th century (Bonanno, 2009; Granek, 2010). The most influential was Freud's essay "Mourning and Melancholia" (1917/1955), in which he noted that both depression and bereavement involve suffering in response to the experience of loss; however, he considered grief a normal response and not a pathological condition like depression and melancholia. He also put forth the idea of "grief work," the process of reclaiming the psychological energy or libido invested in the deceased person by reliving memories, hopes, and longing for the beloved. Freud viewed this painful process as necessary in order to break the bond with the deceased and move on to a resolution of the grief. Following the deaths of his daughter and his favorite grandson, Freud continued to try to understand the intense pain of grief. In the last year of his life, he shared his idea of grief's long-term impact in a letter to Binswanger: "Although we know that after such a loss the acute state of mourning will subside, we also know we shall remain inconsolable and will never find a substitute. No matter what may fill the gap, even if it be filled completely, it nevertheless remains something else. And actually, this is how it should be. It is the only way of perpetuating that love which we do not want to relinquish" (Freud, 1929/1960, p. 386). Thus, Freud refuted his earlier idea that grief work involved the breaking of the bonds of love in order to resolve grief.

From his orientation toward psychobiological medical models, Lindemann, a psychiatrist, viewed grief as a medical–psychiatric problem (Granek, 2010). He was greatly influenced by his well-known and foundational clinical study of a group of bereaved family members whose loved ones had died in the famous Coconut Grove nightclub fire in Boston, as well as from patients in therapy. Lindemann (1944) delineated what he called the *syndrome of acute grief* and described both normal emotional responses of grief and abnormal responses. The syndrome of grief encompassed five striking responses: (a) preoccupation with thoughts of the deceased; (b) guilt; (c) hostility; (d) somatic distress; and (e) loss of usual patterns of behavior. He also suggested that grief could be distorted, delayed, or exaggerated, hypothesizing that such reactions could ultimately have an impact on mental and physical health. Similar to Freud's early work, Lindemann also viewed grief work as the process of emancipating from bondage with the deceased, readjusting to the environment from which the deceased is missing, and the forming of new relationships, placing the responsibility for the resolution of grief on the bereaved individual. His views were largely based on clinical observations; he never conducted further research to validate his views, but they had great influence on subsequent views of grief (Granek, 2010).

Crisis Theory

Building on Lindemann's work and based on his crisis theory, Caplan (1964) proposed that grief triggered a crisis. As such, he hypothesized that the distress of grief generally resolved in 4 to 6 weeks and that individuals who were not improved in this time frame should be referred for psychiatric care. His crisis theory also included the idea that the balance of stressors and resources determines the outcomes of a crisis. Caplan's crisis theory, along with Lindemann's 1944 paper, erroneously gave the impression that the grief response was short-lived; this had a dramatic influence on the research and clinical treatment of the bereaved. Caplan (1974), however, subsequently revised his concept of grief as a single crisis that resolved in 6 to 8 weeks to a series of crises that he called life transitions, which are resolved over a much longer period of time.

Attachment Models

Rooted in psychoanalysis but also influenced by neurophysiology, ethology, and information theory, Bowlby developed theories about attachment and loss. He viewed attachment as a protective biological mechanism and internal motivation that ensures the survival of the individual and the species (Bowlby, 1969). His astute observations of infants and young children separated from their mothers led Bowlby to identify the separation response syndrome, which entails three phases: protest, despair, and detachment (Bowlby, 1980). Working with Parkes, Bowlby (1982) extended his attachment theory to incorporate the grief response of bereaved adults. Bowlby viewed the emotional distress of grief as breaking the bonds of attachment and conceptualized bereavement responses as falling into four phases: (a) numbing; (b) yearning and searching; (c) disorganization and despair; and (d) reorganization. He also proposed factors that can affect the course of mourning, including the identity and role of the deceased, the age and sex of the bereaved, causes and circumstances of the loss, social and psychological circumstances surrounding the loss, and the personality of the bereaved.

Based on research with widows in the United Kingdom, Parkes (1972) at first viewed grief as an acute stress response. Later, he conceptualized grief as a major life transition in which the bereaved person "gradually changes his view of the world and the places and habits by means of which he orients and relates to it" (Parkes, 1970, p. 465). He also provided systematic descriptions of the painful emotional, behavioral, and physical manifestations of grief including acute episodes of severe anxiety and psychological pain, pining for the deceased, preoccupation with thoughts of the deceased, and feelings such as anxiety, guilt, depression, and aimlessness, as well as numerous physical reactions such as sleep disturbances, aches and pains, loss of energy, and appetite changes (Parkes, 1970, 1972). Influenced by Bowlby's attachment theory, Parkes identified several phases in the grief process: numbness, yearning and protest, disorganization, and a phase of reorganization. He noted that the transitions from one phase to another are seldom distinct and features from one phase of grief often persist into the next; therefore, he hypothesized and evaluated in his research antecedent, concurrent, and subsequent variables that influence grief resolution. In his most recent work, Parkes (2006) identified the influence of Bowlby's patterns of childhood attachment, recalled as adults, on reactions to loss in later life.

Integrative Theory

Based on empirical research and psychodynamic grief theories, Sanders (1989) proposed an integrative theory of bereavement. Her model includes five phases of bereavement: (a) shock; (b) awareness of loss; (c) conservation–withdrawal; (d) healing; and (e) renewal. Each phase is characterized by a wide variety of responses that affect three levels of functioning: emotional, biological, and social. A unique perspective of her model is that she proposed that the bereaved individual make a decision, conscious or unconscious, to survive or to remain in perpetual bereavement at the end of the phase of conservation–withdrawal. This decision involves motivation to implement enormous changes to reach renewal. According to Sanders, this inclusion of motivation is what differentiates her theory from earlier models of grief. Sanders further proposed that internally and externally moderated variables interact during the bereavement process and have a significant effect on outcome.

Stage, Task, and Trajectory Models

In the 1970s, grief began to be viewed as a process of experiencing certain reactions or emotions in preset stages or points in time from immediately after the loss to the completion of grief work. Some popular versions of stage theory imply that if the bereaved did not experience each of these stages, grief would be delayed and could become problematic. The most popular stage theory is that of Kübler-Ross (1969). Based on her clinical work with dying adults, she proposed that the terminally ill person experienced five major emotions that occurred in stages: denial, anger, guilt, bargaining, and acceptance. Kübler-Ross further suggested that the individual had to work through the struggles of one stage before moving on to the next. While her original book was based on limited observations of dying patients, clinicians quickly adapted the model to the bereaved, and she later published a book on the stages of grief (Kübler-Ross & Kessler, 2005). Her work was never validated with empirical evidence, and the stages she identified do not include the complex emotions and other reactions of the dying nor those of the grieving survivors. Her book on death and dying, however, was important in focusing attention on the dying process and on the bereaved family. Despite its serious shortcomings, her model continues to be used to guide researchers and clinicians today.

Based on a longitudinal study of the responses of individuals and families to life-threatening illness and suicide, Worden (1982) proposed that four tasks of mourning must be completed in order to resolve grief. The tasks are (a) accepting the reality of the loss; (b) experiencing the pain of grief; (c) adjusting to an environment in which the deceased is missing; and (d) withdrawing emotional energy and reinvesting it in another relationship. He developed his model as a way to understand what grieving people were experiencing and as a guide for grief counseling.

Both Rando (1986) and Walter (1996) countered the dominant models of grief that focused on grief resolution by working through emotions and separating from the deceased. Rando (1986) conceptualized tasks of grief and related them within three phases in the process. During the avoidance phase, grief requires recognizing the loss. During the confrontation phase, the task is to identify, accept, and express reactions to the loss, to realistically review and remember the deceased, and to relinquish old attachments to the deceased and the old assumptive world. During the accommodation phase, the survivor develops a new relationship to the deceased, adopts new ways of being in the world, establishes a new identity, and puts emotional energy into new relationships and goals. Rando's views of grief are related to her extensive experience as a grief counselor. Walter (1996), in his biographical model of grief, also viewed the purpose of grief as the reconstruction of a new identity through talking with others, sharing memories about the deceased, and ultimately creating a new life story that includes the beloved person who died.

Bonanno (2009) described four trajectories of grief: (a) resilience—the ability to maintain stable healthy psychological and physical functioning and a capacity for generative experiences and positive emotions; (b) recovery—subthreshold psychopathology for a period of time; (c) chronic dysfunction—prolonged suffering and inability to function, usually lasting several years or longer; and (d) delayed grief—when adjustment seems normal, but the grief responses surface months later.

Stress Frameworks

Starting in the 1980s, the focus on traumatic and disaster-related losses led to conceptualizations of grief within stress frameworks. Horowitz (1982) proposed a cognitive emotional view of grief in which the response to death was seen as a general stress response syndrome. This response required a change in one's inner psychic models involving the integration of reality and the development of new schemata. During this process, the bereaved exhibit painful emotional responses such as vulnerability, rage, guilt, and sadness, as well as controls to blunt the flood of feelings. In Horowitz's view, the response to death includes an outcry stage, replaced by a vacillation between denial and/or numbing in which reality is avoided and blocked, and intrusion, in which the reality is faced. As the reality and schemata are integrated, the stress response syndrome is resolved. The model is unique in its conceptualization of avoidance and intrusion as primary aspects of grief; however, the model does not account for many aspects of the grief response nor for variables that may have an impact on the process.

More recently, the grief response has been conceptualized as a trauma that may trigger a posttraumatic stress response in some individuals (Simpson, 1997). An outgrowth of posttraumatic stress disorder (PTSD) literature is the conceptualization of posttraumatic growth (PTG), suggesting that the experience of loss and the ensuing grief can lead to personal growth (Tedeschi, Park, & Calhoun, 1998). Davis (2008) suggested that death leads to a shattering of one's views of the world and/or the sense of self. This, in turn, leads to active cognitive processing to find meaning and can lead to new views of the world and direction for one's life. Numerous researchers and clinicians have observed that this search for meaning is an important aspect of the grief process and can lead to resolution and growth (Frantz, Farrell, & Trolley, 2001; Keesee, 2008; Murphy, Johnson, & Lohan, 2003; Neimeyer & Sands, 2011).

PARENTAL GRIEF MODELS

Most of the models conceptualizing grief emerged from the study of adults who were widows and widowers or who had experienced the death of a significant relative or friend. Several authors, however, have conceptualized the process and responses to grief from the unique perspective of parents who have experienced the death of an infant or child.

Miles (1984) proposed a psychodynamic model for understanding parental grief based on the work of Lindemann and Parkes and on observations grounded in clinical practice with bereaved parents. She described three overlapping phases of parental grief responses: (a) numbness and shock, (b) intense grief, and (c) reorganization. Reactions during the phase of intense grief include loneliness and emptiness leading to intense yearning and searching; helplessness leading to anger, guilt, and fear; physical symptoms such as appetite and sleep changes, somatic distress, and the onset of health problems; and symptoms including difficulty concentrating, confused thought processes, disorganization, and, for some, abuse of drugs and alcohol. The search for meaning is a critical element in the grief process in this model (Miles & Crandall, 1983).

Miles and her colleague Demi (1983–1984) further developed a typology of guilt sources from the analysis of open-ended statements from parents of children who died of accidents, chronic disease, or suicide. The most poignant types of guilt were *death causation guilt* arising from parental views about their role in the specific cause of death; *illness-related guilt* arising from perceived failures in the parental role during the child's illness; and *child-rearing guilt* arising from parents' beliefs about perceived failures in child-rearing. For example, a parent might experience guilt over an otherwise positive action such as buying a bicycle for a child that led to a fatal accident, or a parent might experience guilt over hurtful issues such as a poor relationship or abuse. Miles and Demi also hypothesized the process through which feelings of guilt are developed and identified key factors that may impact on guilt responses. Unfortunately, further research to validate and refine this model of parental grief was never conducted.

Based on his extensive clinical experiences with bereaved parents during grief support groups, Klass (1988) viewed the death of a child as unique because parental bonds to a child are strong and deeply rooted in the parent's own psychic life, which is radically changed by the death of the child. New psychic equilibrium is achieved as the inner representations of the child are reformed and incorporated into the bereaved parent's ongoing psychic life. The majority of bereaved parents internalize the dead child by introjection, a process of keeping a sense of the child and their emotional bond with the child intact while transforming the inner representation of the child in such a way that it brings solace (Klass, 1988). The strength of Klass's model of parental bereavement is his attempt to tie the parent's responses to the death of a child to the overall parental role. In doing so, he described some struggles unique to bereaved parents.

Despite the fact that the death of an infant or child involves a family, few models adequately conceptualize grief within a family context. Riches and Dawson (2000) examined the importance of social relationships within and outside the family as important in helping parents as well as siblings adjust to the death of a child. This includes shared remembering in transforming survivors' relationships with the deceased and in helping rebuild their own identity within a family structure that has changed significantly. As part of the process, the family's cultural resources and wider social networks are highly influential in their grieving. Some of the issues that may confront families include a lack of information and communication within the family, especially for siblings; gender issues in expressions of grief such as the invisibility of fathers' grief; the weakening of intimate relationships, particularly between parents and with siblings; and a sense of isolation felt by some family members.

DISCUSSION

Since the 1970s, the interest of clinicians and researchers in understanding processes related to grief has resulted in a highly developed literature on the topic. The literature summarized here supports the view that the manifestations of acute grief include emotional distress as well as physiological, cognitive, spiritual, and social challenges. The concept of grief work leading to "breaking the bonds" with the deceased has been broadened into dialogue about the various ways in which the bereaved reconstruct their relationship or identity with the deceased. There continues to be dialogue about the role of attachment, including the attachment with the deceased and the previous attachment experiences and styles of the bereaved. Although the stage theory of grief has been refuted, grief is understood as a process that develops over time with a lessening of the pain and other manifestations that ultimately lead to reorganization and healing, although the pain of grief can still emerge. The earlier view that grief could or should be resolved within a certain time frame has been refuted, leaving open the question of the temporal aspects of the acute grief experience.

The search for meaning in coping with grief is a current focus of grief theorists and researchers. While the search for meaning often leads to positive growth, it can become problematic if it leads to negative meaning. The vast literature on delayed, prolonged, or complicated grief suggests that some individuals are at risk for enduring distress and dysfunction (Prigerson et al., 2009). Thus, individuals who experience prolonged and/or intense symptoms that interfere with relationships and moving forward in the way one would like to may need the support of a professional counselor or psychotherapist. These symptoms include continued deep, disabling pain, depressive and/or anxiety symptoms, and continuing anger and disorganization, among others.

TOWARD CONCEPTUALIZING THE GRIEF OF PARENTS

So what does this literature tell us about the unique experiences of grieving parents? Attempting to put on paper conceptualizations about the very painful grief experienced by parents when an infant or child dies is complex, sensitive, and challenging. Parents bring into the experience of losing a child a network of critical personal and family history. The death of a child is a specific family crisis causing much distress for individual family members and potentially disrupting family dynamics. The context of perinatal and child death is often complex, and the illness experience may be very prolonged and painful. Moreover, the research exploring the connections between personal and contextual aspects of a child's death and the emotional, behavioral, cognitive, and physical responses from the perspective of bereaved parents remains limited. In this section, the previously reviewed literature is synthesized and earlier conceptualizations about the unique responses and needs of bereaved parents are incorporated. This synthesis is limited in that it does not include the increasingly important research studies with bereaved parents nor the literature on family influences on and experiences with the death of a child.

Many of the author's perspectives about the grief of parents were developed during a period in her professional career when she worked closely with parents who had experienced the death of an infant or child. Although she did conduct some research with bereaved parents then, the approaches to research in the 1970s were not yet well developed. However, the views about parents' grief have been validated in a unique way. In the 1970s, when the author was working with bereaved parents, she learned that they were quite confused and scared by the intensity of their many feelings. Some, especially mothers, shared their worry that they were "going crazy." At the same time, Miles realized there was little written at that time about parental grief that might guide them. Based on what she learned from them and informed by the literature on grief in general, she wrote a pamphlet, *The Grief of Parents. . . .When a Child Dies* (Miles, 1978, 2012) to give to parents. In turn, she got wonderful feedback from grieving parents who said the pamphlet reflected their own pain and dilemmas while grieving for their child. The pamphlet was donated to Compassionate Friends and for more than 30 years has been distributed to bereaved parents across the country.

There is universal agreement that the death of a child is a major life transition for the individual parent and the family. It is devastating and precipitates a profound personal crisis that can have an impact on a parent's identity, shattering core beliefs and assumptions about the world and the expectations about how life should unfold. The intense and complex grief responses of bereaved parents are uniquely linked to their close emotional attachment to their child, their sense of responsibility for the child's well-being, and their personal identity as a parent. Thus, the painful emotions of grief are very intimate and idiosyncratic to the bereaved parent.

Circumstances related to the child's death may complicate parental grief. A stillbirth or neonatal death precludes parenting. Women and their partners who experience a miscarriage or elect pregnancy termination due to a lethal or life-limiting fetal defect often experience their grief alone, because few people may have yet known of the pregnancy or of its loss. Even when others know, the distress of miscarriage or early pregnancy loss may be discounted. Parents of infants or children who die suddenly (e.g., sudden infant death syndrome, an accident, acute illness) are unprepared for their tragic loss. Similarly, a child's suicide or murder is devastating to parents. When infants and children die after a chronic or prolonged illness that required an extended period of parental caregiving, parents may have residual distress about the many treatment decisions they had to make as well as painful memories of their child being sick.

In addition, the unique personal history of parents can influence their grief reactions. This might include a previous loss, concurrent life stressors, mental illness, gender, support resources, spirituality, and personality. The dynamics of the mother–father relationship and the family system can heavily influence their response to grief. The parental and family resilience are very important resources and may pose an interesting area of inquiry for future research.

In this model of parental grief, grief is viewed as a complex and time-consuming process that involves many interrelated emotional, behavioral, cognitive, social, spiritual, and physical responses that occur in varying intensity and frequency over an indeterminate period of time as bereaved parents cope with their painful loss and altered personal identity. The grief process is conceptualized as occurring across three phases. However, these phases of grief may overlap or occur at the same time. The phases are the crisis period, acute grief, and assimilation.

Crisis Period

At the time of the child's death, parents experience a crisis. They may respond with denial, disbelief, shock, or numbness, especially if the death was unexpected. These reactions may help cushion the full impact of the child's death until they are ready to face the devastating reality and the multiple meanings of the child's death for everyone involved. Such reactions may last for only a short time or can last for days or weeks. For some parents, but not all, it is helpful if they can see and/or hold their child after death both to validate the death and to say goodbye to the physical body. When a child dies following a long period of illness, a parent may at some point feel relief that the child is no longer suffering and is at peace. Also during this crisis period, parents exhibit emotional release such as wailing, crying, raging anger, or talking incessantly. This release of feelings is important and should never be discouraged.

Acute Grief

During the months after a child's death, parents enter a period of acute grieving. During this time, they are working on facing the reality and finality of their child's death and the loss of their parental role, leading to a flood of painful emotions that can be confusing and difficult for parents to understand. The emotional pain often leads to physiological, behavioral, spiritual, and social manifestations of grief. These acute grief responses are clustered into three groups: emptiness and yearning for the child; guilt, anger, and vulnerability; and sadness, all of which can lead to physical, cognitive, and behavioral changes.

Emptiness and Yearning

As parents face the huge void in their lives with the absence of their infant or child and losses associated with their parenting role, they experience deep feelings of emptiness or "feeling dead" inside. One mother described her empty feeling: "A child is a part of you in a way that no other human being can ever be. When my child died, a part of me died with him." The emptiness can cause intense yearning—a deep aching desire to see and touch their child again and preoccupation with thinking about their child. Some are troubled by the memory of the child at the time of death or during an acute illness. With a sudden violent death, parents may be haunted by visions of the death scene, whether they were present or not. Parents also may periodically sense the presence of their baby or child. They may report hearing their child cry, seeing their child in a crowd, or feeling their child's presence in the room. Some suddenly feel a sense of panic when they feel they can no longer remember things about their child and desperately attempt to recall the child's appearance, voice, or behaviors. On the other hand, as a way of coping with painful memories and the pain of grief, some parents may try to forget the child by avoiding places that evoke particular memories or by not talking about the child's death.

Guilt, Anger, and Vulnerability

Feelings of guilt may occur as bereaved parents begin to grope for the reasons for their child's death. This may include guilt related to the cause of death if parents blame themselves by thinking that something they did, or neglected to do, may have in some way contributed to the child's death. Mothers of infants who die of various causes may feel guilty for not protecting their fetus during pregnancy or may feel their body failed the infant. Parents of children with a health problem may feel guilty because they think they might have detected the symptoms of the illness earlier or because they signed the operative permit giving their approval for the surgery, which the child did not survive. Some parents may report guilt related to things they failed or wished they had done differently as they cared for their sick child (illness-related guilt). Additionally, guilt related to perceived failures in parenting (child-rearing guilt) may be felt. A father may experience guilt because he did not spend enough time with the infant or child, or a mother may feel guilt because she went back to work. A hidden source of guilt may be moral guilt when a parent feels that the child's death was somehow a punishment for past sins and transgressions such as a pregnancy before marriage, a past abortion, extramarital affairs, or even poor attendance at church. The causes for feelings of guilt are often irrational thoughts that are not based on reality and are difficult to share with others. It is helpful for grieving parents to find a professional counselor with whom they can share these feelings, sort out the various causes of the guilt, and identify the irrational aspects of these feelings, especially if the guilt feelings are intense and prolonged. They may need permission to forgive themselves so they are not consumed by guilt for months or even years.

Some parents experience anger toward a variety of persons or situations. They may feel angry toward the health care team for not saving the child or for poor communication that left them confused and unsupported. A mother who had a miscarriage, stillbirth, or whose infant dies of a birth defect can feel anger toward friends or relatives who, while pregnant, continued risky behavior such as smoking or drinking and still gave birth to a normal infant. It is common to feel anger toward others, especially friends and family members who do not acknowledge the child or who discount parental grief responses and go on as if the child's death did not happen.

Death of a child may shatter parental beliefs and assumptions about the world and often leads to questioning and confusion about spirituality and religious beliefs. This can lead to a period of anger toward God or a higher spiritual being. Feelings of anger can be difficult to deal with because the reasons for that anger may be hard to express, and sharing anger is not socially acceptable in our culture. Anger that is not expressed may lead to a general feeling of irritability that is hard to understand and very hard to overcome. As with guilt, it is important to be able to talk about anger issues with some neutral person such as a counselor who cares and understands.

Encountering the death of one's child, the intense and confusing pain that follows, and the shattered views of the world may cause some parents to feel *vulnerable and fearful* that something else bad might happen to them or their family. This might include increased protectiveness toward other children or intense concerns about a future pregnancy outcome. They may also become fearful about the well-being of their spouse. Some parents may feel concerned and vulnerable because of their confused and painful emotional state and question their own mental health.

Sadness and Depressive Symptoms

As a result of this struggle to come to grips with the feelings that result from the loss of a child, parents experience deep sadness such as feeling blue and unhappy, preoccupation with sad thoughts, continued loss of interest in activities, and crying. Some parents may experience more intense depressive symptoms such as feeling hopeless or worthless, loss of confidence, lack of energy and fatigue, irritability, or agitation. Thoughts of death or suicide may indicate signs of depression requiring medical help.

These intense and deep feelings during acute grief often intensify over the early months after the loss and may cause parents to fear that they have become mentally ill or that they will always be in deep pain. Societal views about grief as a short-lived time of emotional distress may limit the support of others or may cause bereaved parents to hide their feelings and act as if they are feeling better when actually they are struggling to cover their pain.

Physical Symptoms, Cognitive Changes, and Social Challenges

Prolonged sadness and depression may lead to subtle bodily distress and physical symptoms, cognitive changes, and social challenges. It is not unusual for bereaved parents to experience physical symptoms such as loss of appetite (or increased appetite), body aches, deep fatigue, difficulty getting to sleep, oversleeping, or waking up too early. Sexual interest may be greatly diminished for a time after the death of a child.

Cognitive changes that are common include forgetfulness, disorganization, and difficulty in thinking, concentrating, and making decisions. Most grieving persons have a period when they feel disorganized and find it difficult to concentrate on tasks and keep up with work. Mothers may find that their housework is piling up and the other children's needs are often unmet. Working parents may have a hard time managing the demands of their jobs. Grieving parents also may find it difficult to make decisions, even simple ones. One major decision is what to do with the child's room, clothing, toys, and other possessions. Some parents clear them soon after the death because they cause too much pain. Other parents have reported that looking at the child's belongings for a time helped them face the reality of their loss and helped them maintain a connection with their child as they grieved. One of the biggest decisions parents of childbearing age face is often whether and when to have another child. While some parents find decisions difficult to make, it is also possible to begin making decisions impulsively and without foresight and planning. Their attitude may be, "What do I have to lose . . . ?" Thus, important decisions, such as moving, should be made carefully and with deliberate thought and planning.

Social challenges such as relationship difficulties, communication challenges, and isolation can ensue. On the other hand, the support of family, friends, and coworkers can help to ease the distress of a parent. The relationship between mothers and fathers can be strained, especially if they are grieving in different ways and are not sharing their pain and communicating.

In order to cope with the difficult emotional feelings and the nagging physical symptoms, some may turn to the use of drugs or alcohol to help shut out the pain. If a parent turns to drugs or alcohol to help shut out the pain and sadness, he or she should be encouraged to seek professional help.

Assimilation

The death of a child is a life-shattering experience and challenges parents' views of themselves and the world. The death destroys hopes and dreams; it alters their life story, their self-image, and their self-confidence. Over time, most bereaved parents begin to assimilate their child's death into their identity and their views of the world (Davis, 2008). During this process of assimilation, as memories of the child are assimilated into the life story of the parents, the attachment to the child and pain of the child's death remains in the heart. The child can be discussed with more happiness and less pain. In addition, the intense suffering slowly diminishes and good days outnumber bad days. Parents can get reinvolved in life activities and see possibilities for a more positive future. However, parents are never their "old selves" after the death, changed from what they were before. Gradually, over time, the bereaved parent can enjoy life again.

The search for meaning is an important step in the process of assimilation. Early on in the grief process, parents try to make sense of the loss and search for answers: Why did my child die? Why mine? Why do children die? They may focus on why the child died, seeking medical consultation and reading about the cause of the illness. This may or may not answer the question of what might have prevented the death. The search for meaning also leads to struggles to understand shattered views of the world, spirituality, and family relationships. Ultimately, this search may provide an opportunity for positive life changes and personal growth. Bereaved parents have reported feeling closer to their family, stronger, more self-confident, and more sensitive to the needs of others.

Family Considerations

The death of a child is ultimately a family affair, and the shared grief affects each member, family dyads, and relationships among all family members. Children in the family also grieve, and parents often are challenged in how to help the siblings, while also coping with their own intense pain. Of most importance is the relationship between grieving parents. Parental role, personality, communication styles, and gender, among others, shape how parents grieve and how they relate to each other. While it is commonly thought that men are more apt to hide their grief and not want to talk about it, this can also occur in women, such that assumptions should not be made. The unique perspective of fathers has not been adequately studied, nor have the dynamics within the family system.

CONCLUSION

In summary, this model about the grief of parents is incomplete and inadequate. This review is limited in scope. The research on grief was not included nor was the literature on complicated grief or prolonged grief. The literature on family and sibling responses to child death was not included. The author hopes that clinicians and researchers will be stimulated to read and synthesize further the vast new literature focused on grief. There are many gaps to be filled and questions to be asked. Limited research has been conducted to test or advance models of parental grief. Many clinicians in their practice with bereaved parents and researchers use older literature and concepts that have not been validated or have been refuted (e.g., Kübler-Ross's stages of grief). However, the author hopes that clinicians and scholars will move away from simplistic stage models of grief toward a better understanding of the uniqueness and complexity of the grief process experienced by parents when a fetus, infant, or child dies. Also, it is hoped that scholars will build on, reject, and revise the conceptualization put forth here, such that we develop a more intensive understanding of parental grief. It is critical that we work toward sensitive, complex, and valid conceptualizations about the grief process experienced by parents and within families to guide our clinical practice and our research.

CASE STUDY

Jessica and Martin's 11-year-old son, Ira, recently died. They have three other children ages 5, 7, and 9. Since their son died, they have noticed that they are not as close as they once were. Jessica feels that she still needs to work through "the stages of the grief process." Martin shared that he believes things are progressing well, but he sometimes feels very tired and sick. He does not need to talk about their son's death but expresses that "it seems like Jessica wants to talk about Ira all the time." Both Jessica and Martin feel that their other children are doing well. But, they are concerned that their 5-year-old will experience problems when he begins kindergarten in the fall because he has been having nightmares and has temper tantrums more frequently.

FOCUS QUESTIONS

1. What theoretical perspectives would be most helpful in determining the best approach to developing a plan of care for this family?

2. How could Jessica and Martin be encouraged to share their feelings with each other?
3. How has the family system been affected by Ira's death?
4. What concerns might you have about Ira's siblings?

REFERENCES

American Psychiatric Association. (2013). *Diagnostic and statistical manual of mental disorders (DSM-IV,* 5th ed.). Washington, DC: Author.

Arnold, J., & Gemma, P. B. (1983). *A child dies: A portrait of family grief.* Rockville, MD: Aspen Systems Corporation.

Bonanno, G. A. (2009*). The other side of sadness: What the new science of bereavement tells us about life after loss.* New York, NY: Basic Books Group.

Bowlby, J. (1969). *Attachment and loss, Vol. I. Attachment.* New York, NY: Basic Books.

Bowlby, J. (1980). *Attachment and loss, Vol. III. Loss: Sadness and depression.* New York, NY: Basic Books.

Bowlby, J. (1982). Attachment and loss: Retrospect and prospect. *American Journal of Orthopsychiatry, 52,* 664–678.

Caplan, G. (1964). *Principles of preventive psychiatry.* New York, NY: Basic Books.

Caplan, G. (1974). Foreword. In I. Glick, R. Weiss, & C. M. Parkes. *The first year of bereavement* (pp. VII–XIV). New York, NY: John Wiley and Sons.

Chekhov, A. (1886). *Misery.* Retrieved from http://classiclit.about.com/library/bl-etexts/achekhov/bl-achek-misery.htm

Ch'en, M. Y. (1002–1060/1971). On the death of new born child. In K. Rexroth (Eds.), *One hundred poems from the Chinese.* New York, NY: New Directions Book.

Cowles, K. D., & Rodgers, B. L. (1991). The concept of grief: A foundation for nursing research and practice. *Research in Nursing and Health, 14,* 119–227.

Davis, C. G. (2008). Redefining goals and redefining self: A closer look at post-traumatic growth following loss. In M. S. Stroebe, R. O. Hansson, H. Schut, & W. Stroebe (Eds.), *Handbook of bereavement research and practice: Advances in theory and intervention* (pp. 309–325). Washington, DC: American Psychological Association.

Frantz, T. T., Farrell, M. M., & Trolley, B. C. (2001). Positive outcomes of losing a loved one. In R. A. Neimeyer (Ed.), *Meaning reconstruction and the experience of loss.* Washington, DC: American Psychological Association.

Freud, S. (1957). Mourning and melancholia. In J. Strachey (Ed.), *The standard edition of the complete psychological works of Sigmund Freud* (Vol. 14, pp. 237–260). London, England: Hogarth Press and Institute for Psychoanalysis. (Original work published in 1917.)

Freud, S. (1929/1960). Letter to Binswanger. In E. L. Freud (Ed.), *Letters of Sigmund Freud* (p. 386). New York, NY: Basic Books, Inc.

Granek, L. (2010). Grief as pathology: The evolution of grief theory in psychology from Freud to the present. *History of Psychology, 13(1),* 46–73.

Gunther, J. (1949). *Death be not proud* (1998 ed.). New York, NY: Harper Perennial.

Herdman, T. H. (Ed.). (2012). *NANDA International: Nursing diagnoses, definitions, and classifications.* Oxford, England: Wiley-Blackwell.

Horowitz, M. J. (1982). Stress response syndromes and their treatment. In L. Goldbrger & S. Breznitz (Eds.), *Handbook of stress: Theoretical and clinical aspects.* New York, NY: The Free Press.

Howarth, R. A. (2011). Concepts and controversies in grief and loss. *Journal of Mental Health Counseling, 33,* 4–10.

Keesee, N. J. (2008). Predictors of grief following the death of one's child: The contribution of finding meaning. *Journal of Clinical Psychology, 64,* 1–19.

Klass, D. (1988). *Parental grief: Solace and resolution.* New York, NY: Springer Publishing Company.

Kübler-Ross, E. (1969). *On death and dying.* New York, NY: MacMillan, Inc.

Kübler-Ross, E., & Kessler, D. (2005). *On grief and grieving: Finding the meaning of grief through the five stages of loss.* New York, NY: Schribner.

Lamb, C. (1827). On an infant dying as soon as born. *Poetry Foundation.* http://www.poetryfoundation.org/poem/173785#poem

Lindemann, E. (1944). Symptomatology and management of acute grief. *American Journal of Psychiatry, 101,* 141–148.

Miles, M. S. (1978, 2012). *The grief of parents. . . .When a child dies.* Oak Brook, IL: Compassionate Friends, Inc.

Miles, M. S. (1984). Helping adults mourn the death of a child. In H. Wass & C. Corr (Eds.), *Children and death* (pp. 219–241). Washington, DC: Hemisphere Publishing Co.

Miles, M. S., & Crandall, E. K. (1983). The search for meaning and its implication for growth in bereaved parents. *Health Values: Achieving High Level Wellness, 7,* 19–23.

Miles, M. S., & Demi, A. (1983–1984). Toward the development of a theory of bereavement guilt. *Omega, 14,* 299–314.

Moffat, M. J. (Ed.). (1982). *In the midst of winter: Selections from the literature of mourning.* New York, NY: Random House, Inc.

Murphy, S. A., Johnson, L. C., & Lohan, J. (2003). Finding meaning in a child's violent death: A five-year prospective analysis of parents' personal narratives and empirical data. *Death Studies, 27,* 381–404.

Neimeyer, R. A., Harris, D. L., Winokuer, H. R., & Thornton, G. F. (Eds.). (2011). *Grief and bereavement in contemporary society: Bridging research and practice* (pp. 9–22). New York, NY: Routledge.

Neimeyer, R. A., & Sands, D. C. (2011). Meaning reconstruction in bereavement: From principles to practice. In R. A. Neimeyer, D. L. Harris, H. R. Winokuer, & G. F. Thornton (Eds.), *Grief and bereavement in contemporary society: Bridging research and practice* (pp. 9–22). New York: NY: Routledge.

Parkes, C. M. (1970). The first year of bereavement: A longitudinal study of the reaction of London widows to the death of their husbands. *Psychiatry, 33,* 444–467.

Parkes, C. M. (1972). *Bereavement: Studies of grief in adult life.* New York, NY: International Universities Press, Inc.

Parkes, C. M. (2006). *Love and loss: The roots of grief and its complications.* New York, NY: Rutledge.

Prigerson, H. G., Horowitz, M. J., Jacobs, S. C., Parkes, C. M., Aslan, M., Goodkin, K. . . .Maciejewski, P. K. (2009). Prolonged grief disorder: Psychometric validation of criteria proposed for *DSM-5* and ICD-11. *PLos Med, 6(8),* e1000121. doi:10.1371/journal pmed. 1000121

Rando, T. (1986). *Parental loss of a child.* Champaign, IL: Research Press.

Rexroth, K. (1971). *One hundred poems from the Chinese.* New York, NY: New Directions Book.

Riches, G., & Dawson, P. (2000). *An intimate loneliness.* Philadelphia, PA: Open University Press.

Sanders, C. M. (1989). *Grief: The mourning after.* New York, NY: John Wiley & Sons, Inc.

Scheff, T. (2015). Toward defining basic emotions. *Qualitative Inquiry, 21*(2), 111–121. doi:10.1177/1077904414550462

Shakespeare, W. (1606/1623). *Macbeth.* Stratford-upon-Avon, England: Shakespeare Theatre Company.

Shear, M. K. (2011). Complicated grief and related bereavement issues for *DSM-5. Depression and Anxiety, 28*, 103–117.

Simpson, M. A. (1997). Traumatic bereavements and death-related PTSD. In C. R. Figley, B. E. Bride, & N. Mazza (Eds.), *Death and trauma: The traumatology of grieving.* Philadelphia, PA: Taylor and Francis.

Stroebe, M. S., Hansson, R. O., Schut, H., & Stroebe. W. (Eds.). (2008). *Handbook of bereavement research and practice: Advances in theory and intervention* (pp. 309–325). Washington, DC: American Psychological Association Press.

Tedeschi, R. G., Park, C. L., & Calhoun, L. G. (Eds.). (1998). *Posttraumatic growth: Positive changes in the aftermath of crisis.* Mahwah, NJ: Lawrence Erlbaum Associates, Publishers.

Walter, T. (1996). A new model of grief: Bereavement and biography. *Mortality 1,* 7–25.

Weiss, R. S. (2008). The nature and causes of grief. In M. S. Stroebe, R. O. Hansson, H. Schut, & W. Stroebe (Eds.), *Handbook of bereavement research and practice: Advances in theory and intervention* (pp. 29–42). Washington, DC: American Psychological Association Press.

Worden, J. W. (1982). *Grief counseling and grief therapy.* New York, NY: Springer Publishing Company.

CHAPTER 12

Theoretical Perspectives on Pediatric Palliative Care

Rose Steele and Kimberley Widger

*P*ediatric palliative care is both a philosophy and a type of care; it is not synonymous with end-of-life care. Sometimes, it is the sole focus of care; other times, it is provided in combination with treatments aimed at curing the underlying condition (Friebert, 2009). The principles of pediatric palliative care can be used to guide the provision of care for children living with progressive, life-limiting conditions where survival to adulthood is unlikely. Pediatric palliative care also includes children with a life-threatening condition that is no longer considered curable and children who are facing an acute, potentially fatal event. When the diagnosis of a potentially life-threatening condition occurs before birth or when a neonate is born too early, is too sick, or is not responding to treatment, the principles of palliative care are the same as for children and adolescents, but the associated terms refer to when care is provided: prenatally (prior to birth), perinatally (before, at the time of, or shortly following birth), or neonatally (during the first 28 days of life; National Perinatal Association [NPA], 2009). In this chapter, pediatric palliative care encompasses prenatal, perinatal, and neonatal palliative care. In all cases, the child's family is included as the focus of care.

Ideally, pediatric palliative care is offered from the time of diagnosis, even if prior to birth, and may continue for many years, through the end of life and into bereavement. The age range of patients receiving pediatric palliative care, typically 0 to 19 years of age, requires consideration of the child's developmental, relational, educational, social, and recreational needs (Friebert, 2009). The developmental stage of the family must also be considered, regardless of the patient's age.

In this chapter, we discuss the theoretical perspectives that underpin the field of pediatric palliative care, starting with additional definitions of terms and a history of the development of this field. Standards and principles of practice are discussed and models of pediatric palliative care are described. The chapter concludes with information about education and support for health care professionals in pediatric palliative care.

Life-Limiting or Life-Threatening. There is some controversy among pediatric palliative care experts about whether the term *life-limiting* (no realistic hope for cure) or *life-threatening* (cure may be possible) should be used when discussing the conditions appropriate for pediatric palliative care. In this chapter, we use the more inclusive term *life-threatening* because of the prognostic uncertainty associated with most serious illnesses as well as the rapid advances in medicine that are altering the possibility of cure for previously fatal conditions.

Hospice and/or Palliative Care. The term *hospice* has various meanings, often depending on where one lives and whether referring to care that is provided primarily to adults or children. *Hospice* may refer to a philosophy of care that focuses on people who are terminally ill, to a building or unit where dying patients are cared for, or to a program that serves patients in the community. Freestanding hospices for children tend to provide both respite care earlier in the disease trajectory and end-of-life care. Palliative care, particularly for children, is much more encompassing than hospice care; it focuses on care from the time of diagnosis of a life-threatening condition rather than just on the end-of-life period. Pediatric palliative care is also generally understood to include care provided to the family after the child's death, that is, bereavement follow-up.

EVOLUTION OF PEDIATRIC PALLIATIVE CARE

Hospice and palliative care initially developed within the context of adult patients and focused only on cancer. The word *hospice* means *hospitality* or *hospitable* and was used to describe the care provided to the sick and the destitute in the fourth century. The first modern-day freestanding hospice opened in London, England, in 1967. St. Christopher's Hospice was founded by Cecily Saunders, who was a nurse, a social worker, and a physician (Canadian Hospice Palliative Care Association [CHPCA], 2014). In 1973, Balfour Mount, a Canadian urological cancer surgeon, sought to improve the care given to dying patients. Thus, after reading Kübler-Ross's (1969) seminal book, *On Death and Dying*, he arranged to visit St. Christopher's. At the hospice, he learned of approaches to alleviate much of the suffering associated with death and dying that often occurred for patients in his own hospital. On his return to Montreal, Dr. Mount began a pilot project that included a hospital ward for the dying, a consultation team to work with other hospital wards, a home care outreach service, and a bereavement follow-up program. But because the term *hospice* had a negative connotation in French and Canada is a bilingual country, he chose the term *palliative care* instead, as the word *palliate* means to cloak (CHPCA, 2014) or to ease without curing (Rallison, Limacher, & Clinton, 2006). Hence, palliative care

TABLE 12.1 The WHO Definition of Palliative Care

Palliative care is an approach that improves the quality of life of patients and their families facing the problem associated with life-threatening illness, through the prevention and relief of suffering by means of early identification and impeccable assessment and treatment of pain and other problems, physical, psychosocial and spiritual. Palliative care:

- Provides relief from pain and other distressing symptoms
- Affirms life and regards dying as a normal process
- Intends neither to hasten or postpone death
- Integrates the psychological and spiritual aspects of patient care
- Offers a support system to help patients live as actively as possible until death
- Offers a support system to help the family cope during the patient's illness and in their own bereavement
- Uses a team approach to address the needs of patients and their families, including bereavement counselling, if indicated
- Will enhance quality of life, and may also positively influence the course of illness
- Is applicable early in the course of illness, in conjunction with other therapies that are intended to prolong life, such as chemotherapy or radiation therapy, and includes those investigations needed to better understand and manage distressing clinical complications

WHO, World Health Organization.
Reprinted from WHO (2006).

entered the health care lexicon. The World Health Organization's (WHO's) definition of palliative care is included in Table 12.1.

Pediatric palliative care developed about a decade behind the adult counterpart and took a broader approach than cancer because the conditions affecting children were much more heterogeneous. In the second half of the 20th century, the rapidly declining rates of infant mortality and deaths due to infectious diseases led to an increase in life expectancy. Concurrently, advances in medical technology and treatments changed previously fatal conditions, such as childhood cancer and infant prematurity, to ones of survival (Craft, 2004; National Cancer Institute, 2014). As the decades passed, children with genetic, neurodegenerative, and metabolic diseases also were treated with newer medications and technologies that kept the child alive, though not necessarily cured. Increasingly, conditions that had previously been acute and inevitably fatal were now viewed as chronic and requiring a different approach to longer term care. A variety of models were developed to deliver palliative care services to children with these types of conditions and their families in their homes, in hospices, in hospitals, and in other settings. The WHO (2006) also developed a definition of palliative care specifically for children (Table 12.2).

The first freestanding children's hospice, Helen House, opened in Oxford, England, in 1982. The first in North America, Canuck Place in Vancouver, Canada, opened its doors in 1995 (Davies, 1996). Since then, children's hospices have opened in multiple countries, though rarely in the

TABLE 12.2 The WHO Definition of Palliative Care for Children

Palliative care for children represents a special, albeit closely related field to adult palliative care. WHO's definition of palliative care appropriate for children and their families is as follows; the principles apply to other pediatric chronic disorders.

- Palliative care for children is the active total care of the child's body, mind and spirit, and also involves giving support to the family.
- It begins when illness is diagnosed, and continues regardless of whether or not a child receives treatment directed at the disease.
- Health providers must evaluate and alleviate a child's physical, psychological, and social distress.
- Effective palliative care requires a broad multidisciplinary approach that includes the family and makes use of available community resources; it can be successfully implemented even if resources are limited.
- It can be provided in tertiary care facilities, in community health centers and even in children's homes.

WHO, World Health Organization.

Reprinted from WHO (2006).

United States due to its health care funding system. Because of the nature of the children's conditions, pediatric hospices typically provide respite as well as end-of-life care and bereavement services; they do not focus solely on the end of life.

More than half the children who die do so in hospitals and more than 85% of those deaths occur in intensive care units (ICUs), including neonatal ICUs (NICUs) and pediatric ICUs (PICUs; Feudtner, Feinstein, Satchell, Zhao, & Kang, 2007). Hospital-based palliative care programs have now been developed in most children's tertiary centers, and NICU palliative care pathways have been developed and implemented in some NICU settings (Gale & Brooks, 2006; Together for Short Lives, 2013). Excellent perinatal bereavement models have been the standard of care for some time, but comprehensive perinatal palliative care programs are much more recent (Kobler & Limbo, 2011).

It was not until about 2004 that perinatal palliative care programs and hospices started to appear (Munson & Leuthner, 2007), but now, many women's hospitals have a maternal fetal program where women are referred for complicated pregnancies. Such programs may be complemented by a medical genetics program so couples can obtain genetic counseling if they have an ultrasound abnormality, an abnormal maternal serum screen, or a family history of a genetic condition. If a life-threatening fetal condition is detected, then palliative care services may be offered to parents who choose to continue the pregnancy after the prenatal diagnosis (Kobler & Limbo, 2011). The NPA (2009) is in full support of offering palliative care at any time during the pregnancy cycle, both before and after birth.

STANDARDS AND PRINCIPLES OF PRACTICE

The growth in pediatric palliative care over the past few decades has included efforts to develop standards, principles, and a charter of rights to provide details and guidance on what pediatric palliative care is and how it should be delivered. Health professionals must clearly understand the current national standards and recommendations that exist in their own country as well as more local guidelines that may be available in their workplace. Table 12.3 lists some key resources to assist clinicians in identifying and accessing currently available standards from different organizations and parts of the world. In addition, the International Children's Palliative Care Network (ICPCN, 2008) published a Charter of Rights for children with life-limiting or life-threatening conditions. Their goal is to have the charter accepted and ratified by governments and health departments around the world. To date, the charter is available in 25 different languages and can be downloaded from the ICPCN website (ICPCN, 2008). The charter calls for children to receive appropriate palliative care when they need it, care that will promote quality of life and relieve physical, emotional, and spiritual suffering (Table 12.4). Some key principles and values common to the charter and most of the standard documents are described further in the following subsections and include child and family as the unit of care, quality of life, location of care, whole-person approach, attention to child and family culture and religion, goals of care, respite, bereavement, and involvement of an interprofessional team.

TABLE 12.3 Pediatric Palliative Care Standards and Recommendations

- **American Academy of Pediatrics**: http://pediatrics.aappublications.org/content/106/2/351 .full.pdf+html; http://pediatrics.aappublications.org/content/126/2/e488.full.pdf+html
- **Canadian Hospice Palliative Care Association**: http://www.chpca.net/media/7841/Pediatric _Norms_of_Practice_March_31_2006_English.pdf
- **Children's Project on Palliative/Hospice Services (ChiPPS), NHPCO's pediatric leadership council (USA)**: http://www.nhpco.org/quality/nhpco's-standards-pediatric-care
- **European Association for Palliative Care**: http://www.eapcnet.eu/LinkClick.aspx?fileticket=Sh MQyZuTfqU%3d&tabid=284
- **National Hospice and Palliative Care Organization (USA)**: http://www.nhpco.org/sites/ default/files/public/quality/Ped_Pall_Care%20_Standard.pdf.pdf
- **National Perinatal Association (USA)**: http://www.nationalperinatal.org/resources/ palliative%20care%20%2012-12-13.pdf
- **Together for Short Lives (UK)**: http://www.togetherforshortlives.org.uk/assets/0000/5003/ Standards_framework_update_2013.pdf

TABLE 12.4 ICPCN Charter of Rights

1. Every child should expect individualized, culturally and age appropriate palliative care as defined by the World Health Organization (WHO). The specific needs of adolescents and young people shall be addressed and planned for.
2. Palliative care for the child and family shall begin at the time of diagnosis and continue alongside any curative treatments throughout the child's illness, during death and in bereavement. The aim of palliative care shall be to relieve suffering and promote quality of life.
3. The child's parents or legal guardians shall be acknowledged as the primary care givers and recognized as full partners in all care and decisions involving their child.
4. Every child shall be encouraged to participate in decisions affecting his or her care, according to age and understanding.
5. A sensitive but honest approach will be the basis of all communication with the child and the child's family. They shall be treated with dignity and given privacy irrespective of physical or intellectual capacity.
6. Every child or young person shall have access to education and wherever possible be provided with opportunities to play, access leisure opportunities, interact with siblings and friends and participate in normal childhood activities.
7. Wherever possible, the child and the family should be given the opportunity to consult with a pediatric specialist with particular knowledge of the child's condition and should remain under the care of a pediatrician or a doctor with pediatric knowledge and experience.
8. The child and the family shall be entitled to a named and accessible key-worker whose task it is to build, coordinate and maintain appropriate support systems which should include a multidisciplinary care team and appropriate community resources.
9. The child's home shall remain the center of care whenever possible. Treatment outside of this home shall be in a child-centered environment by staff and volunteers, trained in palliative care of children.
10. Every child and family member, including siblings, shall receive culturally appropriate, clinical, emotional, psychosocial and spiritual support in order to meet their particular needs. Bereavement support for the child's family shall be available for as long as it is required.

Reprinted from ICPCN (2008).

Child and Family as Unit of Care

In pediatrics, a child cannot be viewed separately from his family. But family denotes not only a genetic relationship—it also includes anyone who is defined as family by the child and other family members (CHPCA, 2006; European Association for Palliative Care [EAPC], 2007; National Hospice and Palliative Care Organization [NHPCO], 2009). Further, friends, schoolmates, and other people in the child's community may also need support. Therefore, it is important for health care providers to ask the child and family who should be included within the unit of care. Decision making is generally the responsibility of the child's parents, depending on the child's age, the child's capacity or competence, and any legal restrictions based on where the family resides, in collaboration with the interprofessional team. It should occur within a context of open and honest discussion so that the family is given the information they need by the health care providers and the professional team obtains a clear understanding of the family's wishes. At all times, the family needs to be viewed and treated as an integral part of the team.

Siblings should not be overlooked within the unit of care (CHPCA, 2006; NHPCO, 2009). It is important for health care providers to assess and address physical, practical, and emotional needs of siblings. Grief, loss, and bereavement supports are particularly important.

Enhancing Quality of Life

Overall care may include treatments or interventions to try to effect a cure, but the focus of care is on enhancing quality of life for children and their families despite those treatments. Particularly for conditions such as cancer, a very high symptom burden is associated with the treatments aimed at cure. Palliative care during this time is crucial to ensure relief of suffering and good quality of life regardless of the outcome of the disease (Waldman & Wolfe, 2013). Only the child and family can determine the experiences or components that are most important to their quality of life.

Location of Care

While pediatric deaths still occur most often in the hospitals, there has been a rising proportion of deaths occurring at home or in a pediatric hospice (Feudtner, Hexem, & Rourke, 2011; Friebert, 2009). Families often express a preference for being at home with their child because they experience a better quality of life at home; their wishes should be met. However, there also needs to be flexibility to allow families to move between locations (e.g., home, hospital, or hospice) as their needs change. The child's care should not be compromised during such changes of location (EAPC, 2007). Whether in the hospital or in the community, the desired care needs to be coordinated, often with a single point of contact to ensure continuity and child-centered care (EAPC, 2007; Together for Short Lives, 2013). If taking their child home, families should be provided with the resources they need before they leave the hospital (Together for Short Lives, 2013) to ensure that the care provided at home really does enhance the child's and family's quality of life rather than becoming a more stressful situation. Quality of life should be a primary focus of care, regardless of the location of care.

Whole-Person Approach

The concept of whole-person care is central to pediatric palliative care. It demands that health care providers attend to all aspects of the child and family and not just focus on one element such as relief of physical pain. The goals of care are determined in discussions among the child (if possible), the family, and the care team. The plan of care then addresses how children and families can fulfill their physical, psychological, developmental, social, recreational, relational, and spiritual goals. Emotional, spiritual, and psychological support needs to be available when the child or family wants it (Together for Short Lives, 2013). Pain and other symptom management should be available 24/7 and be provided by skilled, competent clinicians (CHPCA, 2006; EAPC, 2007; NHPCO, 2009). Nonpharmacological therapies (e.g., music therapy) are important and should be offered at an age-appropriate level to complement pharmacologic treatments (CHPCA, 2006; NHPCO, 2009), unless they are likely to cause significant harm (CHPCA, 2006).

Attention to Cultural and Religious Background

Families receiving pediatric palliative care services come from diverse cultural and religious backgrounds. It should not be assumed, however, that all families from the same culture or religion will have the same needs, preferences, or rituals around death and dying. Sensitivity to the importance of providing culturally safe and appropriate care is required when offering services. But the most important approach is to treat each family individually and to inquire and learn about that family's specific preferences and practices (CHPCA, 2006; NHPCO, 2009; Together for Short Lives, 2013).

Goals of Care

It is important to understand the goals of care for each individual child (Tamburro, Shaffer, Hahnlen, Felker, & Ceneviva, 2011). Among other areas of concern, goals of care provide direction when considering specific health interventions, location of care, or limitations on interventions for a patient. Advance care planning is one approach to clarifying goals of care. It involves open discussion among the child (if possible), family, and health care professionals when a child has a serious condition in order to articulate and elucidate short- and long-term care goals. Honest, open communication among all parties is essential. Advance care planning can include conversations about treatment options and can also involve the writing of formal plans and orders. The legal and ethical principle that underlies decision making in pediatric palliative care is always that of the child's best interests (NHPCO, 2009).

Though not necessarily legally binding (NHPCO, 2009), advance care planning is an important component of pediatric palliative care, whether in the prenatal period or at another point in the infant's/child's life. The child's and family's wishes and preferences need to be known so that the goals of care and the preferred interventions are clearly documented and can, subsequently, be carried out (Garvie, He, Wang, D'Angelo, & Lyon, 2012). Advance directives might include statements about such areas as resuscitation attempts, place of care, and if/when to withdraw or withhold specific treatments. They also may detail a family's preferences about autopsy or organ donation (CHPCA, 2006; Kobler & Limbo, 2011; Together for Short Lives, 2013). Advance directives may change over time as a child's condition changes or parents acknowledge different possibilities. Therefore, it is important that discussions take place on a regular basis to ensure that advance directives are updated to reflect current preferences and that new directives are written as necessary. The frequency of these discussions is generally dependent on the child's condition. It can be difficult, however, to balance between raising the discussion regularly enough to be sure the directives are up to date and not so often that parents feel their wishes are being questioned (Edwards, Kun, Graham, & Keens, 2012).

Respite

For families who care for their child at home, respite is an essential component of pediatric palliative care (CHPCA, 2006; NHPCO, 2009). Caring for a child with a life-threatening condition is physically and emotionally draining, and families may need a break so they can refresh themselves. Various forms of respite are possible, such as inpatient hospital, hospice, or home respite in the child's home or in someone else's home. Respite can be for a few hours to a couple of weeks at a time depending on the format available (EAPC, 2007). The cost of respite care may be covered by a palliative or hospice program, other community care program, or through some private health insurance programs, but the lack of availability of such resources often limits the amount of respite a family can obtain.

Bereavement Services

Though bereavement care is sometimes viewed as only after-death care, pediatric palliative care affirms that anticipatory loss, grief, and bereavement support should begin from diagnosis and continue for as long as it is needed after death (CHPCA, 2006; EAPC, 2007; NHPCO, 2009). Sibling support should not be overlooked when determining the grief supports a family might need. Detailed information about how to provide support to families who are grieving and suffering from loss is provided in other chapters of this textbook.

Support often includes providing developmentally appropriate information about grief, loss, and death for children, including the dying child, siblings, classmates, and other peers, as well as for parents and other members of the child's community both before and after a child's death. Information may be tailored so it can be given directly to a child, or it may be directed at parents or other adults so they can support a grieving child. Children may be best supported by ensuring that parents learn ways to support their grieving children in the midst of their own grief. Child life therapists and psychologists or other counsellors may provide one-on-one interventions or support groups for children and/or adults.

Health professionals can offer a variety of services around the time of death and after the child dies, such as taking hand molds or pictures. Many programs have a bereavement coordinator whose role is to provide such services and to offer follow-up contact. Some send a card to the family at the first-year anniversary of the child's death, and many other supports are possible, such as hospital or hospice memorial services or health professionals' attendance at the funeral. Follow-up by involved health care professionals after the child's death is considered by many families to be a crucial component of end-of-life care (Widger, Steele, Oberle, & Davies, 2009). Some families experience negative consequences after the child's death, and ongoing support for families may help prevent or alleviate prolonged suffering.

Interprofessional Team

The child and family remain at the center of care while also being equal team members. The array of skills and services that may be required to meet the various needs of the child and family means that the care team must have sufficient expertise to address those needs (EAPC, 2007). The core team often comprises a physician, a nurse, and a social worker. Other members might include professionals such as a child life specialist, a psychologist, or a spiritual adviser. New members may become part of the team for a shorter period of time to meet a specific need (e.g., a respiratory therapist or an occupational therapist in the NICU), or they may join the team on a more permanent basis. One member is normally responsible for being the consistent point of contact and for helping the family navigate the system (CHPCA, 2006).

Unlike a traditional team where the physician is the leader, the goal of an interprofessional team in pediatric palliative care is to ensure that the needs of the child and family are met, regardless of which professional takes the lead at a particular time. There tends to be more blurring of disciplinary lines in pediatric palliative care, and each member of the team and support services is considered equally as important as another (Papadatou,

Bluebond-Langer, & Goldman, 2011). Collaboration within the team and a willingness to acknowledge and defer to the expertise of one's colleagues are key in creating a team that can provide optimal care to the child and family.

MODELS OF PEDIATRIC PALLIATIVE CARE

Models of care can be understood as the more tangible "program"-type models like hospital-based programs, freestanding children's hospice facilities, hospice-based programs, or community agency or long-term care facility-based programs. Or they can be viewed as an approach that guides programs on how to provide optimal pediatric palliative care. In this section, overall approaches for care from two major organizations in North America are discussed because they offer conceptual frameworks for considering palliative care delivery. A third model provides a framework for clinical practice with dying children and their families.

Canadian Hospice Palliative Care Association

In 2002, the CHPCA produced a document that outlined the Canadian national principles and norms of practice for adult hospice palliative care (CHPCA, 2002). The purpose of the document was to promote a consistent, standard approach to hospice palliative care across Canada within a specific model of care, including promoting laws, policies, and regulations to facilitate delivery of hospice palliative care. A subsequent document (CHPCA, 2005) detailed how to apply the model of care if planning a program, evaluating a service, or developing education programs. A recent revision of the 2002 document (CHPCA, 2013) included revision of the norms to emphasize the most relevant aspects of hospice palliative care, based on current practice and experience. The document was also streamlined to focus on the information used most often. All documents are to be used in conjunction with one another. The CHPCA continues to promote a national model to encourage consistency in the development and provision of optimal services as well as the development of professional competencies, curricula, and practices.

When the CHPCA's pediatric interest group, the Canadian Network of Palliative Care for Children, adapted the CHPCA adult guiding principles and norms of practice in 2006 for relevance to pediatric care, the model of care was extended to include children and their families. The 2006 document is expected to be reviewed, now that the adult guide has been revised. In the meantime, key features of the pediatric version have been added to the description of the most recent framework.

Circle of Care

In 2013, the CHPCA affirmed that the most effective delivery of hospice palliative care requires an interprofessional team in a therapeutic relationship with the person and family. The importance of collaboration, continuity, and consistency was emphasized to ensure optimal care. The circle of care comprises the interprofessional team; the person and family; as well as friends, other family members, and anyone the person wants to include. This circle of care begins during the illness and continues through bereavement until it is no longer needed.

Square of Care

The Square of Care (CHPCA, 2005, 2013) is a conceptual framework that identifies the most common issues faced by adults and their families during an illness and the steps in providing care, as well as the associated principles and norms for each step in the process. On the vertical plane, we note common issues, including disease management; physical, psychological, social, spiritual, and practical issues; end of life/death management; and loss/grief. Assessment, information sharing, decision making, care planning, care delivery, and confirmation constitute the process of providing care items on the horizontal plane. The circle of care can use the Square of Care as a tool in identifying issues and the steps needed in providing care.

Square of Organization

The Square of Organization is another conceptual framework that offers a guide to organizational development and function (CHPCA, 2005, 2013). It helps identify the resources needed for a hospice palliative care organization, the main functions of an organization, and the associated principles and norms for those functions. The principal functions are noted on the vertical plane: governance and administration, planning, operations, quality management, and communications/marketing. Resources in the other plane include financial, human, informational, physical, and communal. The Square of Organization can be used to identify the principal activities of an organization and guide the development of its infrastructure. A combination of the Square of Care and the Square of Organization results in a comprehensive model, a square, that when applied by organizations can help patients and families receiving hospice palliative care achieve their goals of care.

Though very similar to the combined Square of Care and Square of Organization, the pediatric adaptation (CHPCA, 2006) expanded the original framework. The child/family is at the core, and fixed characteristics (i.e., age, gender, ethnicity, race, education, and literacy) are identified. The process of providing care includes assessment, information sharing, decision making, therapeutic interventions, care delivery, and evaluation of care. Child and family care focuses on illness/disease management; physical, psychological, social, spiritual, developmental, and practical issues; end of life/preparation for death; and loss, grief, and bereavement. Governance and administration issues are covered on one side of the square. The fourth side includes funding, planning, marketing and advertising, quality management, caregiver support/worklife, and research. This model is also accompanied by principles and norms of practice.

NHPCO's Children's Project on Palliative/Hospice Services

Similar to the CHPCA, the purpose of the Children's Project on Palliative/ Hospice Services model (ChiPPS; NHPCO, 2009) is as a guide for service provision programs to use so they can develop best practices in pediatric palliative care. The model is to be used in conjunction with the NHPCO (2009) standards. The model positions the child, family, and community as the central core of a holistic care approach that emphasizes interrelationships between and among the core and medical, spiritual, and psychosocial services. It also emphasizes the continuum of care that is needed to support children and families as they move between various sites of care and among different systems and interprofessional services. Finally, it situates itself within a context of education, advocacy, quality outcomes, and research.

Supportive Care Model

The Supportive Care Model (Widger et al., 2009) was proposed as a guide for clinicians to use when working with dying children and their families. This model provides suggestions within the areas of *valuing*, *connecting*, *empowering*, *doing for/with*, *finding meaning*, and *preserving integrity* that health professionals can use to optimize the quality of pediatric palliative care delivered to children and their families. The model emphasizes the importance of bereavement follow-up and ongoing connections between families and the health professionals who cared for the ill child. Care provided through this model helps focus attention on the elements that are most important to children and their families, thus contributing to the whole-person yet individualized care that is central to excellent pediatric palliative care.

PEDIATRIC PALLIATIVE CARE SPECIALIZATION

It is recognized that varying levels of pediatric palliative care may be more appropriate for different children depending on their needs, condition, or stage in the illness trajectory. At a minimum (level 1), all health care professionals should appropriately apply a palliative care approach (or principles) when a child has a life-threatening condition. Level 2 is an intermediate level in which some patients and families may benefit from care by health care professionals who have training and experience in palliative care, though their full-time role is not palliative care. The most specialized services, level 3, are provided by clinicians who are well trained in pediatric palliative care and whose main role is palliative care (EAPC, 2007). Sometimes, these specialists are called in to consult (e.g., when a child's pain or other symptom is intractable); other times, they are the primary providers of palliative care.

Education for Pediatric Palliative Care Professionals

Everyone working in pediatric palliative care, including professionals and volunteers, needs comprehensive training and support. In addition, it has been recommended that not only should palliative care training be part of the curriculum for all health care professionals but also that every country should develop a national curriculum for its pediatric palliative care professionals (EAPC, 2007). The ICPCN (2013) has developed a free e-learning program to make pediatric palliative care training accessible and affordable to all who need training. It offers several short courses as part of a longer term strategy to provide e-learning programs on pediatric palliative care (Table 12.5). Though the courses are free, they require access to (a) a computer, (b) the Internet, and (c) a clinical site where the student can undertake the pediatric palliative care clinical assessment that is part of a course. Other organizations also offer online learning, though usually at a cost (e.g., NHPCO, 2013). Some also provide continuing education credits for nurses, social workers, physicians, and counselors. The End-of-Life Nursing Education Consortium (ELNEC) project, available through the American Association of Colleges of Nursing, is a national education initiative to improve palliative care. The ELNEC-Pediatric Palliative Care (ELNEC-PPC) was adapted from the ELNEC-Core curriculum in the early 2000s, and in 2009, the curriculum was updated to include enhanced perinatal and neonatal content (ELNEC-PPC, 2009).

Support for Pediatric Palliative Care Professionals

Support for professionals who work in pediatric palliative care is important because team members may face challenges such as moral distress in

TABLE 12.5 ICPCN's E-Learning Program for Pediatric Palliative Care

- Introduction to palliative care in children
- Pain assessment and management for children: A training module linked to the WHO guidelines for persisting pain
- Communicating with children and emotional issues
- Child development and play in children's palliative care
- End-of-life care in children's palliative care
- Grief and bereavement in children's palliative care

Reprinted from ICPCN (2013).

practice; compassion fatigue; professional grief; and incongruity between one's own beliefs, values, and attitudes and those of one's colleagues and/ or the patient and family (Morgan, 2009). External supports (e.g., access to debriefing in a safe environment) or an employee program that pays for counseling as needed are critical. Individuals also need to develop strong self-care activities, such as meditation, exercise, and other stress management techniques, as an integral component of professional practice in pediatric palliative care.

CONCLUSION

Regardless of their country of origin, standards for pediatric palliative care are based on several shared principles:

- Palliative care should be available from the time of diagnosis of a life-threatening condition, including in the prenatal period, and continued through the course of the illness trajectory into bereavement.
- The unit of care is the child and family, and the family is an integral part of the team.
- The focus of care is on enhancing quality of life for children and their families.
- The care provided aims to assist children and families to fulfill their physical, psychological, developmental, social, and spiritual goals and includes excellent pain and other symptom management.
- Palliative care should be provided by competent caregivers in whatever setting a family chooses (e.g., home, hospital, or hospice) and regardless of their financial or health insurance circumstances.
- Sensitivity to the personal, cultural, and religious values of children and families is critical.
- Respite and bereavement care are essential components of pediatric palliative care services.
- Care is provided through an interprofessional team and support services.

Children and their families facing life-threatening conditions deserve to receive high-quality, innovative, and state-of-the art pediatric palliative care from knowledgeable and competent health professionals. Attention to the underlying principles, standards, frameworks, and models of pediatric palliative care and ensuring they are used to guide care, no matter the location of care or stage of the condition, will help ensure that these children and families receive optimal care.

CASE STUDY

Kaleena is a 4-year-old girl who was diagnosed with leukemia 14 months ago. She has received most of her care at a small, community hospital, but her condition began to decline rapidly over the past 2 months. Three weeks ago, she was transferred to a large research hospital 90 miles away from home for more intensive treatments. Upon admission, Kaleena seemed to respond positively to the new treatment regimen; however, over the past 2 weeks, she has become increasingly lethargic and has lost a significant amount of weight. Kaleena's mother and stepfather are very involved in her care and have worked closely with the health care team since her diagnosis. Kaleena has a 2-year-old stepbrother and a 9-year-old sister who are staying with family members in their hometown. Kaleena has expressed a desire to go home but her mother and stepfather believe that she is just tired of invasive treatments. The health care team will meet with Kaleena's mother and stepfather this week to discuss her condition and goals of care.

FOCUS QUESTIONS

1. Which team members should be present at the family meeting to provide accurate information and emotional support?
2. When meeting with Kaleena's family this week, what topics are most important to discuss?
3. What questions would be most helpful to ask Kaleena's family at the meeting?
4. Which model of care would be most helpful in framing interventions with Kaleena's family? Why?
5. At this point in Kaleena's disease process, would it be more appropriate to discuss curative care, palliative care, hospice care, or a combination of options? Support your response with information from the chapter.

REFERENCES

Canadian Hospice Palliative Care Association (CHPCA). (2002). *A model to guide hospice palliative care: Based on national principles and norms of practice.* Ottawa, Ontario, Canada: Author. Retrieved from http://www.chpca.net/media/7422/a-model-to-guide-hospice-palliative-care-2002-urlupdate-august2005.pdf

Canadian Hospice Palliative Care Association (CHPCA). (2005). *Applying "A model to guide hospice palliative care": An essential companion toolkit for planners, policy makers, caregivers, educators, managers, administrators and researchers.* Ottawa, Ontario, Canada: Author. Retrieved from http://www.chpca.net/media/7458/Applying_a-Model-to-Guide-Hospice-Palliative-Care-Toolkit.pdf

Canadian Hospice Palliative Care Association (CHPCA). (2006). *Pediatric hospice palliative care: Guiding principles and norms of practice.* Ottawa, Ontario, Canada: Author. Retrieved from http://www.chpca.net/media/7841/Pediatric_Norms_of_Practice_March_31_2006_English.pdf

Canadian Hospice Palliative Care Association (CHPCA). (2013). *A model to guide hospice palliative care: Based on national principles and norms of practice* (Rev. & cond. ed.). Ottawa, Ontario, Canada: Author. Retrieved from http://www.chpca.net/media/319547/norms-of-practice-eng-web.pdf

Canadian Hospice Palliative Care Association (CHPCA). (2014). *The Canadian Hospice Palliative Care Association: A history.* Retrieved from http://www.chpca.net/about-us/history.aspx

Craft, A. (2004). Children with complex health care needs: Supporting the child and family in the community. *Child: Care, Health and Development, 30*(3), 193–194.

Davies, B. (1996). Assessment of need for a children's hospice program. *Death Studies, 20*(3), 247–268.

Edwards, J. D., Kun, S. S., Graham, R. J., & Keens, T. G. (2012). End-of-life discussions and advance care planning for children on long-term assisted ventilation with life-limiting conditions. *Journal of Palliative Care, 28*(1), 21–27.

End-of-Life Nursing Education Consortium—Pediatric Palliative Care (ELNEC-PPC). (2009). *ELNEC-Pediatric Palliative Care.* Washington, DC: American Association of Colleges of Nursing. Retrieved from http://www.aacn.nche.edu/elnec/about/pediatric-palliative-care

European Association for Palliative Care (EAPC); Steering Committee of the EAPC task force on palliative care for children and adolescents. (2007). IMPaCCT: Standards for paediatric palliative care in Europe. *European Journal of Palliative Care, 14*(3), 109–114.

Feudtner, C., Feinstein, J. A., Satchell, M., Zhao, H., & Kang, T. I. (2007). Shifting place of death among children with complex chronic conditions in the United States, 1989-2003. *Journal of the American Medical Association, 297*(24), 2725–2732.

Feudtner, C., Hexem, K., & Rourke, M. T. (2011). Epidemiology and the care of children with complex conditions. In J. Wolfe, P. S. Hinds, & B. M. Sourkes (Eds.), *Textbook of interdisciplinary pediatric palliative care* (pp. 7–17). Philadelphia, PA: Elsevier Saunders.

Friebert, S. (2009). *NHPCO facts and figures: Pediatric palliative and hospice care in America.* Alexandria, VA: National Hospice and Palliative Care Organization. Retrieved from http://www.nhpco.org/sites/default/files/public/quality/Pediatric_Facts-Figures.pdf

Gale, G., & Brooks, A. (2006). Implementing a palliative care program in a newborn intensive care unit. *Advances in Neonatal Care, 6*(1), 37–53.

Garvie, P. A., He, J., Wang, J., D'Angelo, L. J., & Lyon, M. E. (2012). An exploratory survey of end-of-life attitudes, beliefs and experiences of adolescents with HIV/AIDS and their families. *Journal of Pain and Symptom Management, 44*(3), 373–385.

International Children's Palliative Care Network (ICPCN). (2008). *The ICPCN Charter of Rights for life limited and life threatened children.* Assagay, South Africa: Author. Retrieved from http://www.icpcn.org/icpcn-charter

International Children's Palliative Care Network (ICPCN). (2013). *ICPCN's e-learning programme.* Assagay, South Africa: Author. Retrieved from http://www.elearnicpcn.org

Kobler, K., & Limbo, R. (2011). Making a case: Creating a perinatal palliative care service using a perinatal bereavement program model. *Journal of Perinatal & Neonatal Nursing, 25*(1), 32–41.

Kübler-Ross, E. (1969). *On death and dying.* New York, NY: Touchstone.

Morgan, D. (2009). Caring for dying children: Assessing the needs of the pediatric palliative care nurse. *Pediatric Nursing, 35*(2), 86-90.

Munson, D., & Leuthner, S. R. (2007). Palliative care for the family carrying a fetus with a life-limiting diagnosis. *Pediatric Clinics of North America, 54,* 787–798.

National Cancer Institute. (2014). *Cancer in children and adolescents.* Retrieved from http://www.cancer.gov/types/childhood-cancers/child-adolescent-cancers-fact-sheet

National Hospice and Palliative Care Organization (NHPCO). (2009). *Standards of practice for pediatric palliative care and hospice.* Alexandria, VA: Author. Retrieved from http://www.nhpco.org/sites/default/files/public/quality/Ped_Pall_Care%20_Standard.pdf.pdf

National Hospice and Palliative Care Organization (NHPCO). (2013). *Pediatric palliative care training series bundle (10 modules).* Alexandria, VA: Author. Retrieved from http://www.nhpco.org/education-online-learning/pediatric-care

National Perinatal Association (NPA). (2009). *Palliative care.* Alexandria, VA: Author. Retrieved from http://www.nationalperinatal.org/resources/palliative%20care%20%2012-12-13.pdf

Papadatou, D., Bluebond-Langer, M., & Goldman, A. (2011). The team. In J. Wolfe, P. S. Hinds, & B. M. Sourkes (Eds.), *Textbook of interdisciplinary pediatric palliative care* (pp. 55–63). Philadelphia, PA: Elsevier Saunders.

Rallison, L., Limacher, L. H., & Clinton, M. (2006). Future echoes in pediatric palliative care: Becoming sensitive to language. *Journal of Palliative Care, 22*(2), 99–104.

Tamburro, R. F., Shaffer, M, L., Hahnlen, N. C., Felker, P., & Ceneviva, G. D. (2011). Care goals and decisions for children referred to a pediatric palliative care program. *Journal of Palliative Medicine, 14*(5), 607–613.

Together for Short Lives. (2013). *Standards framework for children's palliative care* (2nd ed.). Bristol, UK: Author. Retrieved from http://www.togetherforshortlives.org.uk/assets/0000/5003/Standards_framework_update_2013.pdf

Waldman, E., & Wolfe, J. (2013). Palliative care for children with cancer. *Nature Reviews Clinical Oncology, 10*(2), 100–107.

WHO. (2006). *WHO definition of palliative care.* Geneva, Switzerland: Author. Retrieved from http://www.who.int/cancer/palliative/definition/en

Widger, K., Steele, R., Oberle, K., & Davies, B. (2009). Exploring the Supportive Care Model as a framework for pediatric palliative care. *Journal of Hospice and Palliative Nursing, 11*(4), 209–216.

CHAPTER 13

Hope, Hopefulness, and Pediatric Palliative Care

Douglas L. Hill and Chris Feudtner

THEORIES OF HOPE AND HOPEFUL PATTERNS OF THINKING

While there are many different notions of hope, most definitions include an expectation that there will be a desired positive outcome in the future (Dufault & Martocchio, 1985; Godfrey, 1987; Gottschalk, 1974; Herth, 1991; Hinds, 1984; Miller & Powers, 1988; Snyder et al., 1991; Stotland, 1969). At one time, psychologists and medical researchers considered hope as something outside of their domain, a theological topic (Godfrey, 1987) or something that charlatans used to exploit the gullible (Eliott, 2005; Lynch, 1974) as opposed to a topic of legitimate research. In the second half of the 20th century, some philosophers (Fromm, 1968; Godfrey, 1987; Shade, 2001) began to argue that hope was a vital force in everyday life, independent of religion. Psychologists and psychiatrists began to describe hope as an important influence in the lives of individuals, especially in times of despair (Beck, Weissman, Lester, & Trexler, 1974; Erickson, Post, & Paige, 1975; Erikson, 1964; Gottschalk, 1974; Lynch, 1974; Mercer & Kane, 1979; Stotland, 1969; Vaillot, 1970).

Many philosophers, psychologists, and health care providers now agree that hope is important to a person's well-being and quality of life (Fromm, 1968; Rustøen, 1995) and for success in reaching valued goals (Snyder et al., 1991). Hope is related to better psychosocial functioning (Bluvol & Ford-Gilboe, 2004; Gilman, Dooley, & Florell, 2006), diminished stress reactivity and more effective coping (Ong, Edwards, & Bergeman, 2006), global life satisfaction, well-being, better quality of life (Bluvol & Ford-Gilboe, 2004; Gilman et al., 2006), constructive problem solving (Snyder et al., 1991), and growth from adversity (Tennen & Affeck, 1999). Hope is closely related to finding meaning in life and experiencing lower levels of anxiety and depression (Feldman & Snyder, 2005). Goal-specific hope is associated with goal attainment (Feldman, Rand, & Kahle-Wrobleski, 2009). Hope is seen as particularly important in stressful circumstances where an individual faces potential or actual losses (Dufault & Martocchio, 1985), recovery from serious injury (Barnum, Snyder, Rapoff, Mani, & Thompson, 1998; Elliott, Witty, Herrick, & Hoffman, 1991), and taking care of a child with chronic illness (Horton & Wallander, 2001). This chapter explores theories of hope and how they apply to health care settings, particularly in the impending loss of a beloved child.

Early theories and measures conceptualized hope in a very narrow sense as an expectancy that a specific outcome is possible (Erickson et al., 1975; Gottschalk, 1974; Stoner & Keampfer, 1985; Stotland, 1969). Other theories focused on the lack of hope or the lack of power or control over one's life, environment, or health (Beck et al., 1974; Mercer & Kane, 1979; Miller, 1992; Miller & Powers, 1988). Later theories argued that hope can either be linked to a specific outcome expectancy or be conceptualized as a broader sense that positive outcomes are possible in life and that life overall has meaning (Dufault & Martocchio, 1985; Farran, Wilken, & Popovich, 1992).

Hope as the Opposite of Hopelessness

Psychological theories often focused on psychopathology, such as depression and hopelessness, rather than hope. Beck's measure of hopelessness defined hopelessness as the lack of any positive expectations in the future (Beck et al., 1974). Seligman's theory of learned helplessness suggested individuals who learn that negative events are beyond their control are more likely to become depressed (Abramson, Seligman, & Teasdale, 1978; Seligman, 1972).

Mercer and Kane followed this paradigm when they attempted to lower the levels of hopelessness among nursing home residents by giving them more control over their environment (Mercer & Kane, 1979). The authors asked the residents in the intervention condition to choose a plant to take care of and encouraged them to participate in a resident council. The residents in the intervention condition showed lower levels of hopelessness and higher levels of activity after the intervention compared to a control condition. The authors noted that a subset of residents showed higher levels of hopelessness after the intervention and suggested the need to tailor interventions based on the needs of individual patients (Mercer & Kane, 1979).

Snyder's Hope Theory

One of the most popular theories and measures of hope in the field of psychology was developed by C. R. Snyder (Snyder et al., 1991). In Snyder's theory, hope is a set of goal-directed cognitive processes that influence and are influenced by emotion. The theory has two major parts. "Agency" is an individual's sense of being generally successful in meeting goals. "Pathways" is an individual's sense of being able to generate successful plans to achieve those goals (Snyder, 2000; Snyder et al., 1991). High-hope individuals have high levels of both agency and pathways, tend to generate more goals overall, are better at working to achieve their goals, are more likely to think of new ways of achieving a blocked goal, and are more likely to substitute another goal for a blocked goal (Irving, Snyder, & Crowson, 1998; Snyder et al., 1991; Snyder et al., 1996). High-hope individuals experience less negative and more positive emotion when they are unable to achieve a goal. In contrast, low-hope individuals are more likely to experience negative emotions after a setback, are more likely to give up, and are less able to set new goals. Snyder and others have shown that this measure of hope captures something separate from optimism and self-efficacy (Magaletta & Oliver, 1999; Snyder, 2002; Snyder et al., 1991).

Synder's hope theory has been supported by studies finding that high-hope individuals have better psychosocial outcomes after burn injuries (Barnum et al., 1998), report higher levels of well-being after the death of a loved one (Michael & Snyder, 2005), experience better adjustment after spinal cord injuries (Elliott et al., 1991), and are less likely to experience distress when taking care of children with chronic health conditions (Horton & Wallander, 2001).

Interventions to increase hopeful thinking usually take place in the context of individual or group psychotherapy for individuals seeking mental health treatment (Snyder, 1994). However, the theory has also been applied to other populations. In one study, people from the community who were interested in hope completed eight sessions of group therapy based on Snyder's theory of hope and reported higher levels of agency hope, improvements in perceived life meaning, higher self-esteem, and lower depression and anxiety (Cheavens, Feldman, Gum, Michael, & Snyder, 2006). After a 90-minute intervention involving a goal-mapping exercise based on Snyder's hope theory, college students showed a significant increase in hope, life purpose, vocational calling, and greater progress on a self-selected goal 1 month later (Feldman & Dreher, 2012).

HOPE IN HEALTH AND HEALTH CARE

Health care researchers have also recognized hope as an important topic, especially in nursing and oncology (Eliott, 2005; Feudtner et al., 2007; Hammer, Mogensen, & Hall, 2009; Owen, 1989; Poncar, 1994; Rustøen, 1995; Vaillot, 1970). Researchers have studied hope in the context of heart failure, lung cancer, cystic fibrosis, stroke, and many other health conditions (Berendes et al., 2010; Bluvol & Ford-Gilbe, 2004; Rustøen, Howie, Eidsmo,

& Moum, 2005; Rustoen, Wahl, Hanestad, Gjengedal, & Moum, 2004). Some researchers describe hope for seriously ill patients as both a resource and something to be protected, a valuable possession that can be threatened or supported by interactions with others (Eliott & Olver, 2009; Miller, 1991). Hope is described as a buffer for stress and as a prerequisite to effective coping that may predict better psychosocial outcomes while recovering from a serious illness (Herth, 1989; Rideout & Montemuro, 1986). Nurses and oncologists report that part of their role is to help patients and family members maintain hope (Clayton et al., 2008; Herth, 2000; Hinds, 1988; Miller, 1985; Vaillot, 1970). Some researchers have defined hope narrowly as a realistic expectation of recovering from an illness. Other researchers have used a broader definition of hope including aspects such as general well-being, relationships with others, spirituality, and a sense of overall purpose in life.

One of the most influential theories of hope in health care was developed by Dufault and Martocchio based on data from elderly cancer patients (Dufault & Martocchio, 1985). They defined hope as "a multidimensional dynamic life force characterized by confident yet uncertain expectation of achieving a future good which to the hoping person is realistically possible and personally significant" (p. 380). The authors suggested that hope is composed of two spheres (generalized and particularized) having six dimensions (affective, cognitive, behavioral, affiliative, temporal, and contextual). Particularized hopes are more specific hopes linked to a specific outcome, whereas generalized hopes are more of an overall attitude that things will turn out well. The authors suggested that generalized hope might protect a person from despair when a particular hope no longer seems realistic. Generalized hope consists not only of specific hopes but also of at least two dimensions. The affiliative dimension emphasizes that hopes often depend on relationships with others including health care providers, family, and friends, as well as transcendent relationships with a higher power such as God. The contextual dimension emphasizes that hopes often depend on the situation the person is including in his or her current health and well-being.

Miller presented another theory of hope in health care settings, which was influenced both by the work of Dufault and Martocchio and by the concept of powerlessness in chronic illness (Miller, 1992). Miller defined hope as "a state of being characterized by an anticipation for a continued good state, an improved state, or a release from a perceived entrapment" (Miller & Powers, 1988, p. 7). Miller and Powers noted that this anticipation may or may not be realistic and noted that relationships with others, a sense of personal competence, coping ability, psychological well-being, and purpose and meaning in life all play a role in hope (Miller & Powers, 1988). The authors developed a 40-item scale that measured 10 critical elements of hope: (1) mutuality-affiliation; (2) sense of the possible; (3) avoidance of absolutizing; (4) anticipation; (5) achieving goals; (6) psychological well-being and coping; (7) purpose and meaning in life; (8) freedom; (9) reality surveillance-optimism; and (10) mental and physical activation. They conducted a factor analysis that identified three factors: satisfaction with self, others, and life; avoidance of hope threats; and anticipation of a future. Other researchers have used Miller's Patient Power Resources Model (Miller, 1992) to design interventions including a small discussion group intervention for homeless veterans (Tollett & Thomas, 1995). Veterans who completed this intervention showed increased levels of hope, self-esteem, and lower levels of depression.

Hinds (1984, 1988) used grounded theory methodology to develop a theory of hope based on her interviews with well adolescents, adolescents being treated for substance abuse, and adolescents with cancer. Based on the interviews, she put forth a definition of hope as the degree to which an adolescent believes that a personal tomorrow exists for the self and others. She identified four hierarchical levels of hope from forced effort (artificially trying to adopt a positive view) to anticipation of a personal future (identifying specific and positive personal future possibilities) and developed a scale to measure these aspects of hope. Hinds also found that for adolescents in treatment for substance abuse, caring behaviors of nurses were associated with adolescent hopefulness (Hinds, 1988). In a study of adolescents with cancer, Hinds and Martin identified self-sustaining strategies adolescents used to maintain hope including keeping busy, reminding themselves that things could be worse, remembering they had made it this far, looking forward to normalcy, using distractions, relying on God, remembering the past, learning from other cancer survivors, and remembering that others have hope for them (Hinds & Martin, 1988).

The most commonly used measure of hope in health care settings was developed by Herth (Herth, 1991). The Herth Hope Scale is a 30-item scale based closely on Dufault and Martocchio's theory of hope (Herth, 1991). Items include spirituality, support from others, and purpose and meaningfulness of life. The scale measures three factors: temporality and future, positive readiness and expectancy, and interconnectedness. Herth also developed the Herth Hope Index, an abbreviated 12-item version of the Herth Hope Scale, which showed the same three factors (Herth, 1992). Herth found that among adult patients undergoing chemotherapy, hope was associated with coping and those who reported more interference from their family responsibilities reported lower levels of hope and coping (Herth, 1989). Herth and colleagues developed the Hope Intervention Program (HIP) based on this theory of hope. Patients with a first recurrence of cancer met for eight 2-hour group discussion sessions that covered different aspects of hope including seeking social support, value and belief clarification exercises, joy collages, cognitive strategies for maintaining hope, developing manageable goals, and spiritual and transcendent topics (Herth, 2000, 2001). The authors found that the intervention had a significant effect on hope and quality of life even after 9 months (Herth, 2000).

Rustøen and colleagues conducted a similar hope intervention for newly diagnosed cancer patients consisting of eight meetings, each 2 hours per week, and found a significant increase in hope and insignificant trend of increased quality of life (Rustøen & Hanestad, 1998; Rustøen, Wiklund, Hanestad, & Moum, 1998). The authors conducted the same intervention with other cancer patients and found that the hope intervention was associated with lower levels of psychological distress compared to baseline (Rustøen, Cooper, & Miaskowski, 2011).

Other clinicians have argued that hope can play an important role in managing other chronic or progressive illnesses (Kim, 1989; Miller, 1989). One study explored the idea that patients with chronic illness can experience hope in different ways (Kim, Kim, Schwartz-Barcott, & Zucker, 2006). This study classified patients as showing one of five different hope orientations (externalism, pragmatism, reality, future, and internalism) and further classified each orientation on two axes: future versus present and internal versus external (Kim et al., 2006).

Many caregivers report feeling overwhelmed and struggle to make sense of what is happening (Duggleby, Williams, Holtslander, Cunningham, & Wright, 2012). Researchers have argued that family members and caretakers can play an important role both in maintaining or reinforcing the hope of the patient and in maintaining their own hope (Duggleby et al., 2010; Miller, 1991). One study of caregivers of terminally ill patients found that caregivers reported a variety of strategies to maintain hope, that the physical and emotional comfort of the patient was key to maintaining hope among caregivers, and that lack of sleep and high fatigue were associated with lower levels of hope (Herth, 1993). Another study found that hope predicted higher quality of life both for stroke survivors and for their caregivers (Bluvol & Ford-Gilboe, 2004). Levels of caregiver and patient hope are important determinants of the level of burden experienced by caregivers (Lohne, Miaskowski, & Rustøen, 2012; Utne, Miaskowski, Paul, & Rustøen, 2013).

Concerns About False Hope

Some philosophers and clinicians describe hope as having a negative side, arising if hopes are unrealistic (Godfrey, 1987; Sokol, 2006). In the original ancient Greek myth, Pandora opens up a box and lets loose curses and troubles into the world. Hope is the last thing in the box. In the Western Christian–Judaic tradition, this hope is often seen as a gift to mankind to offset the curses. The ancient Greeks had a more jaded perspective on hope, often seeing it as one last curse to torment mankind with misleading illusions (Eliott, 2005; Godfrey, 1987; Shade, 2001). Psychologists have debated about the trade-off between the benefits of positive expectancies and the potential costs of unrealistic goals or wishful thinking (Taylor & Brown, 1988, 1994). Hope researchers have argued that this concern is often misplaced because hopeful thinking is associated with setting and attaining higher goals rather than simple denial and maladaptive wishful thinking (Snyder, Rand, King, Feldman, & Woodward, 2002). Many psychologists now agree that moderate positive expectancies can be beneficial, whereas extreme positive illusions or deep denial of potential negative outcomes could lead to more adverse health and well-being effects.

In the health care context, clinicians worry that unrealistic hopes or expectations for a miracle cure might be dangerous for patients, especially if unrealistic hope sets them up for future disappointment (Beavers & Kaslow, 1981; McGee, 1984; Reder & Serwint, 2009; Sokol, 2006; Tomko, 1985). The dangers of false hopes are particularly relevant to the next topic in this chapter, palliative care.

Hope and Palliative Care

Palliative care situations pose a unique challenge to the idea of promoting hopeful thinking. Patients receiving palliative care are typically not expected to make a full recovery. These patients may be facing a chronic condition that can be managed without ever being completely cured, resulting in a shortened life span, or they may be dying with no curative options left. These difficult circumstances may be when patients and their families are most vulnerable to despair and most in need of hope. But how can health care providers encourage hopeful thinking without misleading patients and their families about the seriousness of their condition?

In one of the most influential books on the experience of dying, Kübler-Ross noted that terminal patients who are still hoping for a cure often live longer and do better than those who have given up all hope (Kübler-Ross, 1970). Kübler-Ross suggests that in some cases, health care providers might appropriately preserve these false hopes for the sake of the patient. Snyder also tells an anecdotal story of a doctor who helps a dying patient achieve a dramatic improvement by deceiving the patient about the potential benefits of an experimental drug. Once the patient discovers that the drug has been proven to be ineffective, he loses hope and quickly dies (Snyder, 1994).

Many doctors once considered this kind of deception acceptable in the paternalistic model of medicine where the doctor was responsible for making the important medical decisions, and information that might upset the patient was normally withheld (Clayton, Butow, Arnold, & Tattersall, 2005). The current approach to medicine, however, places great emphasis on patient autonomy and shared decision making with patients (Davidson et al., 2007; Fiks & Jimenez, 2010; Madrigal et al., 2012; Stacey, Samant, & Bennett, 2008; White & Curtis, 2005), and health care providers can no longer justify deceiving their patients. Health care providers of patients at the end of life often report struggling to find the balance between being honest with their patients and not taking away their hope. Some health care providers emphasize the importance of distinguishing specific unrealistic hopes for a cure from other kinds of hopes that can be beneficial even if a patient is terminal (Clayton et al., 2008). Dying patients and their caregivers are often able to find other ways to be hopeful even after accepting that death is inevitable (Clayton et al., 2005; Clayton et al., 2008; Hexem, Mollen, Carroll, Lanctot, & Feudtner, 2011; Reder & Serwint, 2009). Terminally ill patients, parents of children with cancer, and health care providers agree that there are ways of fostering hope while giving an accurate prognosis and setting realistic goals (Clayton et al., 2005; Clayton et al., 2008; Mack et al., 2007; Salmon et al., 2012). Many patients and family members report appreciating honesty from doctors, finding it more upsetting when they suspect that the doctor is hiding something from them (Hagerty et al., 2005). Under these circumstances, hope changes but does not disappear (Feudtner, 2009). The focus may change from the future to simply "being" in the present (Herth, 1993). Some dying patients refer to hopes of leaving a legacy and maintaining or deepening their relationships with family and other loved ones (Eliott & Olver, 2009).

Clinicians often must find a balance between being honest with patients and their families about the seriousness of the situation and yet not necessarily challenging unrealistic hopes. In some cases, patients and family members may simply need time to adjust to the upsetting new reality. In other cases, patients and their families may have complex reasons for continuing to talk about miracle cures that are extremely unlikely. For example, some patients may talk about unrealistic cures not because they are in denial but because they do not want to let down their family members by giving up (Eliott & Olver, 2009).

Interventions to increase hope among caregivers of adults with terminal illness include having caregivers watch a video of other caregivers talking about strategies for maintaining hope and then having caregivers keep journals about their experiences for 2 weeks (Duggleby, Wright, et al., 2007). The authors reported that initial qualitative results showed higher levels of hope and quality of life for caregivers who participated in the intervention (Duggleby, Degner, et al., 2007). The authors designed a similar intervention for rural caregivers that involved watching a video about hope and caregivers and participating in a 2-week hope activity and reported increased hope and self-efficacy and reduced severity of loss and grief for caregivers (Duggleby et al., 2013).

PEDIATRIC PALLIATIVE CARE

Pediatric palliative care presents unique challenges for patients, families, and health care providers. Parents of seriously ill children confront an extremely difficult and, at times, emotionally overwhelming situation: Their child may die in the near future or live with a severely debilitating chronic condition, become medically fragile, and often require intensive medical treatment and technology to remain stable (Rosenberg et al., 2013). A child's illness can be traumatic to parents and other caregivers in many ways. First, parents must endure suffering associated with seeing the beloved child suffering. Second, parents experience the sadness of knowing the child may never get a chance to grow up and live a normal life. Third, parents feel powerless when they can do little to help their child. Fourth, parents feel they have failed to protect their child and find some way to make things better. Finally, some parents experience high levels of uncertainty when their child lives for years with a serious life-shortening chronic condition that can get worse at any time (Feudtner et al., 2002; Feudtner et al., 2011).

Parents report that hope is an important part of coping with this highly stressful situation (Carroll, Mollen, Aldridge, Hexem, & Feudtner, 2012; Reder & Serwint, 2009; Utne et al., 2013). In a study of both parental and provider hope during a high-risk pregnancy (Roscigno et al., 2012), researchers identified that parents used hope as an emotional motivator providing "energy to cope with recommended treatments" (p. 1236). Pediatric palliative care research has found that hope among parents is not as simple as believing their child's illness will be miraculously cured or being in denial about the severity of the illness. Parents of seriously ill children report wanting information about their child's prognosis even if that information is upsetting (Mack, Wolfe, Grier, Cleary, & Weeks, 2006). Receiving negative information about a child's prognosis does not necessarily lower hope among parents (Mack et al., 2007). Parents report continuing to hope for a miraculous recovery while being quite aware of the severity of the child's illness and sometimes while making practical preparations for the undesired outcome (Feudtner, 2009; Mack et al., 2007; Reder & Serwint, 2009).

Many authors have argued that hope can be a resource for parents of children and adolescents with potentially incurable cancer (Kylma & Juvakka, 2007). One recent study found that parents of children with difficult-to-treat cancer described hope as being both tenacious (they could stick to their hopes, no matter what happened) and tenuous (their hopes were undermined by barriers such as negative effects of the child's illness, negativity of others, and physical and emotional depletion experienced by parents) (Barrera et al., 2013). A study with the same population found that parent hopes changed over time, depending on changes in the child's health (Granek et al., 2013). Parents of children who were doing better than expected shifted to more future-oriented hopes over time, whereas parents of children who were not doing well focused on more immediate hopes such as hoping their child would not suffer or experience complications (Granek et al., 2013).

Pediatric palliative care providers also need to be aware that parents' hopes are influenced by complex factors that are not always obvious (Feudtner, 2007; Hill et al., 2013; Renjilian, Womer, Carroll, Kang, & Feudtner, 2013). Some parents are reluctant to discuss the possibility of withdrawing interventions that are no longer effective, because they perceive that even admitting that there is a possibility that their child may die is a form of giving up. These parents may believe that staying positive is vitally important even as they realize with increasing clarity that their child is unlikely to recover. Some parents report being relieved when someone else brings up the possibility that their child may die because the parents have been thinking about this, but did not want to be the first to say so. Other parents may angrily reject any discussion of their child's death, determined not to give up or risk that their child will receive insufficient care. In addition to wanting the best for their child, many parents are highly motivated by the idea of "doing as a good parent would do," which may include advocating for their child and making sure their child feels loved (Hinds et al., 2009; October, Fisher, Feudtner, & Hinds, 2014).

Hopeful thinking can be important for pediatric palliative care providers also. Pediatric palliative care providers often report experiencing distress as parents ask them to continue interventions that may be increasing the child's suffering, with little chance of benefit (Reder & Serwint, 2009). Some health care providers are uncomfortable discussing end-of-life issues with families and may feel as if they have failed. Health care providers who have higher levels of hopeful thinking themselves may be more comfortable discussing palliative care issues with families (Feudtner et al., 2007).

To our knowledge, there have been no interventions to increase hopeful thinking among parents of children receiving palliative care, but in the next section, we discuss a theoretical model that may lay the foundation for such interventions.

Hopeful Thinking and Regoaling in Pediatric Palliative Care

From our clinical experience of working with parents of children with serious illness, we believe that hopeful thinking and goals play an important role in helping parents cope with both the child's illness and the possibility of the child's death. In particular, hopeful thinking may help parents regoal or shift from one goal (or set of goals) to another goal (or set of goals) over time, investing in these new goals in ways that help positive adaptation to dire circumstances.

Commitment to valued personal goals or strivings that are meaningful and potentially attainable is associated with subjective well-being and life satisfaction (Brunstein, 1993; Emmons, 1986). Goals are also an important part of life schemes, cognitive representations of a person's life that provide a sense of order and purpose (Power, Swartzman, & Robinson, 2011). Individuals are motivated to meet personal goals, and perceived failure to make progress toward important goals can cause negative affect such as feelings of anxiety, dysphoria, or despair (Brunstein, 1993; Carver & Scheier, 1998; Klinger, 1975).

Parent hopes and goals may change over time as the child's condition changes (Granek et al., 2013). Some parents of children with serious illness are confronted with evidence that their initial goals (e.g., curing the condition and restoring their child to full health) are no longer realistic. At that point, these parents face a decision point with two potential paths. On the first path, parents may persist in the pursuit of their initial goals even though they are aware that the attainment of these goals is believed by members of the clinical team to no longer be realistic. On the second path, parents may relinquish their initial goals for the child's medical care and pursue a set of new goals viewed now as more achievable, appropriate, or desirable, such as managing the child's condition with the least amount of treatment-related pain or suffering, limiting exposure to some invasive or extreme interventions, and maintaining the child's quality of life.

We call the process in the second path "regoaling" and have developed a conceptual model of factors that may be relevant to the regoaling process including disengagement from goals, reengagement in new goals, positive and negative affect, and hopeful thinking (Figure 13.1A) (Hill et al., 2014). The model is based on past research findings that (a) individuals experience negative affect when highly valued goals are blocked (Carver & Scheier, 1998; Klinger, 1975); (b) disengaging from unrealistic goals may lead to positive outcomes (Wrosch, Amir, & Miller, 2011; Wrosch, Scheier, Carver, & Schulz, 2003); (c) positive affect can facilitate the ability to think of new ideas (Fredrickson, 2001); and (d) hopeful thinking can facilitate the ability to generate new goals when one goal is blocked (Snyder et al., 1991).

The proposed model suggests there are two processes underlying regoaling (Figure 13.1B): (a) critiquing and letting go of the initial goals (disengagement) and (b) generating new goals (reengagement). The model then identifies several factors that influence the critiquing of initial goals and the generation of new goals, including (a) negative affect, (b) positive affect, and (c) hopeful thinking (Figure 13.1C).

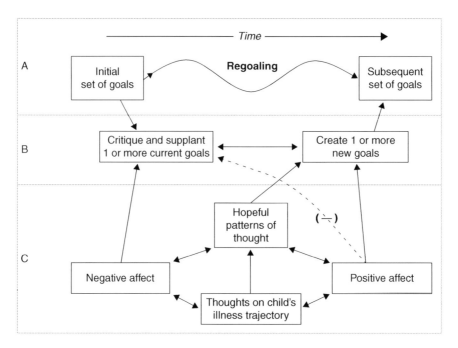

FIGURE 13.1 Regoaling process and underlying influential factors.
Source: Hill, Miller, Walter, Carroll, Morrison, Munson, and Feudtner (2014).

Our model begins with thoughts about the child's current illness trajectory (such as whether the child is getting better or worse; Figure 13.1C). If the child is getting better, the parent will be more likely to experience positive mood and less likely to question the initial set of goals. If the child's condition is getting worse, the parent will experience negative affect and be more likely to question their initial assumptions. Initially, the parents will increase their efforts to meet the initial goals and look for other treatments or approaches that will help the child. If these efforts fail, over time, some of these parents will be more likely to accept that their initial goals are unrealistic and start to disengage from them.

Some level of positive affect and hopeful thinking may help parents of seriously ill children manage the negative affect associated with giving up on a valued goal and help them start to think about new goals. A key assumption of our model is that both negative affect and positive affect are necessary for regoaling. Parents who experience only negative affect are more likely to be overwhelmed with despair and relinquish their initial goals related to their child's care without generating any new goals. Parents who experience only positive affect are unlikely to give up on their initial goals or consider new goals (hence, the negative dashed line between positive affect and critiquing initial goals).

In our model, we suggest that among parents of children with serious illness, parents with higher levels of hopeful thinking are more likely to disengage from initial goals, experience more positive affect, experience less negative affect, and generate new goals. Over time, this will be a reinforcing cycle. Experiencing some level of positive affect will increase hopeful thinking, hopeful thinking will increase the likelihood of generating new goals, and focusing on new goals will help reduce negative affect and increase positive affect, which in turn will increase hopeful thinking. This cycle leads to the transition from the initial set of goals to a new set of goals.

We found preliminary support for this model in a study of parents of children receiving palliative care (Feudtner et al., 2010). We observed that these parents had levels of hope comparable to other populations (i.e., patterns of hopeful thinking do not disappear even in the face of this grim situation; Feudtner et al., 2010). Our key finding was that, as the child's perceived health status worsened, parents with higher levels of hope (compared to parents with lower levels of hope) were more likely to decide to limit interventions, such as by having a do-not-attempt-resuscitation order (DNAR; Feudtner et al., 2010). These findings suggest that hopeful thinking is not a form of denial for these parents, and high-hope parents may be better at transitioning from one set of goals (such as "help my child recover") to another set of goals (such as "keep my child comfortable").

Hopeful Thinking and Bereavement

Parents who experience a balance of positive affect, negative affect, and hopeful thinking may also be better prepared if their child dies. The death of a child is a uniquely traumatic event, which can shatter parents' personal identity and self-concept (Uren & Wastell, 2002), elicit feelings of guilt and parental incompetence for their perceived failure to protect the child (Surkan et al., 2006), disrupt relationships with other family members, and challenge the parents' overall worldviews (Meert, Thurston, & Briller, 2005). Parents who experience the death of a child are at high risk for complicated grief (Field & Behrman, 2003), especially if the parents feel their needs and the needs of their child were not met by health care providers (Meert et al., 2012) or that their grief or sense of loss is not acknowledged by others (Reilly, Hastings, Vaughan, & Huws, 2008).

Research on how people cope with the death of a loved one has found that many individuals have two main coping strategies: sensemaking (trying to make sense of the death or finding meaning in it) and finding benefits (identifying good things that have happened since the loss such as personal growth or being closer to others; Davis & Nolen-Hoeksema, 2001; Davis, Nolen-Hoeksema, & Larson, 1998). Sensemaking seems to help individuals adjust to loss in the first 6 months, whereas benefit finding seems to be more helpful in the longer term (Davis & Nolen-Hoeksema, 2001; Davis et al., 1998). Some parents may experience posttraumatic growth after the death of a child (Picoraro, Womer, Kazak, & Feudtner, 2014).

Parents of deceased children often report a strong need for a continuing bond with the child, a desire to keep the child's memory alive, and attempts to find meaning in the child's death (Davies, 2004; Klass, 1993; Meert et al., 2005). Barrera and colleagues found that some parents were able to maintain their emotional bond with their child and continue to occasionally grieve in private for them without grief interfering with their ongoing lives (integrated grief), whereas other parents reported being overwhelmed by memories and feelings of sadness related to the deceased child that interfered with their lives and, in some cases, their ability to care for their surviving children (complicated grief; Barrera et al., 2007). These overwhelmed parents also reported feeling socially isolated and alone in their grief.

We suggest that hopeful thinking and regoaling may help parents cope with bereavement and experience integrated grief as opposed to complicated grief. Bereaved parents who are higher in patterns of hopeful thinking may be more likely to be able to make sense of their loss and identify benefits or positive things (no matter how small) that have happened since the death of their child. Bereaved caregivers who are able to make positive appraisals about the situation and set long-term goals are more likely to report positive well-being and better recovery 12 months after the death of a partner from AIDS (Stein, Folkman, Trabasso, & Richards, 1997). Research on hopeful thinking suggests that hopeful individuals would be more likely to make positive appraisals and set new long-term goals while experiencing the death of a loved one.

Another approach to helping parents with the bereavement process can unfold when palliative care providers open up a dialogue with parents regarding what the parents feel that they need to do to be a "good parent" in their own self-evaluation and then work with the parents to help them achieve those good parent goals (October et al., 2014). Parents who regret their decisions or feel that they did not do enough for their child may be likely to experience complicated grief. If palliative care providers are able to help parents see how they can meet their goal of being a good parent to their child up to the child's last breath, parents may cope better with the child's death, comforted by the knowledge that their child was loved and that the parents did everything they could for the child.

Many parents report finding hope and comfort in the idea that their child's life touched others and was meaningful. Families make a particular effort to keep the memory of the child alive by participating in ritual, creating and treasuring keepsakes, and helping the child be known by others (Davies, 2004; Klass, 1993). Some parents start nonprofits in memory of their children. Parents who are able to develop and pursue these kinds of long-term positive goals in memory of their child may be less likely to experience complicated grief. Over time, parents may be able to see the loss of their child, while still extremely painful and sad, as part of their life story that made them and others better people.

FUTURE DIRECTIONS

There are several possible strategies for helping parents of children with serious illness cope with this stressful situation and potentially engage in regoaling. One strategy already used by some pediatric palliative care providers is to explore the breadth of hopes that parents hold and gently guide parents toward new goals (Feudtner, 2007, 2009). Providers can do this by providing clear information about the child's condition, giving parents time to accept the news, acknowledging and supporting parents' emotional reactions ("I can see how hard this is"), and creating small positive experiences by praising parents and recognizing how much they are doing ("I can see how much you and your husband care about your son"; Back, Arnold, Baile, Edwards, & Tulsky, 2010). When parents seem ready, providers can carefully prompt them to think about new hopes and goals by asking what they are hoping for, given the current situation. Some parents may immediately identify other goals, such as taking the child home, reducing the number of painful interventions, or having a baptism. Others may need time to think of new goals. Providers may be able to provide suggestions ("What some loving families have done in this situation is . . .") or cocreate goals ("If that doesn't work out, then what would you hope for?"). Once parents start to talk about additional hopes or goals, providers can focus on the most realistic possibilities and offer suggestions of how those goals can be achieved. They can help these parents achieve hopeful thinking by supporting both pathways ("Here are ways you can achieve this goal, and here is how we can help") and agency ("I know this is hard, but you will be able to do this"). In particular, pediatric palliative care providers can help parents identify what it means to them personally to be a good parent to their child in this difficult situation and how they can meet their good parent goals as the child gets closer to death (Hinds et al., 2009; October et al., 2014).

Specific interventions could also be designed to promote hopeful thinking among parents taking care of dying children. Based on Duggleby's work with caregivers of adult patients, parents could be asked to watch a video where other parents of children with serious illness describe their experiences, keep journals about their own experiences, or start a hope collection (Duggleby, Degner, et al., 2007; Duggleby et al., 2013; Duggleby & Williams,

2010; Duggleby, Wright, et al., 2007). Parents could also be asked to complete a goal-mapping exercise where they would identify specific, realistic goals they could achieve and plans of how they would achieve those goals (Feldman & Dreher, 2012).

A more general approach that might be effective with parents in pediatric palliative care settings and other parents of sick children is having them learn strategies for managing their stress such as listening to mindfulness mediation recordings, which have been used successfully with adult patients (Altschuler, Rosenbaum, Gordon, Canales, & Avins, 2012). Parents could also be asked to participate in general well-being interventions that have been used with other populations (Lyubomirsky, Dickerhoof, Boehm, & Sheldon, 2011; Mongrain & Anselmo-Matthews, 2012; Ramachandra, Booth, Pieters, Vrotsou, & Huppert, 2009; Seligman, Steen, Park, & Peterson, 2005). Implementing these kinds of interventions would be challenging, as parents of sick children have very limited time and resources and are often unable to participate in or complete interventions (Drotar, 2005; Hocking et al., 2014).

CONCLUSION

In this chapter, we presented theories that hope and hopeful thinking are an essential part of life, and even more so in the darkest of times when parents face the death of their beloved child. It is difficult to find hope in the face of such a terrible loss, but pediatric palliative care providers may be able to help parents find new forms of hopeful thinking as they are taking care of their child and lay the foundation for a healthier bereavement process in which the memory of the child is cherished rather than a source of despair.

CASE STUDY

Cara is a 4-year-old child who has leukemia and is seriously ill. Cara is hospitalized at a large, metropolitan hospital 2 hours away from her family's home for the eighth time this year. Her mother is becoming increasingly weary due to being far from home and away from her other children. She expressed concern that staying near the hospital is expensive, and she feels alone because her family is not with her. Yet, she is grateful that she has the opportunity to bring Cara to this medical center. Cara's doctors were confident that they were offering her the best chance for recovery and were working with social services to ease the burden on Cara's family. After Cara's last two admissions, however, Cara's medical team became concerned that Cara was not responding to treatments as well as she had previously. The team plans to meet with Cara's mother this afternoon.

FOCUS QUESTIONS

1. What are the most important points of discussion to be raised with Cara's mother during the team meeting?
2. What is the best approach to initiating a conversation with Cara's mother about hopes and goals of care?
3. How can hopes be encouraged in this situation?
4. How can Cara's mother be encouraged to set new hopes/goals and remain hopeful?

REFERENCES

Abramson, L. Y., Seligman, M. E., & Teasdale, J. D. (1978). Learned helplessness in humans: Critique and reformulation. *Journal of Abnormal Psychology, 87*(1), 49–74. doi: http://dx.doi.org/10.1037/0021-843X.87.1.49

Altschuler, A., Rosenbaum, E., Gordon, P., Canales, S., & Avins, A. L. (2012). Audio recordings of mindfulness-based stress reduction training to improve cancer patients' mood and quality of life—a pilot feasibility study. *Supportive Care in Cancer, 20*(6), 1291–1297. doi: 10.1007/s00520-011-1216-7

Back, A. L., Arnold, R. M., Baile, W. F., Edwards, K. A., & Tulsky, J. A. (2010). The art of medicine: When praise is worth considering in a difficult conversation. *The Lancet, 376*(9744), 866–867. doi: http://dx.doi.org/10.1016/S0140-6736(10)61401-8

Barnum, D. D., Snyder, C. R., Rapoff, M. A., Mani, M. M., & Thompson, R. (1998). Hope and social support in the psychological adjustment of children who have survived burn injuries and their matched controls. *Children's Health Care, 27*(1), 15–30. doi: 10.1207/s15326888chc2701_2

Barrera, M., D'Agostino, N. M., Scneiderman, G., Tallett, S., Spencer, L., & Jovcevska, V. (2007). Patterns of parental bereavement following the loss of a child and related factors. *Omega: Journal of Death and Dying, 55*(2), 145–167. doi: http://dx.doi.org/10.2190/OM.55.2.d

Barrera, M., Granek, L., Shaheed, J., Nicholas, D., Beaune, L., D'Agostino, N. M., . . . Antle, B. (2013). The tenacity and tenuousness of hope: Parental experiences of hope when their child has a poor cancer prognosis. *Cancer Nursing, 36*(5), 408–416. doi: 10.1097/NCC.0b013e318291ba7d

Beavers, W. R., & Kaslow, F. W. (1981). The anatomy of hope. *Journal of Marital and Family Therapy, 7*(2), 119–126. doi: http://dx.doi.org/10.1111/j.1752-0606.1981.tb01361.x

Beck, A. T., Weissman, A., Lester, D., & Trexler, L. (1974). The measurement of pessimism: The hopelessness scale. *Journal of Consulting and Clinical Psychology, 42*(6), 861–865. doi: http://dx.doi.org/10.1037/h0037562

Berendes, D., Keefe, F. J., Somers, T. J., Kothadia, S. M., Porter, L. S., & Cheavens, J. S. (2010). Hope in the context of lung cancer: Relationships of hope to symptoms and psychological distress. *Journal of Pain and Symptom Management, 40*(2), 174–182. doi: 10.1016/j.jpainsymman.2010.01.014

Bluvol, A., & Ford-Gilboe, M. (2004). Hope, health work and quality of life in families of stroke survivors. [Research Support, Non-U.S. Gov't]. *Journal of Advanced Nursing, 48*(4), 322–332. doi: 10.1111/j.1365-2648.2004.03004.x

Brunstein, J. C. (1993). Personal goals and subjective well-being: A longitudinal study. *Journal of Personality and Social Psychology, 65*(5), 1061–1070. doi: 10.1037/0022-3514.65.5.1061

Carroll, K. W., Mollen, C. J., Aldridge, S., Hexem, K. R., & Feudtner, C. (2012). Influences on decision making identified by parents of children receiving pediatric palliative care. *AJOB Primary Research, 3*(1), 1–7.

Carver, C. S., & Scheier, M. F. (1998). *On the self-regulation of behavior.* New York, NY: Cambridge University Press.

Cheavens, J. S., Feldman, D. B., Gum, A., Michael, S. T., & Snyder, C. R. (2006). Hope therapy in a community sample: A pilot investigation. *Social Indicators Research, 77*(1), 61–78. doi: http://dx.doi.org/10.1007/s11205-005-5553-0

Clayton, J. M., Butow, P. N., Arnold, R. M., & Tattersall, M. H. (2005). Fostering coping and nurturing hope when discussing the future with terminally ill cancer patients and their caregivers. *Cancer, 103*(9), 1965–1975. doi: 10.1002/cncr.21011

Clayton, J. M., Hancock, K., Parker, S., Butow, P. N., Walder, S., Carrick, S., . . . Tattersall, M. H. (2008). Sustaining hope when communicating with terminally ill patients and their families: A systematic review. *Psycho-Oncology, 17*(7), 641–659. doi: 10.1002/pon.1288

Davidson, J. E., Powers, K., Hedayat, K. M., Tieszen, M., Kon, A. A., Shepard, E., . . . Armstrong, D. (2007). Clinical practice guidelines for support of the family in the patient-centered intensive care unit: American college of critical care medicine task force 2004-2005. *Critical Care Medicine, 35*(2), 605–622. doi: 10.1097/01.CCM.0000254067.14607.EB

Davies, R. (2004). New understandings of parental grief: Literature review. [Review]. *Journal of Advanced Nursing, 46*(5), 506–513. doi: 10.1111/j.1365-2648.2004.03024.x

Davis, C. G., & Nolen-Hoeksema, S. (2001). Loss and meaning: How do people make sense of loss? *American Behavioral Scientist, 44*(5), 726–741. doi: http://dx.doi.org/10.1177/00027640121956467

Davis, C. G., Nolen-Hoeksema, S., & Larson, J. (1998). Making sense of loss and benefiting from the experience: Two construals of meaning. *Journal of Personality and Social Psychology, 75*(2), 561–574. doi: http://dx.doi.org/10.1037/0022-3514.75.2.561

Drotar, D. (2005). Commentary: Involving families in psychological interventions in pediatric psychology: Critical needs and dilemmas. *Journal of Pediatric Psychology, 30*(8), 689–693. doi: 10.1093/jpepsy/jsi056

Dufault, K., & Martocchio, B. C. (1985). Symposium on compassionate care and the dying experience. Hope: Its spheres and dimensions. *The Nursing Clinics of North America, 20*(2), 379–391.

Duggleby, W., Degner, L., Williams, A., Wright, K., Cooper, D., Popkin, D., & Holtslander, L. (2007). Living with hope: Initial evaluation of a psychosocial hope intervention for older palliative home care patients. *Journal of Pain and Symptom Management, 33*(3), 247–257. doi: 10.1016/j.jpainsymman.2006.09.013

Duggleby, W., Holtslander, L., Kylma, J., Duncan, V., Hammond, C., & Williams, A. (2010). Metasynthesis of the hope experience of family caregivers of persons with chronic illness. *Qualitative Health Research, 30*(2), 148–158.

Duggleby, W., & Williams, A. M. (2010). Living with hope: Developing a psychosocial supportive program for rural women caregivers of persons with advanced cancer. *BMC Palliative Care, 9*, 3. doi: 10.1186/1472-684X-9-3

Duggleby, W., Williams, A., Holstlander, L., Cooper, D., Ghosh, S., Hallstrom, L. K., . . . Hampton, M. (2013). Evaluation of the living with hope program for rural women caregivers of persons with advanced cancer. *BMC Palliative Care, 12*(1), 36. doi: 10.1186/1472-684X-12-36

Duggleby, W., Williams, A., Holtslander, L., Cunningham, S., & Wright, K. (2012). The chaos of caregiving and hope. *Qualitative Social Work, 11*(5), 459–469. doi: 10.1177/1473325011404622

Duggleby, W., Wright, K., Williams, A., Degner, L., Cammer, A., & Holtslander, L. (2007). Developing a living with hope program for caregivers of family members with advanced cancer. *Journal of Palliative Care, 23*(1), 24–31.

Eliott, J. A. (2005). What have we done with hope? A brief history. *Interdisciplinary perspectives on hope* (pp. 3–45). Hauppauge, NY: Nova Science Publishers.

Eliott, J. A., & Olver, I. N. (2009). Hope, life, and death: A qualitative analysis of dying cancer patients' talk about hope. [Article]. *Death Studies, 33*(7), 609–638. doi: 10.1080/07481180903011982

Elliott, T. R., Witty, T. E., Herrick, S. M., & Hoffman, J. T. (1991). Negotiating reality after physical loss: Hope, depression, and disability. *Journal of Personality and Social Psychology, 61*(4), 608–613. doi: 10.1037/0033-2909.103.2.193

Emmons, R. A. (1986). Personal strivings: An approach to personality and subjective well-being. *Journal of Personality and Social Psychology, 51*(5), 1058–1068. doi: http://dx.doi.org/10.1037/0022-3514.51.5.1058

Erickson, R. C., Post, R. D., & Paige, A. B. (1975). Hope as a psychiatric variable. *Journal of Clinical Psychology, 31*(2), 324–330. doi: http://proxy.library.upenn.edu:2092/10.1002/1097-4679(197504)31:2

Erikson, E. H. (1964). *Insight and responsibility: Lectures on the ethical implications of psycoanalytic insight.* New York, NY: W.W. Norton and Co.

Farran, C. J., Wilken, C., & Popovich, J. M. (1992). Clinical assessment of hope. *Issues in Mental Health Nursing, 13*, 129–138.

Feldman, D. B., & Dreher, D. E. (2012). Can hope be changed in 90 minutes? Testing the efficacy of a single-session goal-pursuit intervention for college students. *Journal of Happiness Studies, 13*(4), 745–759. doi: http://dx.doi.org/10.1007/s10902-011-9292-4

Feldman, D. B., Rand, K. L., & Kahle-Wrobleski, K. (2009). Hope and goal attainment: Testing a basic prediction of hope theory. *Journal of Social and Clinical Psychology, 28*(4), 479–497. doi: http://dx.doi.org/10.1521/jscp.2009.28.4.479

Feldman, D. B., & Snyder, C. R. (2005). Hope and the meaningful life: Theoretical and empirical associations between goal-directed thinking and life meaning. *Journal of Social and Clinical Psychology, 24*(3), 401–421. doi: http://dx.doi.org/10.1521/jscp.24.3.401.65616

Feudtner, C. (2007). Collaborative communication in pediatric palliative care: A foundation for problem-solving and decision-making. *Pediatric Clinics of North America, 54*(5), 583–607, ix. doi: 10.1016/j.pcl.2007.07.008

Feudtner, C. (2009). The breadth of hopes. *The New England Journal of Medicine, 361*(24), 2306–2307. doi: 10.1056/NEJMp0906516

Feudtner, C., Carroll, K. W., Hexem, K. R., Silberman, J., Kang, T. I., & Kazak, A. E. (2010). Parental hopeful patterns of thinking, emotions, and pediatric palliative care decision making: A prospective cohort study. *Archives of Pediatrics & Adolescent Medicine, 164*(9), 831–839. doi: 10.1001/archpediatrics.2010.146

Feudtner, C., Christakis, D. A., Zimmerman, F. J., Muldoon, J. H., Neff, J. M., & Koepsell, T. D. (2002). Characteristics of deaths occurring in children's hospitals: Implications for supportive care services. *Pediatrics, 109*(5), 887–893.

Feudtner, C., Kang, T. I., Hexem, K. R., Friedrichsdorf, S. J., Osenga, K., Siden, H., . . . Wolfe, J. (2011). Pediatric palliative care patients: A prospective multicenter cohort study. *Pediatrics, 127*(6), 1094–1101. doi: 10.1542/peds.2010-3225

Feudtner, C., Santucci, G., Feinstein, J. A., Snyder, C. R., Rourke, M. T., & Kang, T. I. (2007). Hopeful thinking and level of comfort regarding providing pediatric palliative care: A survey of hospital nurses. *Pediatrics, 119*(1), e186–e192. doi: 10.1542/peds.2006-1048

Field, M. J., & Behrman, R. E. (Eds.). (2003). *When children die: Improving palliative care and end-of-life care for children and their families*. Washington, DC: The National Academies Press.

Fiks, A. G., & Jimenez, M. E. (2010). The promise of shared decision-making in paediatrics. *Acta Paediatrica, 99*(10), 1464–1466. doi: 10.1111/j.1651-2227.2010.01978.x

Fredrickson, B. L. (2001). The role of positive emotions in positive psychology. The broaden-and-build theory of positive emotions. *American Psychologist, 56*(3), 218–226.

Fromm, E. (1968). *The revolution of hope: Towards a humanized technology*. New York, NY: Harper and Row.

Gilman, R., Dooley, J., & Florell, D. (2006). Relative levels of hope and their relationship with academic and psychological indicators among adolescents. *Journal of Social and Clinical Psychology, 25*(2), 166–178. doi: http://dx.doi.org/10.1521/jscp.2006.25.2.166

Godfrey, J. J. (1987). *A philosophy of human hope*. Dordrecht, The Netherlands: Kluwer.

Gottschalk, L. A. (1974). A hope scale applicable to verbal samples. *Archives of General Psychiatry, 30*(6), 779–785. doi: http://dx.doi.org/10.1001/archpsyc.1974.01760120041007

Granek, L., Barrera, M., Shaheed, J., Nicholas, D., Beaune, L., D'Agostino, N., . . . Antle, B. (2013). Trajectory of parental hope when a child has difficult-to-treat cancer: A prospective qualitative study. *Psycho-Oncology, 22*(11), 2436–2444. doi: 10.1002/pon.3305

Hagerty, R. G., Butow, P. N., Ellis, P. M., Lobb, E. A., Pendlebury, S. C., Leighl, N., . . . Tattersall, M. H. (2005). Communicating with realism and hope: Incurable cancer patients' views on the disclosure of prognosis. *Journal of Clinical Oncology 23*(6), 1278–1288. doi: 10.1200/JCO.2005.11.138

Hammer, K., Mogensen, O., & Hall, E. O. (2009). The meaning of hope in nursing research: A meta-synthesis. *Scandinavian Journal of Caring Sciences, 23*(3), 549–557. doi: 10.1111/j.1471-6712.2008.00635.x

Herth, K. (1989). The relationship between level of hope and level of coping response and other variables in patients with cancer. *Oncology Nursing Forum, 16*(1), 67–72.

Herth, K. (1991). Development and refinement of an instrument to measure hope. *Scholarly Inquiry for Nursing Practice, 5*(1), 39–51; discussion 53–36.

Herth, K. (1992). Abbreviated instrument to measure hope: Development and psychometric evaluation. *Journal of Advanced Nursing, 17*(10), 1251–1259.

Herth, K. (1993). Hope in the family caregiver of terminally ill people. *Journal of Advanced Nursing, 18*, 538–548.

Herth, K. (2000). Enhancing hope in people with a first recurrence of cancer. *Journal of Advanced Nursing, 32*(6), 1431–1441.

Herth, K. (2001). Development and implementation of a hope intervention program. *Oncology Nursing Forum, 28*(6), 1009–1017.

Hexem, K. R., Mollen, C. J., Carroll, K., Lanctot, D. A., & Feudtner, C. (2011). How parents of children receiving pediatric palliative care use religion, spirituality, or life philosophy in tough times. *Journal of Palliative Medicine, 14*(1), 39–44. doi: 10.1089/jpm.2010.0256

Hill, D. L., Miller, V. A., Hexem, K. R., Carroll, K. W., Faerber, J. A., Kang, T., & Feudtner, C. (2013). Problems and hopes perceived by mothers, fathers and physicians of children receiving palliative care. *Health Expectations.* Retrieved from http://www.ncbi.nlm.nih.gov/pmc/articles/PMC3796017/pdf/nihms475464.pdf. doi: 10.1111/hex.12078

Hill, D. L., Miller, V., Walter, J. K., Carroll, K. W., Morrison, W. E., Munson, D. A., . . . Feudtner, C. (2014). Regoaling: A conceptual model of how parents of children with serious illness change medical care goals. *BMC Palliative Care, 13*(1), 9. doi: 10.1186/1472-684X-13-9

Hinds, P. S. (1984). Inducing a definition of 'hope' through the use of grounded theory methodology. *Journal of Advanced Nursing, 9*(4), 357–362.

Hinds, P. S. (1988). The relationship of nurses' caring behaviors with hopefulness and health care outcomes in adolescents. *Archives of Psychiatric Nursing, 2*(1), 21–29.

Hinds, P. S., & Martin, J. (1988). Hopefulness and the self-sustaining process in adolescents with cancer. *Nursing Research, 37*(6), 336–340.

Hinds, P. S., Oakes, L. L., Hicks, J., Powell, B., Srivastava, D. K., Spunt, S. L., . . . Furman, W. L. (2009). "Trying to be a good parent" as defined by interviews with parents who made phase 1, terminal care, and resuscitation decisions for their children. *Journal of Clinical Oncology, 27*(35), 5979–5985. doi: 10.1200/JCO.2008.20.0204

Hocking, M. C., Kazak, A. E., Schneider, S., Barkman, D., Barakat, L. P., & Deatrick, J. A. (2014). Parent perspectives on family-based psychosocial interventions in pediatric cancer: A mixed-methods approach. *Supportive Care in Cancer, 22*(5), 1287–1294. doi: 10.1007/s00520-013-2083-1

Horton, T. V., & Wallander, J. L. (2001). Hope and social support as resilience factors against psychological distress of mothers who care for children with chronic physical conditions. *Rehabilitation Psychology, 46*(4), 382–399. doi: 10.1037/0090-5550.46.4.382

Irving, L. M., Snyder, C. R., & Crowson, J. J. (1998). Hope and coping with cancer by college women. *Journal of Personality, 66*(2), 195–214. doi: 10.1111/1467-6494.00009

Kim, D. S., Kim, H. S., Schwartz-Barcott, D., & Zucker, D. (2006). The nature of hope in hospitalized chronically ill patients. *International Journal of Nursing Studies, 43*, 547–556.

Kim, T. S. (1989). Hope as a mode of coping in amyotrophic lateral sclerosis. *The Journal of Neuroscience Nursing, 21*(6), 342–347.

Klass, D. (1993). Solace and immortality: Bereaved parents' continuing bond with their children. *Death Studies, 17*(4), 343–368. doi: http://dx.doi.org/10.1080/07481189308252630

Klinger, E. (1975). Consequences of commitment to and disengagement from incentives. *Psychological Review, 82*(1), 1–25.

Kübler-Ross, E. (1970). *On death and dying.* New York, NY: Collier Books/Macmillan Publishing Co.

Kylma, J., & Juvakka, T. (2007). Hope in parents of adolescents with cancer-factors endangering and engendering parental hope. *European Journal of Oncology Nursing, 11*(3), 262–271. doi: 10.1016/j.ejon.2006.06.007

Lohne, V., Miaskowski, C., & Rustoen, T. (2012). The relationship between hope and caregiver strain in family caregivers of patients with advanced cancer. *Cancer Nursing, 35*(2), 99–105.

Lynch, W. F. (1974). *Images of hope.* Notre Dame, IN: University of Notre Dame Press.

Lyubomirsky, S., Dickerhoof, R., Boehm, J. K., & Sheldon, K. M. (2011). Becoming happier takes both a will and a proper way: An experimental longitudinal intervention to boost well-being. *Emotion, 11*(2), 391–402. doi: http://dx.doi.org/10.1037/a0022575

Mack, J. W., Wolfe, J., Cook, E. F., Grier, H. E., Cleary, P. D., & Weeks, J. C. (2007). Hope and prognostic disclosure. *Journal of Clinical Oncology, 25*(35), 5636–5642. doi: 10.1200/JCO.2007.12.6110

Mack, J. W., Wolfe, J., Grier, H. E., Cleary, P. D., & Weeks, J. C. (2006). Communication about prognosis between parents and physicians of children with cancer: Parent preferences and the impact of prognostic information. *Journal of Clinical Oncology, 24*(33), 5265–5270. doi: 10.1200/JCO.2006.06.5326

Madrigal, V. N., Carroll, K. W., Hexem, K. R., Faerber, J. A., Morrison, W. E., & Feudtner, C. (2012). Parental decision-making preferences in the pediatric intensive care unit. *Critical Care Medicine, 40*(10), 2876–2882. doi: 10.1097/CCM.0b013e31825b9151

Magaletta, P. R., & Oliver, J. M. (1999). The hope construct, will, and ways: Their relations with self-efficacy, optimism, and general well-being. *Journal of Clinincal Psychology, 55*(5), 539–551.

McGee, R. F. (1984). Hope: A factor influencing crisis resolution. *Advances in Nursing Science, 6*(4), 34–44.

Meert, K. L., Templin, T. N., Michelson, K. N., Morrison, W. E., Hackbarth, R., Custer, J. R., . . . Thurston, C. S. (2012). The bereaved parent needs assessment: A new instrument to assess the needs of parents whose children died in the pediatric intensive care unit. *Critical Care Medicine, 40*(11), 3050–3057. doi: 10.1097/CCM.0b013e31825fe164

Meert, K. L., Thurston, C. S., & Briller, S. H. (2005). The spiritual needs of parents at the time of their child's death in the pediatric intensive care unit and during bereavement: A qualitative study. *Pediatric Critical Care Medicine, 6*(4), 420–427. doi: 10.1097/01.PCC.0000163679.87749.CA

Mercer, S., & Kane, R. A. (1979). Helplessness and hopelessness among the institutionalized aged: An experiment. *Health and Social Work, 4*(1), 90–116.

Michael, S. T., & Snyder, C. R. (2005). Getting unstuck: The roles of hope, finding meaning, and rumination in the adjustment to bereavement among college students. *Death Studies, 29*(5), 435–458. doi: 10.1080/07481180590932544

Miller, J. F. (1985). Inspiring hope. *The American Journal of Nursing, 85*(1), 22–25.

Miller, J. F. (1989). Hope-inspiring strategies of the critically ill. *Applied Nursing Research, 2*(1), 23–29.

Miller, J. F. (1991). Developing and maintaining hope in families of the critically ill. *AACN Clinical Issues in Critical Care Nursing, 2*(2), 307–315.

Miller, J. F. (1992). *Coping with chronic illness: Overcoming powerlessness* (2nd ed.). Philadelphia, PA: F.A. Davis.

Miller, J. F., & Powers, M. J. (1988). Development of an instrument to measure hope. *Nursing Research, 37*(1), 6–10.

Mongrain, M., & Anselmo-Matthews, T. (2012). Do positive psychology exercises work? A replication of Seligman et al. (2005). *Journal of Clinical Psychology, 68*(4), 382–389. doi: http://dx.doi.org/10.1002/jclp.21839

October, T. W., Fisher, K. R., Feudtner, C., & Hinds, P. S. (2014). The parent perspective: "Being a good parent" when making critical decisions in the picu. *Pediatric Critical Care Medicine, 15*(4), 291–298. doi: 10.1097/PCC.0000000000000076

Ong, A. D., Edwards, L. M., & Bergeman, C. S. (2006). Hope as a source of resilience in later adulthood. *Personality and Individual Differences, 41*(7), 1263–1273. doi: http://dx.doi.org/10.1016/j.paid.2006.03.028

Owen, D. C. (1989). Nurses' perspectives on the meaning of hope in patients with cancer: A qualitative study. *Oncology Nursing Forum, 16*(1), 75–79.

Picoraro, J. A., Womer, J. W., Kazak, A. E., & Feudtner, C. (2014). Posttraumatic growth in parents and pediatric patients. *Journal of Palliative Medicine, 17*(2), 209–218. doi: 10.1089/jpm.2013.0280

Poncar, P. J. (1994). Inspiring hope in the oncology patient. *Journal of Psychosocial Nursing and Mental Health Services, 32*(1), 33–38.

Power, T. E., Swartzman, L. C., & Robinson, J. W. (2011). Cognitive-emotional decision making (cedm): A framework of patient medical decision making. *Patient Education and Counseling, 83*(2), 163–169. doi: 10.1016/j.pec.2010.05.021

Ramachandra, P., Booth, S., Pieters, T., Vrotsou, K., & Huppert, F. A. (2009). A brief self-administered psychological intervention to improve well-being in patients with cancer: Results from a feasibility study. *Psycho-Oncology, 18*(12), 1323–1326. doi: 10.1002/pon.1516

Reder, E. A., & Serwint, J. R. (2009). Until the last breath: Exploring the concept of hope for parents and health care professionals during a child's serious illness. *Archives Pediatrics & Adolescent Medicine, 163*(7), 653–657. doi: 10.1001/archpediatrics.2009.87

Reilly, D. E., Hastings, R. P., Vaughan, F. L., & Huws, J. C. (2008). Parental bereavement and the loss of a child with intellectual disabilities: A review of the literature. *Intellectual and Developmental Disabilities, 46*(1), 27–43. doi: http://dx.doi.org/10.1352/0047-6765(2008)46%5B27:PBATLO%5D2.0.CO;2

Renjilian, C. B., Womer, J. W., Carroll, K. W., Kang, T. I., & Feudtner, C. (2013). Parental explicit heuristics in decision-making for children with life-threatening illnesses. *Pediatrics, 131*(2), e566–e572. doi: 10.1542/peds.2012-1957

Rideout, E., & Montemuro, M. (1986). Hope, morale and adaptation in patients with chronic heart failure. *Journal of Advanced Nursing, 11*(4), 429–438.

Roscigno, C. I., Savage, T. A., Kavanaugh, K., Moro, T. T., Kilpatrick, S. J., Strassner, H. T., . . . Kimura, R. E. (2012). Divergent views of hope influencing communications between parents and hospital providers. *Qualitative Health Research, 22*(9), 1232–1246. doi: 10.1177/1049732312449210

Rosenberg, A. R., Dussel, V., Kang, T., Geyer, J. R., Gerhardt, C. A., Feudtner, C., & Wolfe, J. (2013). Psychological distress in parents of children with advanced cancer. *JAMA Pediatrics, 167*(6), 537–543. doi: 10.1001/jamapediatrics.2013.628

Rustøen, T. (1995). Hope and quality of life, two central issues for cancer patients: A theoretical analysis. *Cancer Nursing, 18*(5), 355–361.

Rustøen, T., Cooper, B. A., & Miaskowski, C. (2011). A longitudinal study of the effects of a hope intervention on levels of hope and psychological distress in a community-based sample of oncology patients. *European Journal of Oncology Nursing, 15*(4), 351–357. doi: 10.1016/j.ejon.2010.09.001

Rustøen, T., & Hanestad, B. R. (1998). Nursing intervention to increase hope in cancer patients. *Journal of Clinical Nursing, 7*, 19–27.

Rustøen, T., Howie, J., Eidsmo, I., & Moum, T. (2005). Hope in patients hospitalized with heart failure. *American Journal of Critical Care, 14*(5), 417–425.

Rustøen, T., Wahl, A. K., Hanestad, B. R., Gjengedal, E., & Moum, T. (2004). Expressions of hope in cystic fibrosis patients: A comparison with the general population. *Heart & Lung: The Journal of Critical Care, 33*(2), 111–118. doi: 10.1016/j.hrtlng.2003.12.003

Rustøen, T., Wiklund, I., Hanestad, B. R., & Moum, T. (1998). Nursing intervention to increase hope and quality of life in newly diagnosed cancer patients. *Cancer Nursing, 21*(4), 235–245.

Salmon, P., Hill, J., Ward, J., Gravenhorst, K., Eden, T., & Young, B. (2012). Faith and protection: The construction of hope by parents of children with leukemia and their oncologists. *The Oncologist, 17*(3), 398–404. doi: 10.1634/theoncologist.2011-0308

Seligman, M. E. (1972). Learned helplessness. *Annual Review of Medicine, 23*(1), 207–412.

Seligman, M. E., Steen, T. A., Park, N., & Peterson, C. (2005). Positive psychology progress: Empirical validation of interventions. *American Psychologist, 60*(5), 410–421. doi: http://dx.doi.org/10.1037/0003-066X.60.5.410

Shade, P. (2001). *Habits of hope: A pragmatic theory.* Nashville, TN: Vanderbilt University Press.

Snyder, C. R. (1994). *The psychology of hope: You can get there from here.* New York, NY: The Free Press.

Snyder, C. R. (2002). Hope theory: Rainbows in the mind. *Psychological Inquiry, 13*(4), 249–275. doi: 10.1037/0021-843x.87.1.49

Snyder, C. R. (Ed.). (2000). *Handbook of hope: Theory, measures, and applications.* San Diego, CA: Academic.

Snyder, C. R., Harris, C., Anderson, J. R., Holleran, S. A., Irving, L. M., Sigmon, S. T., . . . Harney, P. (1991). The will and the ways: Development and validation of an individual-differences measure of hope. *Journal of Personality and Social Psychology, 60*(4), 570–585.

Snyder, C. R., Rand, K. L., King, E. A., Feldman, D. B., & Woodward, J. T. (2002). "False" hope. *Journal of Clinical Psychology, 58*(9), 1003–1022. doi: http://dx.doi.org/10.1002/jclp.10096

Snyder, C. R., Sympson, S. C., Ybasco, F. C., Borders, T. F., Babyak, M. A., & Higgins, R. L. (1996). Development and validation of the state hope scale. *Journal of Personality and Social Psychology, 70*(2), 321–335.

Sokol, D. K. (2006). What is false hope? *The Journal of Clinical Ethics, 17*(4), 367–368.

Stacey, D., Samant, R., & Bennett, C. (2008). Decision making in oncology: A review of patient decision aids to support patient participation. *CA: A Cancer Journal for Clinicians, 58*(5), 293–304. doi: 10.3322/CA.2008.0006

Stein, N., Folkman, S., Trabasso, T., & Richards, T. A. (1997). Appraisal and goal processes as predictors of psychological well-being in bereaved caregivers. *Journal of Personality and Social Psychology, 72*(4), 872–884. doi: http://dx.doi.org/10.1037/0022-3514.72.4.872

Stoner, M. H., & Keampfer, S. H. (1985). Recalled life expectancy information, phase of illness and hope in cancer patients. *Research in Nursing & Health, 8*(3), 269–274.

Stotland, E. (1969). *The psychology of hope.* San Francisco, CA: Jossey-Bass Publishers.

Surkan, P. J., Kreicbergs, U., Valdimarsdottir, U., Nyberg, U., Onelov, E., Dickman, P. W., & Steineck, G. (2006). Perceptions of inadequate health care and feelings of guilt in parents after the death of a child to a malignancy: A population-based long-term follow-up. *Journal of Palliative Medicine, 9*(2), 317–331. doi: http://dx.doi.org/10.1089/jpm.2006.9.317

Taylor, S. E., & Brown, J. D. (1988). Illusion and well-being: A social psychological perspective on mental health. *Psychological Bulletin, 103*(2), 193–210.

Taylor, S. E., & Brown, J. D. (1994). Positive illusions and well-being revisited: Separating fact from fiction. *Psychological Bulletin, 116*(1), 21–27.

Tennen, H., & Affeck, G. (1999). Finding benefits in adversity. In C. R. Snyder (Ed.), *Coping: The psychology of what works* (pp. 279–304). New York, NY: Oxford University Press.

Tollett, J. H., & Thomas, S. P. (1995). A theory-based nursing intervention to instill hope in homeless veterans. *Advances in Nursing Science, 18*(2), 76–90.

Tomko, B. (1985). The burden of hope. *Hospice Journal, 1*(3), 91–97. doi: http://dx.doi.org/10.1300/J011v01n03_06

Uren, T. H., & Wastell, C. A. (2002). Attachment and meaning-making in perinatal bereavement. *Death Studies, 26*(4), 279–308. doi: http://dx.doi.org/10.1080/074811802753594682

Utne, I., Miaskowski, C., Paul, S. M., & Rustoen, T. (2013). Association between hope and burden reported by family caregivers of patients with advanced cancer. *Supportive Care in Cancer, 21*(9), 2527–2535. doi: 10.1007/s00520-013-1824-5

Vaillot, M. (1970). Hope: The restoration of being. *The American Journal of Nursing, 70*(2), 268–273. doi: 10.2307/3421157

White, D. B., & Curtis, J. R. (2005). Care near the end-of-life in critically ill patients: A North American perspective. *Current Opinions in Critical Care, 11*(6), 610–615. doi: 00075198-200512000-00018 [pii]

Wrosch, C., Amir, E., & Miller, G. E. (2011). Goal adjustment capacities, coping, and subjective well-being: The sample case of caregiving for a family member with mental illness. *Journal of Personality and Social Psychology, 100*(5), 934–946. doi: 10.1037/a0022873

Wrosch, C., Scheier, M. F., Carver, C. S., & Schulz, R. (2003). The importance of goal disengagement in adaptive self-regulation: When giving up is beneficial. *Self and Identity, 2*(1), 1–20. doi: 10.1037/0022-006x.49.4.508

CHAPTER 14

Grieving the Traumatic Death of a Child

Wendy G. Lichtenthal, Geoffrey W. Corner,
Corinne Sweeney, and Kailey E. Roberts

The loss of a child is one of the most profoundly painful experiences a parent can endure. When the circumstances of the death are perceived as traumatic, the grief experience can become all the more excruciating and complex. Parents not only struggle with the loss of their cherished and beloved child but are also forced to grapple with the often incomprehensible, seemingly senseless, and violent circumstances of the death. How parents come to make meaning of their experiences plays a central role in adaptation. In this chapter, we give substantial attention to research, including our own, on meaning-making in bereaved parents.

As we consider what constitutes a traumatic death, we acknowledge that what is considered traumatic is based on the perception and experience of the individual. This being said, traumatic deaths often tend to be the result of circumstances that are violent, sudden, or unexpected. This chapter, therefore, discusses bereavement by suicide, homicide, motor vehicle accident, or a sudden and unexpected medical complication. It also focuses on the experience of bereaved parents, though it is important to acknowledge that the traumatic death of a child often has devastating effects that reverberate throughout the entire family and community.

We begin by describing research on parents' common reactions to the traumatic death of a child, as well as more impairing grief and traumatic stress responses. Next, we cover theoretical models through which we can view and understand reactions to a traumatic loss, including meaning-making and reconstruction, life transition theory, and continuing bonds theory. We then discuss physical health and mortality risks in traumatic bereavement and how the cause and circumstances of a child's death may influence the parent's bereavement experience. Pre- and postloss factors that may increase risk for negative bereavement outcomes are then described. Finally, we provide guidelines for health care and support providers and detail specific interventions for mental health clinicians working with traumatically bereaved parents.

PSYCHOLOGICAL RESPONSES TO THE TRAUMATIC LOSS OF A CHILD

Much like the larger bereaved parent population, parents bereaved by traumatic circumstances often face numerous mental health challenges, including depression, anxiety, somatization, hostility, and paranoid ideation, in the wake of their loss (Johnson, Murphy, & Dimond, 1996; Miles, 1985). Traumatically bereaved parents may also experience survivor's guilt, which is characterized by feelings that they did not do enough to save the child, feelings of guilt or responsibility for the death, or feeling they do not deserve to continue their own life after their child's death (Clements, Garzon, & Milliken, 2006). There is evidence to suggest that parents who have experienced the loss of a child, particularly a traumatic loss, report higher incidence of suicidal thoughts, plans, and attempts than their nonbereaved peers (Feigelman, Jordan, McIntosh, & Feigelman, 2012). In their study of parents bereaved primarily by suicide or drug-related deaths, Feigelman and colleagues (2012) found that although rates of suicidal thoughts, plans, and attempts decreased at 3 years after the loss, they remained higher than the general population.

Perhaps most prominent among the challenges that bereaved parents face is a profound sense of grief, yearning, and longing for their child, which commonly lasts a lifetime. This, of course, is not unique to parents bereaved by traumatic circumstances, but it often dominates their experience as grieving parents. In an effort to better characterize the distinction between pathological and nonpathological responses to the traumatic death of a child, Oliver and Fallat (1995) conducted interviews with 29 parents from 20 families that lost a child at a pediatric trauma center. Causes of death included motor vehicle accidents, burns, falls, blows to the head, and other fatal injuries, and all children died within 14 days of being admitted to the hospital. Interview assessments were based on work by Worden (1991) and Demi and Miles (1987), and they focused on processes, characteristics, behaviors, and symptoms that these previous studies identified as helpful in adjustment to bereavement. These included whether or not parents had accepted the reality of their loss and how they were working through the pain of grief and adjusting to life without their child. Based on the success parents had in accomplishing these tasks, the authors found that more than three quarters of the parents they interviewed exhibited pathological grief reactions and severe challenges coping with their loss (Oliver & Fallat, 1995).

Notably, the authors observed that parents who conceptualized their child's death as unfair seemed to be having greater difficulty that those who did not. Oliver and Fallat (1995) pointed out, though, that some grief symptoms were less diagnostic of psychopathology in traumatically bereaved parents, such as the intensity of the initial emotional shock of the loss, which commonly lasted for months. Parents typically expressed that their loss was not only the most devastating challenge they have personally experienced but also the worst kind of suffering anyone can possibly experience. As a result, many indicated they no longer feared their own death as much as they once had (Oliver & Fallat, 1995). Harper, O'Connor, Dickson, and O'Carroll (2011) similarly noted that traumatically bereaved mothers in their study felt ambivalent about their own mortality, with some expressing outright pre-occupation with death and suicidal ideation. These mothers viewed death as a way to end their painful grief and to potentially be reunited with their deceased child in the afterlife. Caring for surviving children was described as both a reason for living as well as a challenging responsibility that was difficult to effectively fulfill, particularly in the more immediate aftermath of their loss (Harper et al., 2011).

Oliver and Fallat (1995) highlighted that one of parents' most common concerns was that their child would not be remembered, although they described different ways of coping with this fear. Some viewed their painful grief as a way to keep their child in their memory, which resulted in a fear that dissipation of their grief would mean they were forgetting their child. All married parents stressed the impact of the death on their relationship, which faced considerable strain under the shared grief experience (Oliver & Fallat, 1995). That being said, while some research has substantiated the commonly held belief that bereaved parents face marital strain and an elevated divorce risk, other studies have found no such risk, and patterns of both improvement and ongoing struggle have been observed in bereaved parents' relationships (Alam, Barrera, D'Agostino, Nicholas, & Schneiderman, 2012; Eilegård & Kreicbergs, 2010; Rogers, 2008; Schwab, 1998).

Pathological Grief and Traumatic Stress Responses

As noted in the preceding text, Oliver and Fallat (1995) offered a qualitative description of the features and signs of what they describe as "pathological mourning" in parents bereaved by traumatic causes. Another important conceptualization of pathological grief focuses on the persistence of grief-related symptoms and their impact on the bereaved individual's ability to function. Among bereaved parents, it is common to experience yearning for their lost child throughout their entire life. Though this pain frequently persists, parents do often find a way to adapt and coexist with their grief. For some parents, however, the intensity of the yearning along with other symptoms, such as avoidance, disbelief, difficulty accepting the reality of the death and moving forward with life, role confusion, and loss of a sense of meaning in life, are debilitating and impairing. In the general bereaved population, this syndrome of "stuckness" is referred to as prolonged grief disorder (PGD), which has been empirically distinguished from bereavement-related depression, characterized by sadness, anhedonia, and somatic symptoms; and anxiety, characterized by fear of a threatening situation (Lichtenthal, Cruess, & Prigerson, 2004; Prigerson et al., 2009). Other diagnostic criteria have been proposed for PGD and a similar syndrome, complicated grief (CG) (Maercker & Lalor, 2012; Shear et al., 2011).

To stimulate research on the topic of debilitating, protracted grief reactions, the latest version of the *Diagnostic and Statistical Manual for Mental Disorders, Fifth Edition* (*DSM-5*) added a disorder characterized by several of the proposed PGD and CG symptoms, persistent complex bereavement disorder (PCBD), to the appendices as a condition for further research (American Psychiatric Association, 2013). Of note, PCBD includes a "with traumatic bereavement" specifier for those who were bereaved by homicide or suicide and are experiencing persistent preoccupations related to the circumstances of death (e.g., the deceased's last moments, degree of suffering, or mutilating injury; or the malicious or intentional nature of the death; American Psychiatric Association, 2013). Given the limited research on how these diagnostic criteria may be used in clinical practice, our team is currently investigating the clinical utility of the diagnostic criteria of bereavement-related mental disorders.

Traumatic circumstances also place parents at greater risk for posttraumatic stress disorder (PTSD; Murphy et al., 1999a). To meet the technical diagnostic criteria for PTSD, a parent must have been a direct witness to the death of his or her child, or if he or she learned about the death, it "must have been violent or accidental" (American Psychiatric Association, 2013). Although witnessing a death can be unthinkably horrifying, the moment that a parent who was not physically present at the time of a violent or accidental death learns of it is also utterly devastating. In fact, studies have shown that parents who lost a child in a motor vehicle accident have levels of peritraumatic stress and dissociation that are similar to those in individuals who themselves were in serious motor vehicle accidents (Allenou et al., 2010; Vaiva et al., 2003).

An important body of work has demonstrated the distinction between PGD and PTSD symptoms (Boelen & van den Bout, 2005; Boelen, van den Bout, & de Keijser, 2003; Prigerson et al., 1995; Prigerson et al., 1996). We have previously noted how symptoms that appear to overlap, such as intrusive thoughts, avoidance, and increased arousal, are often qualitatively different (Lichtenthal et al., 2004). Specifically, we posited that (a) intrusive thoughts in PTSD are focused on the traumatic event and related emotions, while they are typically images of the deceased in PGD; (b) bereaved individuals exhibiting PGD symptoms may actually seek out reminders of their loved one and may exhibit avoidance as denial of and dissociation from the loss of their loved one and/or as avoidance of their painful grief; and (c) while PTSD exhibits increased arousal through feelings of threatened safety, hypervigilance in PGD is typically associated with a search for reminders of the deceased and proximity seeking. Maercker and Lalor (2012) similarly explained how a key difference between PTSD and PGD is the emotional valence of intrusive and recurrent trauma-related memories; with PTSD, these memories are uniformly negative, while with PGD, they can have both positive and negative components, resulting in something that could potentially be described as somewhat "bittersweet." This being said, it is not uncommon for traumatically bereaved parents to experience comorbid PTSD and PGD (American Psychiatric Association, 2013; Simon et al., 2011). A neurological connection between PTSD and protracted grief has even been proposed by Nakajima, Ito, Shirai, and Konishi (2012), who posited that deficits in the functioning of the anterior cingulate cortex and medial prefrontal cortex demonstrated in individuals with PTSD may contribute to pathological grieving through dysfunctional emotional regulation in conjunction with the activation of the amygdala and feelings of sadness and separation distress (Bremner et al., 1999; Freed, Yanagihara, Hirsch, & Mann, 2009; Lanius et al., 2001; Phan et al., 2005).

Additionally, there is some conceptual overlap between grieving and traumatic experiences when considering the theoretical framework of "shattered assumptions" (Janoff-Bulman, 2010). The traumatic death of a child, which represents a life event that is chronologically "out of order," commonly challenges parents' existing beliefs, such as assumptions that the world is benevolent and meaningful and that the self is worthy (Janoff-Bulman, 2010). As individuals naturally attempt to make sense of the universe, parents who lose a child under traumatic circumstances may struggle to believe that they are good people worthy of good things in a rational and caring world that will treat them as such (Beder, 2004). Thus, providers should carefully consider that for some bereaved parents, particularly those who lose their child in violent or traumatic circumstances, trauma and grief symptoms are often intrinsically tied.

Psychological Responses Over Time

Grieving is understood as a process, and thus, there are anticipated changes over time. That being said, there are no firmly established timelines detailing when we should expect certain reactions to emerge or abate for bereaved parents. Researchers examining the trajectory of emotional reactions in bereaved parents have suggested that any differences associated with or explained by cause of death tend to diminish between 3 and 5 years after the loss (Feigelman, Jordan, & Gorman, 2008). A study of parents who lost a child in the pediatric intensive care unit (PICU) found that CG symptoms (i.e., PGD) typically improved approximately 6 to 18 months out from the loss, but it was noted that many parents were still significantly struggling at 18 months after loss (Meert et al., 2011). Another study by Murphy and colleagues (1999b) had similar findings, with parents showing the most improvement in mental distress between 4 and 12 months. Generally speaking, context (e.g., parent, child, and relationship characteristics; circumstances of death) needs to be taken into consideration in understanding a given parent's grief reaction over time.

The trajectory of PTSD symptoms in bereaved parents has also received empirical attention. For instance, Allenou and colleagues (2010) demonstrated that levels of peritraumatic distress were associated with PTSD symptoms in traumatically bereaved mothers 1 and 5 weeks after the loss of their child, a finding that suggests that initial levels of trauma-related distress may be associated with the maintenance or development of PTSD symptoms. In an effort to understand factors that affect the trajectory of PTSD over time, Murphy, Johnson, Chung, and Beaton (2003a) conducted a 5-year follow-up with 173 parents who were initially assessed soon after the traumatic death of their child. They examined the role that nine specific factors played in the trajectory of PTSD symptoms: (1) the child's cause of death, (2) the parents' gender, (3) self-esteem, (4) active coping, (5) repressive coping, (6) affective coping, (7) perceived social support, (8) level of distress, and (9) receipt of early bereavement intervention. Although many of these factors were related to levels of PTSD at baseline (e.g., gender, self-esteem, repressive coping, affective coping, perceived social support, and distress), only two were significantly related to how PTSD changed over time in latent growth models: parents' gender and perceived social support. Mothers' PTSD symptoms were more persistent than those of fathers, and parents who believed that they had high levels of social support typically had their PTSD symptoms improve more rapidly (Murphy et al., 2003a). Murphy and colleagues (1999b) also found differences between mothers and fathers in the trajectory of general mental distress, with mothers showing improvement in the second year of bereavement while fathers experienced some worsening of distress. Clinicians might therefore be mindful of potential gender differences and of the importance of strong support networks in traumatically bereaved parents.

THEORETICAL MODELS OF ADJUSTMENT

To better understand the psychological reactions described by researchers and outlined in the preceding subsection, it is helpful to contextualize them using existing theoretical models of adjustment to the loss of a loved one.

Several bereavement models have been proposed and, here, we focus on those that theorists and researchers have discussed specifically in the context of experiencing the traumatic loss of a child.

Meaning-Making and Reconstruction

Given the obvious challenges that bereaved parents face in making sense of and finding any significant meaning in the untimely loss of a child, our work and the work of others have focused on meaning reconstruction models. Meaning reconstruction, most notably described by psychologist Robert Neimeyer (2011), involves reconstructing or transforming one's worldview assumptions, sense of meaning in life, and sense of identity and purpose in the face of loss. Neimeyer (2011) explained how the "search for meaning" takes place at several levels: the practical level, the relational level, and the spiritual or existential level. Practically, parents may search for or contemplate the specific details surrounding their child's death, striving to understand precisely how their child passed away. Relationally, parents seek to assimilate their new sense of identity in the wake of this devastating and impactful loss; they need to redefine themselves in light of what their child's death changes about the persons they are and want to be. Finally, parents spiritually and existentially pursue an understanding of why this death occurred, whether it was the will of God, the prescription of fate, or simply the result of bad luck (Neimeyer, 2011).

These types of meaning-making processes have been further categorized into "sensemaking" and "benefit finding" (Davis, Wortman, Lehman, & Silver, 2000). Sensemaking involves constructing a reason or explanation for a loss and is typically related to an individual's worldview and beliefs (Davis et al., 2000). Thus, as the theory of shattered assumptions (Janoff-Bulman, 2010) described earlier suggests, sensemaking can be particularly challenging if an individual experiences a disruption in his or her worldview and may be struggling simultaneously to make sense of the loss and reconstruct the sense of meaning in life (Lichtenthal, Currier, Neimeyer, & Keesee, 2010). Parents may make sense of the loss of their child in many ways, including believing the death was God's will, believing the child was better off in the afterlife, and conceptualizing all life as fleeting (Lichtenthal et al., 2010). Benefit finding is defined as the process of identifying the value of an event in the context of one's life and frequently is characterized by recognizing positive changes to one's life (Davis et al., 2000). Following the loss of a child, benefit finding also may take many forms, such as a new desire to help others, increased appreciation for life, and strengthening of relationships (Lichtenthal et al., 2010). Though parents who experience the loss of a child are sometimes able to make sense of their loss, there is evidence to suggest that parents bereaved by the violent loss of a child may find sense-making significantly more challenging than parents who lost their child to natural causes (Lehman, Wortman, & Williams, 1987; Lichtenthal, Neimeyer, Currier, Roberts, & Jordan, 2013; Murphy & Johnson, 2003). However, our research suggests that cause of death may not impact benefit finding in the same way, because rates of benefit finding among parents bereaved by violent and nonviolent causes are quite similar (Lichtenthal et al., 2013).

Meaning-making also takes place within the family system. Various family members may understand how and why the death occurred in different ways and may experience disparate challenges from role shifts. Nadeau (2008) described this process as *family meaning-making*. Coconstruction of meaning occurs through the development of family narratives, as individual family members may have different understandings of how and why the death occurred (Gudmundsdottir & Chesla, 2006). Though family meaning-making can be an adaptive process, negative meanings assigned by family members can complicate how they grieve, particularly when guilt and blame are involved, which may be particularly relevant to traumatic losses (Nadeau, 2008). Other factors that may hinder the meaning-making process within families include inhibition of discussing sensitive topics, absence of family rituals, physical and emotional distance, and avoidance of discussing the death in order to protect family members (i.e., protectionism; Nadeau, 1998, 2008).

Life Transition Theory

Another framework that was applied to the study of traumatically bereaved parents by Kachoyeanos and Selder (1993) is the life transition theory (LTT). Originally established in a spinal cord injury population, LTT seeks to describe how people respond to life events that permanently change their day-to-day reality (Schmitt, 1982). In LTT, an individual experiences "trigger events," which draw attention to and force an individual to accept the permanent change that has occurred. These trigger events are categorized as irrevocability, reactivation, and missed options. Subsequently, the individual must adapt to this change, which occurs through four significant processes: comparative testing, competency testing, normalization, and minimizing missed options (Kachoyeanos & Selder, 1993).

Kachoyeanos and Selder (1993) conducted qualitative analysis of transcripts from semistructured interviews with 27 parents of children who had mostly died in accidents (ages ranging from 4 to 24, time since loss ranging from 18 months to 14 years) in order to understand life transitions in parents coping with the unexpected loss of their child. They noted differences between mothers and fathers. Generally, fathers believed that they were expected to be "stoic and strong" through the loss for their wives and wanted to "put the loss behind them"; mothers were "expected to cry and encouraged to grieve" and emphasized the importance of remembering and staying connected with their lost child (Kachoyeanos & Selder, 1993, pp. 46–47). Table 14.1 summarizes the authors' findings and defines trigger events and adaptation processes in the context of traumatic parental bereavement (Kachoyeanos & Selder, 1993).

There are clearly areas of overlap between meaning reconstruction and LTT. In addition to exploring LTT processes, Kachoyeanos and Selder (1993) identified the act of finding meaning as important, stressing ways in which bereaved parents are able to find a new purpose in life, particularly through charitable acts or engagement in causes related to their child's death.

TABLE 14.1 Life Transition Processes in Traumatically Bereaved Parents

Trigger Events	
Irrevocability	Parents are forced to understand that this change, the loss of their child, is permanent. Initially hearing about the loss in a sensitive way and viewing the child's body can help with this process.
Reactivation	Parents can have their loss be reactivated in a negative, traumatic way or in a positive, nostalgic way. One mother who lost her daughter described a reactivation experience in a shopping center parking lot: "I heard . . . brakes screeching, a loud crash, and then glass breaking. I froze. Suddenly I thought of [my daughter]. I imagined how horrible those last few minutes must have been for her. I started to shake violently" (Kachoyeanos & Selder, 1993, p. 45).
Missed options	Over time, the missed options that parents identify transition from (a) the presence of the child to (b) the child's unique characteristics (e.g., humor, laughter), and finally to (c) achievements or life milestones that the child will never reach (e.g., graduation, marriage).
Structuring a New Reality	
Comparative testing	In comparing themselves to expectations about how bereavement and coping "should" look, parents report the importance and value of speaking with individuals who have suffered the same kind of loss.
Competency testing	In the case of traumatically bereaved parents, "competency" tended to refer to their abilities and capabilities as parents. This was both evaluated retrospectively in the case of the lost child and manifested in how parents treated their surviving children.
Normalization	Normalization occurs through reintegration within society and returning to typical activities of daily living such as employment and social interactions.
Minimizing missed options	Parents reported coping with perceived missed options with an act called "presencing." This was a way to maintain a strong connection with the child, keeping him or her in their thoughts, and often even imagining or feeling his or her physical presence.

Adapted from Kachoyeanos and Selder (1993).

Continuing Bonds

Any discussion of bereaved parents, regardless of the circumstances of their child's death, should note the important role that continued connection to the child plays in parents' adjustment (Harper et al., 2011; Parker & Dunn, 2011). Continuing bonds theory is based on Bowlby's (1980) attachment theory of grief, which asserts that bereavement consists of "protest" and "despair" phases in which bereaved individuals alternately attempt to avoid the reality of the death, and then despair upon realizing the deceased individual is truly not returning (Field, Gao, & Paderna, 2005). According to Bowlby (1980), during the protest phase, a parent who lost a child might seek out physical connection (e.g., sleeping in the child's bed, seeing visions of the child) with the deceased child to alleviate separation distress. However, when these connections prove insufficient, and they realize the permanence of the loss, bereaved parents may feel a sense of despair and attempt to avoid connecting to the deceased child (e.g., avoiding the child's favorite places or activities; Field et al., 2005). Field and colleagues (2005) suggested that bereaved individuals may despair after attempting to maintain a connection to the deceased through physical or behavioral means such as using the child's possessions because these expressions of continuing bond are not internally felt as a deeper, secure bond. Thus, bereaved parents who are able to transform their bond with their child into a more transcendent, meaningful connection may experience less separation distress and a greater sense of peace (Field et al., 2005).

Neimeyer, Baldwin, and Gillies (2006) found evidence that individuals who successfully engage in meaning reconstruction are also able to transform their bond with the deceased, facilitating both the significant need to maintain an attachment to the deceased and adaptation to the loss. In contrast, individuals who struggle with sensemaking and maintain a strong, unchanged attachment to the deceased have been found to experience challenges in their bereavement in the form of CG and separation distress (Neimeyer et al., 2006). The ways in which parents may transform and continue a bond with their child vary and can include visiting the gravesite (Parker & Dunn, 2011), engaging in spiritual connections (e.g., belief in the afterlife; Klass, 2013; Parker & Dunn, 2011), or symbolically connecting with the child (e.g., viewing a butterfly or bird as symbolic of the child; Harper et al., 2011).

CAUSE OF DEATH: DOES IT MATTER?

Given how the nuances of the circumstances of death can vary, researchers and clinicians should be cautious about making generalizations about how the cause of death or the manner in which a child dies impacts grief responses. That being said, researchers have sought to understand trends to help us learn the best ways to support parents. For example, one study of bereaved mothers who were, on average, approximately 22 months post-loss and were recruited from a hospital found that levels of grief were higher among parents who suddenly lost a child when compared to those who anticipated their loss (Seecharan, Andresen, Norris, & Toce, 2004).

Similarly, our own research showed that, on average, parents bereaved by a violent death had significantly higher levels of PGD symptoms than those who lost a child to nonviolent causes (Lichtenthal et al., 2013). We also found some evidence that the cause of death differentially impacts how parents make meaning of their loss. In a mixed methods study, we surveyed 155 parents bereaved by a variety of causes and asked them whether they had made sense of (sensemaking) or found any positive sequelae of their loss (benefit finding) and, if so, how. We qualitatively coded their open-ended responses and found that those bereaved by a violent death generally faced greater challenges in making sense of the loss than those bereaved by a nonviolent death (Lichtenthal et al., 2013). Specifically, while 62% of the parents who lost a child to nonviolent causes reported at least one way of making sense of their loss, less than half (44%) of the parents who lost a child to violent causes reported a way that they were able to make sense of their child's death.

Further, among the parents who expressed they found a way to make sense of their loss, there were a number of differences, depending on cause of death, in the ways they were able to make meaning (Lichtenthal et al., 2013). For example, parents bereaved by violent death were significantly more likely than those bereaved by nonviolent death to describe explanations for the death related to their existential worldviews (e.g., belief in the imperfection of the world or the brevity of life), whereas a greater number of parents bereaved by nonviolent loss expressed that they believed their child's death was God's will. Despite their challenges with sensemaking, parents bereaved by violent and nonviolent causes demonstrated a striking ability to derive and acknowledge positive sequelae of their loss experience (73% and 75%, respectively). However, parents who lost a child to violent causes were less likely than parents bereaved by nonviolent deaths to report improved coping or decreased sense of fear as benefits. Instead, survivors of suicide were more likely to report a change in priorities, and survivors of homicide were more likely to describe finding a greater appreciation of life and relationships (Lichtenthal et al., 2013). These findings highlight how different causes of death may uniquely influence the types of meanings made following the loss of a child, though again, we view these trends as particular to the specific sample we examined, and we expect that a given parent may make meaning in his or her own unique ways that differ from these patterns.

Researchers have also described different patterns of grief reactions among traumatically bereaved parents based on the cause of death. Miles (1985) compared parents bereaved by an accident to those bereaved by a chronic illness and did not find group differences in the incidence of psychological symptoms, including somatization, interpersonal sensitivity, obsessiveness, anxiety, and depression. Comparing the impact of different types of sudden losses, Feigelman, Jordan, and Gorman (2008) demonstrated that parents bereaved by suicide experienced significantly higher levels of grief than those bereaved by accidental deaths, homicide, ambiguous deaths, or natural causes. However, when experiencing more postloss personal growth, parents bereaved by suicide tended to report fewer mental health challenges (Feigelman, Jordan, & Gorman, 2009). Among parents bereaved by nonsuicide deaths, natural deaths were associated with lower levels of grief than accidental/ambiguous deaths and homicides, although this difference was not statistically significant. However, as the amount of time since the loss increased, differences between the groups appeared to diminish; in particular, 3 to 5 years out from the loss was identified as a turning point at which levels of grief were similar across different types of losses (Feigelman et al., 2008). Kovarsky (1989) also showed that the trajectory of negative outcomes in bereavement may differ by cause of death, with grief and loneliness rising over time in parents who have lost a child to suicide and declining over time among survivors of an accident. In contrast, other research has shown that parental suicide survivors initially exhibit greater depressive symptoms than parents who lost a child in an accident, but that these differences were no longer present at a second time point, farther out from the loss (Seguin, Lesage, & Kiely, 1995).

Another study from Norway, however, found no differences in distress between parents bereaved by suicide and accidents, although both of these groups were significantly more distressed than parents in the sample who lost a child to sudden infant death syndrome (SIDS; Dyregrov, Nordanger, & Dyregrov, 2003). Despite the differences found, these authors concluded that equal attention should be paid to all types of sudden and traumatic losses and posited that individual characteristics that serve as risk factors should instead be the focus in targeting bereavement services (Dyregrov et al., 2003).

This latter point is well taken, but still, it is notable that findings in this literature have been mixed. A review article comparing bereavement outcomes in parents who lost a child to suicide with those who experienced other types of loss determined that differences that have been observed were largely contingent upon the particular outcome receiving attention, which could explain the sometimes contradictory findings in the literature (Murphy, Johnson, & Lohan, 2003b). Thus, the complex relationship between time since loss, specific negative outcomes, and cause of death can complicate any efforts to parse out variances in coping between parents facing different types of traumatic death.

Several authors have importantly noted experiences that are unique and common to parents bereaved by specific causes, such as homicide and suicide. For example, Kashka and Beard (1999) discussed the distinctive aspects of losing a child to homicide, a very personal topic for these authors, as Kashka lost her daughter in one of a number of unsolved murders in 1984, and Beard lost her son in a 1988 burglary of his home. They proposed a model for understanding parental bereavement in homicide survivors that emphasizes the complex interactions between the private grief experience, the public nature of the loss, and the role of the criminal justice system in its effort to punish those responsible for the murder. The authors described the way that parents' private experiences are impacted by the death being sudden, inconceivable, violent, and intentional, and they highlighted how it results in a loss of trust in the social fabric and challenges the spiritual belief system (Kashka & Beard, 1999). They also noted how public coverage of a child's murder and interactions with the criminal justice system can shape and often even intensify bereavement.

Several unique aspects of bereavement by suicide have been described as well. Maple, Edwards, Plummer, and Minichiello (2010) highlighted how parents who lose a child to suicide often report feeling unable to share or discuss their loss with others. This isolation stems from the parents' own reactions (e.g., beliefs that others will not understand, concerns about social image) and the reactions of those around them (e.g., avoiding social interaction with the bereaved parent, reluctance or lack of a desire to discuss the loss). This can challenge adaptive grieving because it may limit the use of social support and emotional expression as coping strategies (Maple et al., 2010; Parker & Dunn, 2011).

In sum, the specific circumstances surrounding a child's death can influence how a parent suffers and grieves in complex ways. Therefore, it is extremely important for providers treating traumatically bereaved parents to be mindful of reactions that are common to losing a child to a specific cause while simultaneously considering the ways in which each individual parent's story and journey through grief are unique and personal.

PHYSICAL HEALTH AND MORTALITY

In addition to mental health challenges, traumatically bereaved parents also face deficits in and risks to their physical health. In an effort to explore the general relationship between psychological stress and heart health, Li, Hansen, Mortensen, and Olsen (2002) conducted a follow-up study with a large sample of parents who lost a child under the age of 18 between 1980 and 1996, identified from Danish national registers. The authors conceptualized parental bereavement as an example of extreme stress and examined its relationship to risk for myocardial infarction (MI) later in life. Their findings suggest that these parents experienced high relative risk for MI, and further, parents who lost a child unexpectedly, particularly to SIDS, had an even higher relative risk. More recent research corroborates the finding that bereaved parents may be at risk for poor physical health, demonstrating high postloss incidences of medical and stress-related hospitalizations; increases in dosage of or additions or changes to cardiac medications; and development of chronic illnesses (e.g., angina, hypertension, arthritis, and asthma, although chronic mental health conditions were also considered) in a sample of 249 parents who lost an infant or young child in the neonatal or pediatric intensive care unit, although it was unclear what proportion of these deaths would be characterized as traumatic (Youngblut, Brooten, Cantwell, del Moral, & Totapally, 2013). The authors noted, though, that mothers who suffered an unexpected loss reported significantly more postloss chronic health conditions than mothers who suffered an expected loss, although this comparison also included chronic mental health conditions such as depression (Youngblut et al., 2013). These differences in chronic health conditions and hospitalizations could potentially be related to compromised immune functioning (i.e., increased T-lymphocyte helper/suppressor ratio), which has been found in bereaved parents who experience the sudden loss of a child when compared with nonbereaved controls (Spratt & Denney, 1991). Such findings suggest the need for more research in this area.

In addition to and perhaps as a result of physical health problems that appear to be prevalent in those losing a child, research has demonstrated increased mortality in bereaved parents relative to the general population. Using the same large sample of bereaved parents identified from Danish national registers in the aforementioned study of MI prevalence, Li, Precht, Mortensen, and Olsen (2003) examined mortality in mothers and fathers up to 18 years after bereavement. They found increased mortality from unnatural causes in both mothers (throughout bereavement, most notably in the first 3 years) and fathers (only close to the loss). The authors also noted higher mortality rates among mothers who unexpectedly lost a child (Li et al., 2003). These findings were similarly noted in high relative risk of mortality in a Swedish population of bereaved parents, with mothers unexpectedly losing a younger child appearing to face the highest increased mortality risk (Rostila, Saarela, & Kawachi, 2012). Overall, there is a complex relationship between postloss mental health disturbances, physical health impairment, and increased mortality risk in bereaved parents, and these negative outcomes are likely interrelated.

RISK FACTORS

A number of factors may increase a parent's vulnerability to developing severe and persistent mental health challenges in the face of traumatic loss. Systematic reviews of risk factors for bereavement-related mental health challenges in the general population have identified three main categories of risk: *background factors*, including attachment style and demographics; *death-related factors*, including witnessing violent death; and *bereavement-related factors*, including decreased sense of meaning (Burke & Neimeyer, 2012; Lobb et al., 2010). These risk factors similarly predict a number of mental health challenges in bereaved individuals, including PGD, PTSD, and major depressive disorder (MDD; Burke & Neimeyer, 2012). Though the risk factors presented in the following subsections have each been associated independently with a greater incidence of negative bereavement outcomes, when assessing individuals bereaved by traumatic loss, mental health providers should recognize that a combination of factors tends to put individuals at greater risk (Burke & Neimeyer, 2012) and that many of the risk factors themselves may be interrelated, dynamic, and influenced by cultural norms, life stressors, and insufficient social support (Burke & Neimeyer, 2012; Ellifritt, Nelson, & Walsh, 2003; Oliver & Fallat, 1995; Ott, 2003).

Background Risk Factors

Background risk factors for negative bereavement outcomes include demographics, personal characteristics, and characteristics of the relationship between the bereaved parent and the child that were present prior to the loss.

Demographics

While bereaved mothers and fathers have been found to be at greater risk for mental health problems than nonbereaved individuals (Li, Precht, Mortensen, & Olsen, 2003; Murphy et al., 1999b), mothers appear to have higher risk than fathers in many cases. In their systematic review of risk factors associated with bereavement, Burke and Neimeyer (2012) found that 42% of the studies identified gender as a risk factor for poor grief outcomes, with mothers being at greater risk than fathers. This gender difference appears to be consistent across bereavement-related mental health challenges. For example, following traumatic loss, mothers have been found to be at greater risk for postloss MDD and for a higher rate of depression recurrence (Brent, Moritz, Bridge, Perper, & Canobbio, 1996). Similarly, Murphy and colleagues (2003a) found that 5 years after the loss, mothers were more likely to meet diagnostic criteria for PTSD than fathers. Finally, there is some evidence to suggest that mothers are at risk of experiencing a high intensity of grief regardless of whether the unexpected loss of their child occurs in infancy or during childhood years (Michon, Balkou, Hivon, & Cyr, 2003).

While some studies have found that mothers who have experienced the traumatic loss of a child appear to be at higher risk for negative bereavement outcomes, it is important to consider the societal influences on gender presentation and how this relates to the expression of distress. Because of the potential that this gender difference in risk is partially due to gender role presentations and norms rather than an essential trait, it is important for mental health providers to be aware that mothers may be at more risk but that fathers may also be underreporting distress and to accordingly take care in assessment and treatment planning (Stroebe, Stroebe, & Schut, 2001). As Stroebe and colleagues (2001) stated, "The confusion enters when absolute risks are interpreted as relative risks" (p. 78) and vice versa. Statistically, women may be at higher risk, but the meaning of risk in this context and in other demographic categories may be complicated and not reflect a direct, predictive relationship.

There is also evidence to suggest that non-Caucasian bereaved individuals may be at increased risk for negative bereavement outcomes. However, these findings are mixed and they suggest the importance of considering additional variables that may contribute to racial disparities (Burke & Neimeyer, 2012). Burke and Neimeyer (2012) found that 50% of the studies assessed in their systematic review observed a relationship between racial identity and PGD, with evidence suggesting that African American individuals may be at particular risk. Most recently, Youngblut and colleagues (2013) found that 6 months after the loss of their child, mothers identified as African American and Hispanic showed higher levels of MDD and PTSD, although different results were found among fathers. This finding in particular demonstrates that a combination of risk factors may put bereaved individuals at an even greater risk for distress. Further, as with gender, when considering race as a risk factor for negative bereavement outcomes, it is essential to have an understanding of societal influences that contribute to making race a risk factor, including associations with lower income and systematic oppression.

Personal and Relational Characteristics

Beyond demographic factors, a number of personal and relational characteristics can put individuals at greater risk for intense psychological distress following the traumatic loss of a child. Individuals who have a history of experiencing a mental disorder tend to be at greater risk for developing bereavement-related distress (Ellifritt et al., 2003; Lobb et al., 2010).

Likewise, having a history of prior loss and/or trauma puts individuals at risk for mental health challenges when they face a subsequent traumatic loss (Jordan, Baker, Matteis, Rosenthal, & Ware, 2005; Lobb et al., 2010; Seguin et al., 1995). Certain personality and relational tendencies have been associated with negative bereavement outcomes, including insecure attachment style (Field & Filanosky, 2010; Fraley & Bonanno, 2004; van der Houwen et al., 2010), dependency (Burke & Neimeyer, 2012; Lobb et al., 2010), and low self-esteem and self-efficacy (Murphy et al., 1999a).

Characteristics of the family can impact how family members react to a traumatic loss, as well. Unstable family dynamics can put parents at risk not only for mental health challenges, but also for other risk factors, such as guilt over the loss (Shanfield & Swain, 1984). For both parents and siblings, the closeness of their relationship with a child or adolescent who commits suicide can predict a greater incidence of CG and physical problems (Mitchell, Kim, Prigerson, & Mortimer-Stephens, 2004). Finally, parents who lose their child to suicide are at more risk for mental health problems if they had a negative relationship with their child, and similarly, those experiencing strained family relationships after the loss of a child to suicide may have more grief-related difficulties (Feigelman, Gorman, & Jordan, 2009; Feigelman et al., 2008).

Death-Related Factors

As noted in the preceding text, violent or sudden traumatic death has been found to be a highly predictive risk factor for poor bereavement outcomes (Burke, Neimeyer, & McDevitt-Murphy, 2010; Currier, Holland, & Neimeyer, 2006; Keesee, Currier, & Neimeyer, 2008; Lichtenthal et al., 2013; Lobb et al., 2010; Zisook, Chentsova-Dutton, & Shuchter, 1998). Sudden death (suicide or accident) of an adult child has been associated with an even higher mortality risk (Pitman, Osborn, King, & Erlangsen, 2014; Rostila et al., 2012) and grief symptoms (Dyregrov et al., 2003; Seecharan et al., 2004) than deaths due to disease or chronic conditions. Parents grieving the suicide of their child or adolescent may be at an especially high risk for depression, physical disorders, loneliness, and hospitalization for mental distress (Bolton et al., 2013; Kovarsky, 1989; Omerov et al., 2013; Pitman et al., 2014).

Bolton and colleagues (2013) also found that parents bereaved by suicide tended to have preloss traits that put them at further risk for high rates of certain negative outcomes (e.g., depression and mental health hospitalization) in comparison with parents bereaved by an automobile accident. Findings reported by Feigelman, Jordan, and Gorman (2011) suggest that the association between suicide bereavement and negative outcomes may be influenced by the stigmatization of suicide, indicating that parents who lost a child to a drug-related cause, another stigmatized death, may also be more at risk for mental health problems than parents whose child died from an accident. Finally, though evidence suggests that suicide loss puts parents at higher risk for general mental health challenges than other causes of death, losing a child to homicide specifically places parents at risk for developing PTSD when compared with any other cause of death (Murphy et al., 1999a).

While a violent or unexpected cause of death can significantly impact the mourning process, the circumstances under which the death occurs and those immediately after the death can also put individuals at risk for negative outcomes, particularly in the case of PTSD. For example, peritraumatic distress and dissociation have been found to be associated with PTSD in mothers whose child experienced a motor vehicle accident (Allenou et al., 2010). Additionally, as described earlier in this chapter, the level of stigmatization associated with traumatic death can put bereaved parents at risk for mental health challenges, including depression, ongoing grief, and suicidal ideation (Feigelman et al., 2009).

Bereavement-Related Factors

Studies have also found that the way individuals process the death, particularly the degree to which an individual experiences feelings of regret or self-blame (Foa, Ehlers, Clark, Tolin & Orsillo, 1999) and makes sense of the death (Keesee et al., 2008), can also place them at risk for negative bereavement outcomes. As with other risk factors, bereavement-related risk factors are highly individualized and can be impacted by other factors, such as personality, life stressors, and cultural beliefs. It is important for mental health providers to consider these intersecting influences, particularly when assisting bereaved individuals in navigating the process of making meaning of the loss of a child.

Coping Style

The manner in which an individual copes with the traumatic death of his or her child can have a significant impact on the trajectory of the individual's grief. There is also evidence to suggest that coping styles can be adaptive or maladaptive depending upon the cause of death and time since the loss. For example, Anderson and colleagues (2005) found that among mothers who had unexpectedly lost a child approximately 4 years ago, mothers who took an emotional approach to coping (e.g., self-criticism, anxiety, anger) were more likely to have more intense grief experiences, while mothers who took an avoidant approach to coping had less intense grief reactions.

The authors suggested that an avoidant approach may therefore be more effective farther out from the time of death. In contrast, Oliver and Fallat (1995) and Harper, O'Connor, and O'Carroll (2013) found that avoidance predicted negative bereavement outcomes in parents bereaved by traumatic death. In addition to coping styles, emotions associated with the loss, most notably guilt and shame, can contribute to mental health struggles after the traumatic loss of a child (Clements et al., 2006; Seguin et al., 1995; Shanfield & Swain, 1984).

Meaning-Making

As noted earlier, meaning-making processes can play an important role in coping with the traumatic death of a child (Lichtenthal et al., 2010; Lichtenthal et al., 2013). Individuals who struggle to find meaning after a traumatic loss may be at increased risk for mental and physical health problems and marital distress (Murphy & Johnson, 2003). The process of making meaning of the loss of a child can be significantly impacted by spirituality and religion in both positive and negative ways (Burke & Neimeyer, 2012; Wortmann & Park, 2008). As such, spirituality and religion have been found to be both protective (Bonanno et al., 2002) and risk factors for intense grief reactions (Kersting et al., 2011).

The way individuals utilize religion in the context of traumatic child loss can impact their mental health outcomes. For example, Oliver and Fallat (1995) found that traumatically bereaved parents who viewed God as punishing were more likely to have intense bereavement-related distress. Similarly, in their study of Christian adults, some of whom were traumatically bereaved parents, Lichtenthal, Burke, and Neimeyer (2011) demonstrated that negative religious coping was associated with higher levels of PGD symptoms. Moreover, individuals who experienced a crisis in faith following their loss had greater difficulties with meaning-making, which in turn was associated with prolonged grief reactions (Lichtenthal et al., 2011).

SUPPORTING TRAUMATICALLY BEREAVED PARENTS

The time directly prior to, during, and immediately following the traumatic death of a child is typically excruciatingly painful for parents; it is also a time of shock and utter disbelief. Losing a child suddenly often involves parent interactions with emergency services (i.e., police, ambulance services, emergency departments). In a study examining support needs of parents who lost a child unexpectedly to an accident or illness, Dent, Condon, Blair, and Fleming (1996) found that the majority of parents were satisfied with the care provided by emergency services workers, though some wished for a greater level of sensitivity. Parents have expressed that these initial contacts should be unhurried, conducted in a private location, and approached with respect and compassion (Finlay & Dallimore, 1991). Parents also appreciate being provided with information and updates about their child's medical status during the crisis stage. Some parents have reported feeling underinformed about events in the emergency room, such as progress with resuscitation efforts, which may be alienating and distressing (Finlay & Dallimore, 1991).

Parents who have lost a child to traumatic circumstances may also need to meet with a coroner to identify their child's body or to discuss circumstances surrounding the death, all of which should be approached sensitively (Dent et al., 1996). Parents have expressed appreciation when these interviews are conducted with careful attention to being warm and supportive rather than businesslike or cold (Finlay & Dallimore, 1991). When coroners or other medical providers express their own sadness over the loss, parents feel further validated.

Postmortem examination, or autopsy, is an additional area in which parents commonly desire support and information. Research shows that traumatically bereaved parents are often interested in autopsy both for altruistic reasons and to gain a better understanding of their child's death (Snowden, Elbourne, & Garcia, 2004). Despite these potential benefits, many parents are never approached about autopsy (Ahrens, Hart, & Maruyama, 1997; Finlay & Dallimore, 1991; Oliver, Sturtevant, Scheetz, & Fallat, 2001). The desire to obtain medical explanation may be amplified among families whose loss occurred very suddenly or seemingly without reason, and not having an autopsy may become a source of regret later on (Ahrens et al., 1997; Finlay & Dallimore, 1991; Oliver et al., 2001). Parents who lose children to SIDS, in particular, report feeling especially distressed with the lack of medical explanation (Dent et al., 1996). Additionally, they may feel frustrated or confused about not being approached about organ donation, which they often do not know is not an option for SIDS deaths (Dent et al., 1996). In a study of parents bereaved by SIDS, participants indicated their desire for specific and concrete information delivered in understandable language about autopsy or tissue donation options (Dent et al., 1996). Parents should be approached in a supportive, neutral, and culturally sensitive manner. Clearly explaining what autopsy entails, including the type of procedure performed, the autopsy timeline, and the types of information that may be garnered from results will help parents make informed decisions when electing to have their child's body undergo an autopsy. In addition to answering all questions, support providers should check for understanding to ensure parents comprehend their answers, both prior to and following any postmortem examinations. Many parents report not understanding the answers provided to questions surrounding autopsy findings (Dent et al., 1996).

Parents have also expressed that follow-up contact or meetings with any hospital personnel or pediatricians who may have been involved in their child's care after their child has died can be helpful (Dent et al., 1996; Finlay & Dallimore, 1991). Home visits by support providers have also been identified as especially useful. These contacts may include offering condolences, facilitating access to professional support services, or answering of outstanding questions about their child's death. Parents also frequently desire specific recommendations about connecting with support services, such as psychotherapy or support groups, and how to help surviving siblings (Back, 1991; Dent et al., 1996). In their study of parents bereaved by a variety of causes, including suicide, drug-related death, accident, and some natural causes, Feigelman et al. (2012) found that parents reported seeking out a variety of services, including professional counseling, support groups, psychics, and clergy. The authors additionally noted that parents rated support groups as the most helpful psychosocial resource (Jordan & McIntosh, 2012; Feigelman et al., 2012).

Health care professionals should consider several guidelines in order to provide the most comprehensive and useful support to parents during this difficult stage. First, as noted in the preceding text, delivering timely and clear information to parents is extremely important (Back, 1991). Having support providers available to families during pronouncement of the death is paramount. Blame reduction and guilt alleviation is particularly valuable among traumatic deaths, for which parents may feel responsible for some aspect of their child dying (Back, 1991). Additionally, media coverage about the child's death, which may be inaccurate or insensitive, can be particularly upsetting to parents, and so it is important to be mindful of this when offering support (Dent et al., 1996).

Spending time with the child after death has been consistently identified as immensely meaningful by bereaved parents (Ahrens et al., 1997; Back, 1991; Dent et al., 1996; Finlay & Dallimore, 1991). In fact, in a study of parents who lost children unexpectedly, nearly all parents expressed a desire for this, even if their child's body was mutilated from his or her death (Finlay & Dallimore, 1991). Only one parent in this study reported regretting the decision to see her daughter's body, while a greater number expressed deep regrets for not doing so (Finlay & Dallimore, 1991). Many parents may also desire a memento, such as a lock of hair, footprint, or photograph of their child, though this is infrequently offered (Dent et al., 1996). Personal items, such as clothes or shoes, also maintain value for parents, who appreciate the return of these items after the loss (Finlay & Dallimore, 1991). Given the empirical evidence supporting the importance of offering mementos and time with the child's body (Ahrens et al., 1997; Rudd & D'Andrea, 2013; Shearer & Davidhizar, 1993), support providers should accommodate this process as much as possible while remaining respectful of any decision parents make about seeing their child. These moments may be particularly meaningful in instances of sudden or unexpected deaths when parents or families were not prepared for the loss of their child. Rudd and D'Andrea (2013) noted that this time together may facilitate the transition from denial to understanding the reality of the loss. Spending time with the child also provides an opportunity for saying good-bye (Back, 1991). Preparing parents for potential physical changes in their child's body and managing expectations for altered physical appearance, especially if death is due to injury or violence, may minimize any distress that spending time with the body could otherwise cause (Back, 1991). Allowing parents to touch, hold, or spend time with their child at the time of death or shortly thereafter may be helpful to some parents. Medical personnel should respect this private time and allow parents as long as they need (Shearer & Davidhizar, 1993).

The death of a child, particularly one that is sudden, comes with a substantial decision-making responsibility. Parents face decisions surrounding autopsy, funeral arrangements, and notifying other family members. Providers may offer support or, when appropriate, clarify available options (Back, 1991; Shearer & Davidhizar, 1993). Providing concrete information about timelines and follow-up procedures or processes helps prepare parents and establish some expectations in this otherwise unknown situation (Rudd & D'Andrea, 2013).

Finally, continued acknowledgment and outreach demonstrate ongoing concern for parents' well-being. Back (1991) recommends a 24-hour check-in phone call to parents to convey sympathy. This phone call may also be a time to reassure parents that everything medically possible was done to save their child, reiterate the fact that the parent is not to blame, and express that the medical staff care about their loss (Ahrens et al., 1997). Pediatricians or physicians who were not directly involved medically at the time of death but have a relationship with the family should also reach out following death to acknowledge the loss and offer support (Wender, 2012). These contacts are also important for helping families connect with resources or professional support. Medical personnel may make referrals for providers in the community or other potentially useful organizations (Shearer & Davidhizar, 1993). This can include providing referrals for surviving siblings or other family members (Rudd & D'Andrea, 2013). Care for siblings in the cases of suicide is a particularly neglected area (Lindqvist, Johansson, & Karlsson, 2008); thus, it is important to attempt to connect siblings with available resources. Overall, communication marked by compassion and concern is essential during this sensitive time (Shearer & Davidhizar, 1993). Parents have indicated that receiving support that is empathic and validating in nature is vital throughout the loss and grief process (Rudd & D'Andrea, 2013).

In addition to support services at the time of death, parents desire sustained outreach extending out after their loss. Continued communication and follow-up are essential, particularly for connecting parents with desired support resources (Rudd & D'Andrea, 2013; Wisten & Zingmark, 2007). Some parents may not feel prepared to engage with support providers immediately following their loss; therefore, multiple contacts to offer services are often appreciated. Further, parents may feel abandoned, frustrated, or angry if medical personnel fail to follow up after the loss.

One method of extending this contact is through a follow-up meeting with parents or families. Cook, White, and Ross-Russell (2002) provided guidelines for conducting follow-up meetings after the sudden or unexpected death of a child in the pediatric intensive care unit. Meetings should be attended by parents, the physician, and a counselor and should be delayed until approximately 8 to 12 weeks after the loss to allow time for families to reflect and for postmortem results to become available. New information should be shared and discussed with the family, and parents should have the opportunity to ask outstanding questions. Cook and colleagues (2002) also noted that assuring parents that their child's death was not a result of their actions is critical for reducing blame often felt by families who lose a child suddenly. In addition, screening for pathological grief responses and providing information about available resources is imperative to identifying and meeting parent support needs. Finally, the location of the meeting is also of extreme importance. Returning to the hospital where their child died can be upsetting for families; for others, viewing the ward where their child died may provide closure. Of course, this topic should be approached with a great deal of sensitivity.

In addition to meetings, other types of continued contact, such as research or advocacy opportunities, may also be helpful for some parents. Research participation provides both a means to remain connected to the institute where the child was treated or died and a chance to help advance science. Dyregrov (2004) examined the research participation experiences of parents who lost a child by suicide, accident, or SIDS. While the majority of parents reported that it was painful to discuss their loss through research participation, all parents indicated that they found the experience to be positive and that they did not regret participating. This study used qualitative, in-depth interviews with parents, which may be a particularly appealing format to parents because it provides ample time to tell their story (Dyregrov, 2004).

Advocacy efforts may be an additional means of maintaining contact with parents bereaved by traumatic loss. In a study conducted with parents who lost children to accidental injuries, Girasek (2003) found that all participants thought it was appropriate to contact bereaved parents about taking part in accident prevention campaigns. Reasons cited for engaging in advocacy work included those focused on saving other children's lives or preventing other parents from experiencing grief, as well as reasons related to promoting their own healing or honoring their child. It is important to note that parents believed these types of approaches should be delayed until after the most acute stages of grief have passed.

Psychosocial Interventions

Given the multitude of negative outcomes associated with the traumatic death of a child described earlier in this chapter, psychosocial interventions may be useful to support traumatically bereaved parents and to facilitate their adjustment. These include both hospital-based bereavement care programs and more targeted interventions for the various psychological challenges that are associated with losing a child suddenly or violently. One specific area that is important for interventions for traumatically bereaved parents to consider is survivor's guilt. Interventions may address survivor's guilt through incorporation of several key components, including actualizing the loss, challenging irrational guilt, providing education on grief processes, normalizing reactions, imaginal conversation, and facilitating creative outlets. Early identification and intervention may ameliorate the detrimental role survivor's guilt sometimes plays in the bereavement process (Clements et al., 2006).

We now consider some specific interventions that have targeted traumatically bereaved parents or may be considered when working with this population.

Bereavement Intervention Program

The bereavement intervention program (BIP; Oliver et al., 2001) was designed at a pediatric trauma center for parents who lost a child unexpectedly. BIP consists of contact with a chaplain at the time of death, a brief home visit, an educational meeting with the parents and other supporters within 2 months of the loss, and an in-home interview around 1 year after the loss. The vast majority of parents participating in this program reported that the chaplain visit was helpful and answered questions regarding their child's care. Additionally, parents believed that supporters who attended the educational meeting remember their child; accept the adjustment time for grief; and call, visit, or write more (Oliver et al., 2001). Therefore, there are many beneficial consequences of a structured and systematic intervention program such as BIP, and continued outreach for a year following the death in a variety of formats addresses many of parents' critical support needs.

Parent Bereavement Project

The parent bereavement project (PBP; Murphy, 1996, 2000; Murphy et al. 1998) was developed for parents who have lost a child by accident, homicide, or suicide. The program has five main intervention targets: mental distress, trauma, grief, physical health, and marital functioning. It is implemented in a group format. In a study examining the impact of this intervention, a community-based sample of 261 parents was recruited from medical examiner files and randomized to either a 12-week PBP intervention or a control group. Married couples or partners were assigned to the same treatment condition. Intervention sessions were conducted by trained clinicians and took place in a community setting. Long-term follow-up findings revealed differential results for mothers compared to fathers and depended on the cause of death, which speaks to the necessity of individualizing interventions to the greatest extent possible to best meet parent needs (Murphy, 2000). Overall, though, results showed that the majority of parents felt positive about the program format.

Meaning-Centered Grief Therapy

Meaning-centered grief therapy (MCGT) is a 16-week intervention we designed for bereaved parents to address existential challenges and help support adaptive meaning-making following the loss of a child (Lichtenthal & Breitbart, 2012; Neimeyer & Lichtenthal, in press). After losing a child, parents' sense of meaning, purpose, and identity are often shaken to their core. MCGT aims to assist parents in finding meaning in their own existence, as well as in their child's life and death. Adapted from meaning-centered psychotherapy, a treatment that applies principles of Viktor Frankl's (1955, 1959, 1969, 1975) logotherapy to enhance meaning in the lives of advanced cancer patients (Breitbart et al., 2012; Breitbart et al., 2010), MCGT emphasizes the core principle that when confronted with unthinkable tragedy and pain, we still retain the power to choose our attitude in the face of suffering (Lichtenthal & Breitbart, 2012). It also incorporates psychoeducation on grief reactions and cognitive schemas, cognitive-behavioral techniques, and meaning reconstruction approaches. MCGT is designed to facilitate meaning-making processes and improve parents' sense of meaning and purpose by assisting parents with creating a coherent life narrative for themselves and their child; maintaining a continued adaptive bond with their child; understanding how their child's legacy and their own legacy are intertwined; and enhancing connections with various creative, experiential, historical, and attitudinal sources of meaning. Each session involves brief didactics and experiential exercises, with open-ended questions to help guide discussions. Additionally, parents complete a "Living Legacy Project" as a way of supporting their continued connection to their child and/or other sources of meaning. To refine the MCGT treatment manual and evaluate the feasibility and promise of this approach, this intervention is currently being tested in a pilot clinical trial with bereaved parents reporting elevated symptoms of prolonged grief.

Restorative Retelling

After a child dies in a violent manner, the story is often told and retold as a narrative. This process can become burdensome and upsetting to parents, though, as the pain associated with their child's death is rekindled again and again, and increased attention is paid to the way the child died rather than to the life actually lived. Retelling the story of a traumatic death can be particularly upsetting because of the violent and dramatic nature of the loss, occasionally at the hands of another person (Rynearson, 2001). Restorative retelling is a therapeutic process by which parents retell and reframe their story, emphasizing the active role the parent played, as opposed to that of a helpless witness, and highlighting important memories of the child's lived life (Rynearson, 2001). This intervention allows parents to step back from the ceaseless storytelling as they look for answers to answerless questions. Repeatedly wondering "Why did this happen?" or "How could I have prevented this?" leaves parents unsatisfied and exhausted, as no true, rational answer for these questions exists (Rynearson, 2001). Restorative retelling changes the way parents retell the story so they may disengage from irrational questioning.

Developed by Rynearson and colleagues (2001, 2006, 2011), this psychotherapeutic process is typically conducted in a small group setting and follows a structured format. Early sessions begin with a parent telling his or her story as the therapist aids in reframing it to emphasize remembrance of the deceased rather than simple recounting of the death. Other goals of this intervention include reconnection to life, recommitment to living, and revising the relationship between the bereaved individual and the deceased, moderating distress. Family support is also fostered as bereaved members begin to reengage with life (Rynearson, 2006). A recent open clinical trial examining restorative retelling in a group format with survivors of violent loss demonstrated initial promise for this intervention (Saindon et al., 2014). Following treatment, participants showed reductions in depression, trauma symptoms, and prolonged grief symptoms.

Complicated Grief Therapy

Complicated grief therapy (CGT) was developed by Shear and colleagues (2001, 2005) in response to the increasing need for an intervention targeting the symptoms of CG, which have been identified as distinct from depression and other bereavement-related mental disorders (Lichtenthal et al., 2004; Prigerson et al., 2009; Shear et al., 2001). CGT is a three-phase, 16-session, manualized individual intervention that integrates components of interpersonal therapy (IPT) for depression and cognitive behavioral therapy (CBT) for PTSD (Shear et al., 2001). Applying CBT techniques, each session involves setting an agenda, engaging in an in-session exercise, and assigning homework to prepare for the next session (Wetherell, 2012). The three phases of CGT are intended to address the emotional, cognitive, and behavioral symptoms of CG in an integrated manner. Essential to the efficacy of the middle phase of the intervention is an introductory phase in which the focus is on building a therapeutic alliance, psychoeducation about normal and CG, exploration of the client's interpersonal relationships, and the client's personal goals for the therapy (Shear, Frank, Houck, & Reynolds, 2005; Wetherell, 2012).

Additionally, the therapist provides a description of Stroebe and Schut's (1999) dual processes model, which proposes that individuals experience a dual process of coping through loss orientation (emotion focused) and restoration orientation (problem focused; Shear et al., 2005). During the second phase of treatment, the focus moves to exploring these two processes with the client through exercises done in session and outside of session. Exercises typically include writing and reviewing a "grief monitoring diary," engaging in imaginal and in vivo exposure to address trauma symptoms (Foa & Rothbaum, 1998), and planning personal goals to encourage reengagment in life (Shear et al., 2005; Wetherell, 2012). Imaginal and in vivo exposure exercises are based on techniques developed by Foa and Rothbaum (1998) to reduce symptoms of PTSD and can involve situational revisiting (e.g., visiting a location associated with the child's death or life), imaginal visualization, and expression of the moments leading up to the death and the time of death itself (Wetherell, 2012). In order to effectively and supportively engage a client in this type of work, a number of components are essential to establish prior to the exercises, including the development of a strong therapeutic alliance, discussion of strategies for managing negative emotions, and planning of rewards for engaging in the exercises (Wetherell, 2012). The third and last phase of the intervention involves reviewing progress, reinforcing strategies and topics learned in the previous sessions, and exploring feelings about termination (Shear et al., 2005).

A randomized controlled trial comparing CGT to IPT demonstrated that, while both were effective in improving CG symptoms, CGT had a greater response rate than IPT, providing preliminary evidence for the efficacy of CGT (Shear et al., 2005). Additionally, there is some evidence that CGT may be more effective when provided in tandem with psychopharmacological treatment, possibly due to the intense nature of the imaginal and in vivo exposure exercises (Simon et al., 2008). Because CGT integrates several important components of IPT and CBT and exposure techniques for PTSD, this intervention can be particularly helpful in addressing the complexity and intensity of symptoms that may be experienced by parents following the traumatic loss of a child.

Interventions for Coping With Suicide Loss

Interventions for parents bereaved by suicide typically address common reactions, such as feelings of rejection or anger, intense shame, and guilt or responsibility. Hatton and Valente (1981) describe a supportive group therapy for parents whose children committed suicide. Core components of this intervention included (a) parents sharing their stories and accompanying emotions while offering mutual support, (b) examination of the parenting role, and (c) discussion of stigma and alienation. Following the group, parents reported decreased levels of depression and emotional lability and improved concentration and occupational functioning (Hatton & Valente, 1981). Kaslow and Aronson (2004) provided recommendations for family-based interventions for those who lost a loved one to suicide, highlighting the importance of addressing the painful emotions that arise, dealing with stigma, discussion of family dynamics and coping strategies, and creating a suicide story. This approach aims to help the survivors of suicide come to terms with the loss, with an emphasis on enhancing family relationships. Group formats have been consistently recommended for suicide survivors because of their emphasis on normalization, education, and understanding (Girard & Silber, 2011; Hatton & Valente, 1981). More recently, innovative approaches to forming groups for parents bereaved by suicide delivered through the Internet have been explored. In one study comparing bereaved parents participating in web-based support groups with those attending face-to-face group sessions, Internet support group attendees were found to report greater stigmatization related to the suicide of their child from the rest of their family than from their in-person counterparts, suggesting that web-based groups may provide an important and useful method for over-coming stigma-related barriers to accessing support services (Feigelman, Gorman, Beal, & Jordan, 2008).

CONCLUSION

The traumatic loss of a child commonly results in a cascade of painful bio-psychosocial sequelae. To find meaning in an untimely, unthinkable death may seem near impossible, and yet research has demonstrated that some traumatically bereaved parents can make meaning of their loss, and that those who do report less severe grief and traumatic stress reactions. While trends associated with various causes of death have been described, it bears repeating that it is important for clinicians to remember that each parent's bereavement experience is unique. Providers should be mindful of risk factors of poor bereavement outcomes so that those parents who may need additional support can be better identified. Given the range of psychosocial complexities the traumatic death of a child often yields, providers would do well to familiarize themselves with multiple theoretical models and intervention approaches so that support can be tailored to a given parent's needs.

CASE STUDY

Frank, a 16-year-old high school student, was killed in a motor vehicle accident that occurred when his friend, the driver, lost control of the car after an evening of heavy drinking. Frank's parents were called to the hospital after the accident to identify the body. In the year since the loss occurred, Frank's father, Jack, age 51, has experienced a heart attack and has been in a nonserious car accident. Frank's mother, Aubrey, age 48, has been diagnosed with major depression, gastroesophageal reflux disorder, hypertension, and new-onset diabetes.

FOCUS QUESTIONS

1. Describe the major theoretical concepts that would help a clinician understand Jack's and Aubrey's grief.
2. What aspects of Frank's death complicate his parents' ability to cope with his loss?

3. Discuss how the traumatic loss of a child can contribute to physical decline in parents.
4. What supportive interventions would be most helpful for Jack and Aubrey?

REFERENCES

Ahrens, W., Hart, R., & Maruyama, N. (1997). Pediatric death: Managing the aftermath in the emergency department. *Journal of Emergency Medicine, 15*(5), 601–603.

Alam, R., Barrera, M., D'Agostino, N., Nicholas, D. B., & Schneiderman, G. (2012). Bereavement experiences of mothers and fathers over time after the death of a child due to cancer. *Death Studies, 36*(1), 1–22.

Allenou, C., Olliac, B., Bourdet-Loubere, S., Brunet, A., David, A. C., Claudet, I., . . . Birmes, P. (2010). Symptoms of traumatic stress in mothers of children victims of a motor vehicle accident. *Depression and Anxiety, 27*(7), 652–657.

American Psychiatric Association. (2013). *Diagnostic and statistical manual of mental disorders: DSM-5.* Washington, DC: American Psychiatric Pub Incorporated.

Anderson, M. J., Marwit, S. J., Vandenberg, B., & Chibnall, J. T. (2005). Psychological and religious coping strategies of mothers bereaved by the sudden death of a child. *Death Studies, 29*(9), 811–826.

Back, K. J. (1991). Sudden, unexpected pediatric death: Caring for the parents. *Pediatric Nursing, 17*(6), 571–575.

Beder, J. (2004). Loss of the assumptive world—How we deal with death and loss. *Omega-Journal of Death and Dying, 50*(4), 255–265.

Boelen, P. A., & van den Bout, J. (2005). Complicated grief, depression, and anxiety as distinct postloss syndromes: A confirmatory factor analysis study. *American Journal of Psychiatry, 162*(11), 2175–2177.

Boelen, P. A., van den Bout, J., & de Keijser, J. (2003). Traumatic grief as a disorder distinct from bereavement-related depression and anxiety: A replication study with bereaved mental health care patients. *American Journal of Psychiatry, 160*(7), 1339–1341.

Bolton, J. M., Au, W., Leslie, W. D., Martens, P. J., Enns, M. W., Roos, L. L., . . . Sareen, J. (2013). Parents bereaved by offspring suicide: A population-based longitudinal case-control study. *JAMA Psychiatry, 70*(2), 158–167.

Bonanno, G. A., Wortman, C. B., Lehman, D. R., Tweed, R. G., Haring, M., Sonnega, J., . . . Nesse, R. M. (2002). Resilience to loss and chronic grief: A prospective study from preloss to 18-months postloss. *Journal of Perspectives in Psychology, 83*(5), 1150–1164.

Bowlby, J. (1980). *Attachment and loss.* New York, NY: Basic Books.

Breitbart, W., Poppito, S., Rosenfeld, B., Vickers, A. J., Li, Y., Abbey, J., . . . Cassileth, B. R. (2012). Pilot randomized controlled trial of individual meaning-centered psychotherapy for patients with advanced cancer. *Journal of Clinical Oncology, 30*(12), 1304–1309.

Breitbart, W., Rosenfeld, B., Gibson, C., Pessin, H., Poppito, S., Nelson, C., . . . Olden, M. (2010). Meaning-centered group psychotherapy for patients with advanced cancer: A pilot randomized controlled trial. *Psychooncology, 19*(1), 21–28.

Bremner, J. D., Staib, L. H., Kaloupek, D., Southwick, S. M., Soufer, R., & Charney, D. S. (1999). Neural correlates of exposure to traumatic pictures and sound in Vietnam combat veterans with and without posttraumatic stress disorder: A positron emission tomography study. *Biological Psychiatry, 45*(7), 806–816.

Brent, D. A., Moritz, G., Bridge, J., Perper, J., & Canobbio, R. (1996). The impact of adolescent suicide on siblings and parents: A longitudinal follow-up. *Suicide and Life Threatening Behavior, 26*(3), 253–259.

Burke, L. A., & Neimeyer, R. A. (2012). Prospective risk factors for complicated grief. In M. Stroebe, H. Schut & J. van den Bout (Eds.), *Complicated grief: Scientific foundations for health care professionals* (pp. 145–161). New York, NY: Routledge.

Burke, L. A., Neimeyer, R. A., & McDevitt-Murphy, M. E. (2010). African American homicide bereavement: Aspects of social support that predict complicated grief, PTSD, and depression. *Omega (Westport), 61*(1), 1–24.

Clements, P. T., Garzon, L., & Milliken, T. F. (2006). Survivors' guilt following sudden traumatic loss: Promoting early intervention in the critical care setting. *Critical Care Nursing Clinics of North America, 18*(3), 359–369.

Cook, P., White, D. K., & Ross-Russell, R. I. (2002). Bereavement support following sudden and unexpected death: Guidelines for care. *Archives of Diseases in Childhood, 87*(1), 36–38.

Currier, J. M., Holland, J. M., & Neimeyer, R. A. (2006). Sense-making, grief, and the experience of violent loss: Toward a mediational model. *Death Studies, 30*(5), 403–428.

Davis, C. G., Wortman, C. B., Lehman, D. R., & Silver, R. C. (2000). Searching for meaning in loss: Are clinical assumptions correct. *Death Studies, 24*(6), 497–540.

Demi, A. S., & Miles, M. S. (1987). Parameters of normal grief: A Delphi study. *Death Studies, 11*(6), 397–412.

Dent, A., Condon, L., Blair, P., & Fleming, P. (1996). A study of bereavement care after a sudden and unexpected death. *Archives of Diseases in Childhood, 74*(6), 522–526.

Dyregrov, K. (2004). Bereaved parents' experience of research participation. *Social Science and Medicine, 58*(2), 391–400.

Dyregrov, K., Nordanger, D., & Dyregrov, A. (2003). Predictors of psychosocial distress after suicide, SIDS and accidents. *Death Studies, 27*(2), 143–165.

Eilegård, A., & Kreicbergs, U. (2010). Risk of parental dissolution of partnership following the loss of a child to cancer: A population-based long-term follow-up. *Archives of Pediatric and Adolescent Medicine, 164*(1), 100–101.

Ellifritt, J., Nelson, K. A., & Walsh, D. (2003). Complicated bereavement: A national survey of potential risk factors. *American Journal of Hospice Palliative Care, 20*(2), 114–120.

Feigelman, W., Gorman, B. S., Beal, K. C., & Jordan, J. R. (2008). Internet support groups for suicide survivors: A new mode for gaining bereavement assistance. *Omega (Westport), 57*, 217–243.

Feigelman, W., Gorman, B. S., & Jordan, J. R. (2009). Stigmatization and suicide bereavement. *Death Studies, 33*(7), 591–608.

Feigelman, W., Jordan, J. R., & Gorman, B. S. (2008). How they died, time since loss, and bereavement outcomes. *Omega (Westport), 58*(4), 251–273.

Feigelman, W., Jordan, J. R., & Gorman, B. S. (2009). Personal growth after a suicide loss: Cross-sectional findings suggest growth after loss may be associated with better mental health among survivors. *Omega (Westport), 59*(3), 181–202.

Feigelman, W., Jordan, J. R., & Gorman, B. S. (2011). Parental grief after a child's drug death compared to other death causes: Investigating a greatly neglected bereavement population. *Omega (Westport), 63*(4), 291–316.

Feigelman, W., Jordan, J. R., McIntosh, J. L., & Feigelman, B. (2012). *Devastating losses: How parents cope with the death of a child to suicide or drugs.* New York, NY: Springer Pub.

Field, N. P., & Filanosky, C. (2010). Continuing bonds, risk factors for complicated grief, and adjustment to bereavement. *Death Studies, 34*(1), 1–29.

Field, N. P., Gao, B., & Paderna, L. (2005). Continuing bonds in bereavement: An attachment theory based perspective. *Death Studies, 29*(4), 277–299.

Finlay, I., & Dallimore, D. (1991). Your child is dead. *BMJ, 302*(6791), 1524–1525.

Foa, E. B., Ehlers, A., Clark, D. M., Tolin, D. F., & Orsillo, S. M. (1999). The Posttraumatic Cognitions Inventory (PTCI): Development and validation. *Psychological Assessment, 11*(3), 303–314.

Foa, E. B., & Rothbaum, B. O. (1998). *Treating the trauma of rape: Cognitive-behavioral therapy for PTSD.* New York, NY: Guilford Press.

Fraley, R. C., & Bonanno, G. A. (2004). Attachment and loss: A test of three competing models on the association between attachment-related avoidance and adaptation to bereavement. *Perspectives in Social Psychology Bulletin, 30*(7), 878–890.

Frankl, V. F. (1955). *The doctor and the soul.* New York, NY: Random House.

Frankl, V. F. (1959). *Man's search for meaning.* Boston, MA: Beacon Press.

Frankl, V. F. (1969). *The will to meaning: Foundations and applications of logotherapy.* New York, NY: Penguin Books.

Frankl, V. F. (1975). *Man's search for ultimate meaning.* New York, NY: Plenum Press.

Freed, P. J., Yanagihara, T. K., Hirsch, J., & Mann, J. J. (2009). Neural mechanisms of grief regulation. *Biological Psychiatry, 66*(1), 33–40.

Girard, G. A., & Silber, T. J. (2011). The aftermath of adolescent suicide: Clinical, ethical, and spiritual issues. *Adolescent Medicine: State of the Art Reviews, 22*(2), 229–239, ix.

Girasek, D. C. (2003). Parents of fatally injured children discuss taking part in prevention campaigns: An exploratory study. *Death Studies, 27*(10), 929–937.

Gudmundsdottir, M., & Chesla, C. A. (2006). Building a new world: Habits and practices of healing following the death of a child. *Journal of Family Nursing, 12*(2), 143–164.

Harper, M., O'Connor, R., Dickson, A., & O'Carroll, R. (2011). Mothers continuing bonds and ambivalence to personal mortality after the death of their child—an interpretative phenomenological analysis. *Psychology, Health & Medicine, 16*(2), 203–214.

Harper, M., O'Connor, R. C., & O'Carroll, R. E. (2013). Factors associated with grief and depression following the loss of a child: A multivariate analysis. *Psychology, Health & Medicine, 19*(3), 247–252.

Hatton, C. L., & Valente, S. M. (1981). Bereavement group for parents who suffered a suicidal loss of a child. *Suicide and Life Threatening Behavior, 11*(3), 141–150.

Janoff-Bulman, R. (2010). *Shattered assumptions.* New York, NY: Free Press.

Johnson, L. C., Murphy, S. A., & Dimond, M. (1996). Reliability, construct validity, and subscale norms of the Brief Symptom Inventory when administered to bereaved parents. *Journal of Nursing Measurement, 4*(2), 117–127.

Jordan, J. R., Baker, J., Matteis, M., Rosenthal, S., & Ware, E. S. (2005). The grief evaluation measure (GEM): An initial validation study. *Death Studies, 29*(4), 301–332.

Kachoyeanos, M. K., & Selder, F. E. (1993). Life transitions of parents at the unexpected death of a school-age and older child. *Journal of Pediatric Nursing, 8*(1), 41–49.

Kashka, M. S., & Beard, M. T. (1999). The grief of parents of murdered children: A suggested model for intervention. *Holistic Nursing Practice, 14*(1), 22–36.

Kaslow, N. J., & Aronson, S. G. (2004). Recommendations for family interventions following a suicide. *Professional Psychology: Research and Practice, 35*(3), 240–247.

Keesee, N. J., Currier, J. M., & Neimeyer, R. A. (2008). Predictors of grief following the death of one's child: The contribution of finding meaning. *Journal of Clinical Psychology, 64*(10), 1145–1163.

Kersting, A., Brahler, E., Glaesmer, H., & Wagner, B. (2011). Prevalence of complicated grief in a representative population-based sample. *Journal of Affective Disorders, 131*(1–3), 339–343.

Klass, D. (2013). *The spiritual lives of bereaved parents.* New York, NY: Routledge.

Kovarsky, R. S. (1989). Loneliness and disturbed grief: A comparison of parents who lost a child to suicide or accidental death. *Archives of Psychiatric Nursing, 3*(2), 86–96.

Lanius, R. A., Williamson, P. C., Densmore, M., Boksman, K., Gupta, M. A., Neufeld, R. W., . . . Menon, R. S. (2001). Neural correlates of traumatic memories in posttraumatic stress disorder: A functional MRI investigation. *American Journal of Psychiatry, 158*(11), 1920–1922.

Lehman, D. R., Wortman, C. B., & Williams, A. F. (1987). Long-term effects of losing a spouse or child in a motor vehicle crash. *Journal of Perspectives in Social Psychology, 52*(1), 218–231.

Li, J., Hansen, D., Mortensen, P. B., & Olsen, J. (2002). Myocardial infarction in parents who lost a child: A nationwide prospective cohort study in Denmark. *Circulation, 106*(13), 1634–1639.

Li, J., Precht, D. H., Mortensen, P. B., & Olsen, J. (2003). Mortality in parents after death of a child in Denmark: A nationwide follow-up study. *Lancet, 361*(9355), 363–367.

Lichtenthal, W. G., & Breitbart, W. (2012). Finding meaning through the attitude one takes. In R. A. Neimeyer (Ed.), *Techniques in grief therapy: Creative strategies for counseling the bereaved* (pp. 161–164). New York, NY: Routledge.

Lichtenthal, W. G., Burke, L. A., & Neimeyer, R. A. (2011). Religious coping and meaning-making following the loss of a loved one. *Counseling and Spirituality, 30*, 113–136.

Lichtenthal, W. G., Cruess, D. G., & Prigerson, H. G. (2004). A case for establishing complicated grief as a distinct mental disorder in *DSM-5*. *Clinical Psychology Review, 24*(6), 637–662.

Lichtenthal, W. G., Currier, J. M., Neimeyer, R. A., & Keesee, N. J. (2010). Sense and significance: A mixed methods examination of meaning making after the loss of one's child. *Journal of Clinical Psychology, 66*(7), 791–812.

Lichtenthal, W. G., Neimeyer, R. A., Currier, J. M., Roberts, K., & Jordan, N. (2013). Cause of death and the quest for meaning after the loss of a child. *Death Studies, 37*(4), 311–342.

Lindqvist, P., Johansson, L., & Karlsson, U. (2008). In the aftermath of teenage suicide: A qualitative study of the psychosocial consequences for the surviving family members. *BMC Psychiatry, 8*, 26.

Lobb, E. A., Kristjanson, L. J., Aoun, S. M., Monterosso, L., Halkett, G. K., & Davies, A. (2010). Predictors of complicated grief: A systematic review of empirical studies. *Death Studies, 34*(8), 673–698.

Maercker, A., & Lalor, J. (2012). Diagnostic and clinical considerations in prolonged grief disorder. *Dialogues in Clinical Neurosciences, 14*(2), 167–176.

Maple, M., Edwards, H., Plummer, D., & Minichiello, V. (2010). Silenced voices: Hearing the stories of parents bereaved through the suicide death of a young adult child. *Health & Social Care in the Community, 18*(3), 241–248.

Meert, K. L., Shear, K., Newth, C. J., Harrison, R., Berger, J., Zimmerman, J., . . . Nicholson, C. (2011). Follow-up study of complicated grief among parents eighteen months after a child's death in the pediatric intensive care unit. *Journal of Palliative Medicine, 14*(2), 207–214.

Michon, B., Balkou, S., Hivon, R., & Cyr, C. (2003). Death of a child: Parental perception of grief intensity-end-of-life and bereavement care. *Paediatrics & Child Health, 8*(6), 363–366.

Miles, M. S. (1985). Emotional symptoms and physical health in bereaved parents. *Nursing Research, 34*(2), 76–81.

Mitchell, A. M., Kim, Y., Prigerson, H. G., & Mortimer-Stephens, M. (2004). Complicated grief in survivors of suicide. *Crisis, 25*(1), 12–18.

Murphy, S. A. (1996). Parent bereavement stress and preventive intervention following the violent deaths of adolescent or young adult children. *Death Studies, 20*(5), 441–452.

Murphy, S. A. (2000). The use of research findings in bereavement programs: A case study. *Death Studies, 24*(7), 585–602.

Murphy, S. A., Braun, T., Tillery, L., Cain, K. C., Johnson, L. C., & Beaton, R. D. (1999a). PTSD among bereaved parents following the violent deaths of their 12- to 28-year-old children: A longitudinal prospective analysis. *Journal of Traumatic Stress, 12*(2), 273–291.

Murphy, S. A., Das Gupta, A., Cain, K. C., Johnson, L. C., Lohan, J., Wu, L., & Mekwa, J. (1999b). Changes in parents' mental distress after the violent death of an adolescent or young adult child: A longitudinal prospective analysis. *Death Studies, 23*(2), 129–159.

Murphy, S. A., Johnson, C., Cain, K. C., Das Gupta, A., Dimond, M., Lohan, J., & Baugher, R. (1998). Broad-spectrum group treatment for parents bereaved by the violent deaths of their 12- to 28-year-old children: A randomized controlled trial. *Death Studies, 22*(3), 209–235.

Murphy, S. A., & Johnson, L. C. (2003). Finding meaning in a child's violent death: A five-year prospective analysis of parents' personal narratives and empirical data. *Death Studies, 27*(5), 381–404.

Murphy, S. A., Johnson, L. C., Chung, I. J., & Beaton, R. D. (2003a). The prevalence of PTSD following the violent death of a child and predictors of change 5 years later. *Journal of Traumatic Stress, 16*(1), 17–25.

Murphy, S. A., Johnson, L. C., & Lohan, J. (2003b). Challenging the myths about parents' adjustment after the sudden, violent death of a child. *Journal of Nursing Scholarship, 35*(4), 359–364.

Nadeau, J. W. (1998). *Families making sense of death.* Thousand Oaks, CA: Sage Publications.

Nadeau, J. W. (2008). Meaning-making in bereaved families: Assessment, intervention, and future research. In M. S. Stroebe, R. O. Hansson, H. Schut, & W. Stroebe (Eds.), *Handbook of bereavement research and practice: Advances in theory and intervention* (pp. 511–530). Washington, DC: American Psychological Association.

Nakajima, S., Ito, M., Shirai, A., & Konishi, T. (2012). Complicated grief in those bereaved by violent death: The effects of post-traumatic stress disorder on complicated grief. *Dialogues in Clinical Neurosciences, 14*(2), 210–214.

Neimeyer, R. A. (2011). Reconstructing meaning in bereavement. *Rivista di Psichiatria, 46*(5–6), 332–336.

Neimeyer, R. A., Baldwin, S. A., & Gillies, J. (2006). Continuing bonds and reconstructing meaning: Mitigating complications in bereavement. *Death Studies, 30*(8), 715–738.

Neimeyer, R. A., & Lichtenthal, W. G. (in press). The presence of absence: The struggle for meaning in the death of a child. In G. Cox & R. Stevenson (Eds.), *Children and death.* Amityville, NY: Baywood Publishing.

Oliver, R. C., & Fallat, M. E. (1995). Traumatic childhood death: How well do parents cope? *Journal of Trauma, 39*(2), 303–307.

Oliver, R. C., Sturtevant, J. P., Scheetz, J. P., & Fallat, M. E. (2001). Beneficial effects of a hospital bereavement intervention program after traumatic childhood death. *Journal of Trauma, 50*(3), 440–446; discussion 447–448.

Omerov, P., Steineck, G., Nyberg, T., Runeson, B., & Nyberg, U. (2013). Psychological morbidity among suicide-bereaved and non-bereaved parents: A nationwide population survey. *BMJ Open, 3*(8), e003108.

Ott, C. H. (2003). The impact of complicated grief on mental and physical health at various points in the bereavement process. *Death Studies, 27*(3), 249–272.

Parker, B. S., & Dunn, K. S. (2011). The continued lived experience of the unexpected death of a child. *Omega (Westport), 63*(3), 221–233.

Phan, K. L., Fitzgerald, D. A., Nathan, P. J., Moore, G. J., Uhde, T. W., & Tancer, M. E. (2005). Neural substrates for voluntary suppression of negative affect: A functional magnetic resonance imaging study. *Biological Psychiatry, 57*(3), 210–219.

Pitman, A., Osborn, D., King, M., & Erlangsen, A. (2014). Effects of suicide bereavement on mental health. *Lancet Psychiatry, 1*(1), 86–94.

Prigerson, H. G., Bierhals, A. J., Kasl, S. V., Reynolds, C. F., 3rd, Shear, M. K., Newsom, J. T., & Jacobs, S. (1996). Complicated grief as a disorder distinct from bereavement-related depression and anxiety: A replication study. *American Journal of Psychiatry, 153*(11), 1484–1486.

Prigerson, H. G., Frank, E., Kasl, S. V., Reynolds, C. F., 3rd, Anderson, B., Zubenko, G. S., . . . Kupfer, D. J. (1995). Complicated grief and bereavement-related depression as distinct disorders: Preliminary empirical validation in elderly bereaved spouses. *American Journal of Psychiatry, 152*(1), 22–30.

Prigerson, H. G., Horowitz, M. J., Jacobs, S. C., Parkes, C. M., Aslan, M., Goodkin, K., . . . Maciejewski, P. K. (2009). Prolonged grief disorder: Psychometric validation of criteria proposed for *DSM-5* and ICD-11. *PLOS Medicine, 6*(8), e1000121.

Rogers, C. H. (2008). Long-term effects of the death of a child on parents' adjustment in midlife. *Journal of Family Psychology, 22*(2), 203–211.

Rostila, M., Saarela, J., & Kawachi, I. (2012). Mortality in parents following the death of a child: A nationwide follow-up study from Sweden. *Journal of Epidemiology and Community Health, 66*(10), 927–933.

Rudd, R. A., & D'Andrea, L. M. (2013). Professional support requirements and grief interventions for parents bereaved by an unexplained death at different time periods in the grief process. *International Journal of Emergency Mental Health, 15*(1), 51–68.

Rynearson, E. K. (2001). *Retelling violent death.* New York, NY: Routledge.

Rynearson, E. K. (Ed.). (2006). *Violent death: Resilience and intervention beyond the crisis.* New York, NY: Routledge.

Rynearson, E. K., & Salloum, A. (2011). Restorative retelling: Revisiting the narrative of violent death. In R. A. Neimeyer, D. Harris, H. Winokuer, & G. Thornton (Eds.), *Grief and bereavement in contemporary society: Bridging research and practice* (pp. 177–188). New York, NY: Routledge.

Saindon, C., Rheingold, A. A., Baddeley, J., Wallace, M. M., Brown, C., & Rynearson, E. K. (2014). Restorative retelling for violent loss: An open clinical trial. *Death Studies, 38*, 251–258.

Schmitt, F. E. (1982). *The structuring of a life transition following a spinal cord injury* (Dissertation). University of Illinois at the Medical Center, Chicago, IL.

Schwab, R. (1998). A child's death and divorce: Dispelling the myth. *Death Studies, 22*(5), 445–468.

Seecharan, G. A., Andresen, E. M., Norris, K., & Toce, S. S. (2004). Parents' assessment of quality of care and grief following a child's death. *Archives of Pediatric and Adolescent Medicine, 158*(6), 515–520.

Seguin, M., Lesage, A., & Kiely, M. C. (1995). Parental bereavement after suicide and accident: A comparative study. *Suicide and Life Threatening Behavior, 25*(4), 489–492.

Shanfield, S. B., & Swain, B. J. (1984). Death of adult children in traffic accidents. *Journal of Nervous and Mental Disorders, 172*(9), 533–538.

Shear, K., Frank, E., Houck, P. R., & Reynolds, C. F., 3rd. (2005). Treatment of complicated grief: A randomized controlled trial. *JAMA, 293*(21), 2601–2608.

Shear, M. K., Frank, E., Foa, E., Cherry, C., Reynolds, C. F., 3rd, Vander Bilt, J., & Masters, S. (2001). Traumatic grief treatment: A pilot study. *American Journal of Psychiatry, 158*(9), 1506–1508.

Shear, M. K., Simon, N., Wall, M., Zisook, S., Neimeyer, R., Duan, N., . . . Keshaviah, A. (2011). Complicated grief and related bereavement issues for *DSM-5*. *Depression & Anxiety, 28*(2), 103–117.

Shearer, R., & Davidhizar, R. (1993). Shock and disbelief: Supporting parents who experience the sudden death of their child. *Pennsylvania Nurse, 48*(3), 14–15, 22.

Simon, N. M., Shear, M. K., Fagiolini, A., Frank, E., Zalta, A., Thompson, E. H., . . . Silowash, R. (2008). Impact of concurrent naturalistic pharmacotherapy on psychotherapy of complicated grief. *Psychiatry Research, 159*(1–2), 31–36.

Simon, N. M., Wall, M. M., Keshaviah, A., Dryman, M. T., LeBlanc, N. J., & Shear, M. K. (2011). Informing the symptom profile of complicated grief. *Depression & Anxiety, 28*(2), 118–126.

Snowden, C., Elbourne, D. R., & Garcia, J. (2004). Perinatal pathology in the context of a clinical trial: Attitudes of bereaved parents. *Archives of Disease in Childhood- Fetal and Neonatal Edition, 89*, F208–F211.

Spratt, M. L., & Denney, D. R. (1991). Immune variables, depression, and plasma cortisol over time in suddenly bereaved parents. *Journal of Neuropsychiatry and Clinical Neurosciences, 3*(3), 299–306.

Stroebe, M., & Schut, H. (1999). The dual process model of coping with bereavement: Rationale and description. *Death Studies, 23*(3), 197–224.

Stroebe, M. S., Stroebe, W., & Schut, H. (2001). Gender differences in adjustment to bereavement an empirical and theoretical review. *Review of General Psychology, 5*(1), 62–83.

Vaiva, G., Brunet, A., Lebigot, F., Boss, V., Ducrocq, F., Devos, P., . . . Goudemand, M. (2003). Fright (effroi) and other peritraumatic responses after a serious motor vehicle accident: Prospective influence on acute PTSD development. *Canadian Journal of Psychiatry, 48*(6), 395–401.

van der Houwen, K., Stroebe, M., Stroebe, W., Schut, H., van den Bout, J., & Wijngaards-de Meij, L. (2010). Risk factors for bereavement outcome: A multivariate approach. *Death Studies, 34*(3), 195–220.

Wender, E. (2012). Supporting the family after the death of a child. *Pediatrics, 130*(6), 1164–1169.

Wetherell, J. L. (2012). Complicated grief therapy as a new treatment approach. *Dialogues in Clinical Neuroscience, 14*(2), 159–166.

Wisten, A., & Zingmark, K. (2007). Supportive needs of parents confronted with sudden cardiac death: An qualitative study. *Resuscitation, 74*(1), 68–74.

Worden, J. W. (1991). *Grief counseling and grief therapy: A handbook for the mental health practitioner.* New York, NY: Springer Publishing Company.

Wortmann, J. H., & Park, C. L. (2008). Religion and spirituality in adjustment following bereavement: An integrative review. *Death Studies, 32*(8), 703–736.

Youngblut, J. M., Brooten, D., Cantwell, G. P., del Moral, T., & Totapally, B. (2013). Parent health and functioning 13 months after infant or child NICU/PICU death. *Pediatrics, 132*(5), e1295–e1301.

Zisook, S., Chentsova-Dutton, Y., & Shuchter, S. R. (1998). PTSD following bereavement. *Annals of Clinical Psychiatry, 10*(4), 157–163.

CHAPTER 15

Remembering the "Forgotten Bereaved": Understanding and Caring for Siblings of Completed Suicide Victims

Rebecca Kabatchnick and Beth Perry Black

*T*his chapter provides a thorough discussion on the problem of the "forgotten bereaved." Shneidman (1972) captured the struggle of suicide survivors with his metaphor: "The person who commits suicide puts his psychological skeleton in the survivor's emotional closet." Despite carrying heavy emotional, social, and even physical burdens, siblings of completed suicide victims are deemed "forgotten bereaved" throughout the bereavement literature (Rostila, 2012). Siblings of completed suicide victims suffer devastating psychological sequelae, including depression, suicidality, and posttraumatic stress disorder (PTSD), yet a gap in the literature exists regarding the most efficient interventions for these siblings (Brent, Moritz, Bridge, & Perper, 1996). McIntosh and Wrobleski (1988) initially reported limited research addressing children and adolescents losing siblings to suicide, calling them the "forgotten mourners." Although the bereavement literature addresses depression in these siblings, a significant lack of psychological support and untreated or undiagnosed depression, stress, and anxiety remains prevalent in this population (Brent et al., 1993).

At the same time mothers of completed suicide victims may be coping with severe depression, their surviving sons and daughters suffer from a lack of family support and loss of familial and social relationships (Brent et al., 1996). With the highest mortality rate subsequent to familial death, siblings should no longer remain one of the least-studied familial relationships in the bereavement literature (Rostila, 2012). Considering the risks of suicidality and elevated mortality rates among these surviving siblings, appropriate, timely, and efficient interventions are critical and may be lifesaving.

Although sibling grief may remain "forgotten" in the bereavement literature, health care providers and community members must reach out with early, evidence-based interventions to ensure that the grief of this at-risk group does not remain disenfranchised and hidden. The sibling relationship is complex, one of the most complicated in families; the death of a sibling under any circumstances, especially when young, defies expectations that siblings will live into adulthood (Dickens, 2014). Little is known about sibling grief and bereavement (Barrera, Alam, D'Agostino, Nicholas, & Schneiderman, 2013). A brother or sister's suicide is particularly devastating and can have far-reaching and long-lasting effects on the lives of surviving siblings. Further research is critical to address the profound sorrow and distress of these siblings in order to develop appropriate interventions and approaches to therapy.

Throughout this chapter, we intentionally use the term *completed suicide* rather than the more common term *committed suicide*. Hunt and Hertlein (2015) provided a compelling explanation regarding this topic:

> . . . survivors are not grieving the death of someone who "committed suicide." They are grieving death from or by suicide. . . .People only commit crimes or sins—to say commit suicide implies that it is both and increases the shame and stigma. (p. 24)

COMPLETED SUICIDE AND ITS AFTERMATH: BACKGROUND

Definitions

Disenfranchised grief is the feeling of the loss of the right to grieve because grief is not acknowledged or recognized by society (White, 2006). *Completed suicide* is defined as "death caused by self-directed injurious behavior with any intent to die as a result of the behavior," as compared to a *suicide attempt*, which is a "non-fatal, self-directed potentially injurious behavior with any intent to die as a result of the behavior" (CDC Definitions, 2012). *Sibling suicide survivors* include siblings who have lost a brother or sister to completed suicide.

Statistics

When 38,364 individuals completed suicide in 2010, suicide ranked as the tenth leading cause of death for all ages in the United States (CDC Suicide Facts, 2012). Although the overall rate of suicide in the United States that year was 11.3 per 100,000 individuals, 11 people attempted suicide for every 1 completed suicide victim, and an average of 105 persons completed suicide each day. In the United States, males are more likely to complete suicide (79%) and use firearms (56%), as opposed to females, who more often have suicidal thoughts and complete suicide through poisoning (37.4%). Suicide is the second leading cause of death among American Indians/Alaska Natives aged 15 to 24 years, at a rate 2.5 times higher than the national average in that age range. Suicide is the third leading cause of death in the 15- to 24-year-old age group, with an estimated 100 to 200 suicide attempts for every completed suicide. In 16 states participating in the National Violent Death Reporting System (NVDRS) in 2010, 20% to 30% completed suicide victims tested positive for alcohol, antidepressants, and opiates including prescription painkillers and heroin (CDC Suicide Facts, 2012). In 2014, the Centers for Disease Control and Prevention (CDC) received funding to expand the NVDRS to 32 states, an initiative to assist participating states in designing and implementing tailored prevention and intervention efforts (CDC, 2015).

Silent and Invisible Surviving Siblings

Most siblings suffer from a significantly complicated grief response resulting from their brother or sister's completed suicide (Demi & Howell, 1991). Siblings may be considered the "forgotten" bereaved because they often grieve in silence and out of the eye of the public (Rostila, 2012). Notably, the author of a recent continuing education article on suicide provided an example by prominently omitting siblings in a list of those "left in [suicide's] wake—wives, husbands, partners, children, parents, and friends—all of whom are left wondering why and what might have been done. Even bystanders can suffer lasting emotional repercussions" (Church, 2015, p. 277).

The disenfranchised nature of sibling grief often exacerbates the already detrimental psychological consequences of their brother or sister's suicide (Dyregrov & Dyregrov, 2005). Siblings often take responsibility for supporting their grieving parents, a task they are usually not emotionally capable of while coping with their own grief (Dyregrov & Dyregrov, 2005). This in turn means that some siblings must hide their grief not only from society, but also from their own family. Some families do not discuss the death as a suicide due to fear of societal stigma. Siblings often hesitate before sharing information and feelings about suicide with peers, because the siblings fear others may become uncomfortable during such conversation (Demi & Howell, 1991).

Although the risks for depression and PTSD after sibling suicide increase drastically for the first 6 months following the event, the rates of depression return to their pre-exposure levels by the 3-year mark after the suicide (Brent et al., 1996); however, depression and other coexisting affective illnesses contribute to a higher rate of suicidal behavior among the surviving siblings (Brent et al., 1993). Importantly, completed sibling suicide also increases the surviving sibling's mortality rate and can significantly impact future relationships with parents, children, and other family members (Rostila, 2012).

REVIEWING THE LITERATURE ON SIBLINGS OF COMPLETED SUICIDE VICTIMS

The purpose of this review of the literature is to explore the sequelae and support of surviving siblings of completed suicide victims in the United States. We addressed two issues: the implications of disenfranchised grief and other sequelae in siblings of completed suicide victims and how health care providers can provide effective care for siblings of completed suicide victims.

To address these questions, we conducted a systematic review of the literature using CINAHL, PubMed, and PsycInfo. Search parameters were purposefully wide because we recognized that the literature is small; constraining the search would have likely yielded few results. We used these search terms: *sibling and suicide; sibling and death; suicide and reaction; suicide and response*; and *family and suicide*. We limited the language to English and searched for the literature published between the years 1980 and March 2015. The criteria for inclusion were that the siblings must have experienced the loss of a biological brother or sister to completed suicide, and were adolescents or young adults when the suicide took place. Most of the research was conducted in the United States, Norway, or Sweden.

Disenfranchised Grief and Hidden Feelings

Demi and Howell (1991) spearheaded studies of the psychological sequelae experienced by sibling suicide survivors, and although their research findings were published over two decades ago, their studies have been cited frequently throughout the bereavement literature. The researchers found the surviving siblings were at risk of complicated grief reactions and delayed resolution of grief related to the following: close relationships with the deceased, young ages of the deceased, and modes of suicide. Bereavement following the suicide of a family member invoked significant stress among the sibling survivors due to the stigma, guilt, and rejection associated with such a death. The quality and intensity of relationships with the suicide victim were of particular importance for bereavement outcomes. The researchers described the contrast between recognition of the strength of the often-underestimated sibling bond as opposed to a parent–child bond. Age and level of maturity affected bereavement outcomes of the siblings, and researchers found that the death of a sibling had long-term effects (Demi & Howell, 1991).

In a grounded theory study of young adults whose siblings had completed suicide, Demi and Howell (1991) explored the long-term effects of suicide upon siblings and parents. Participants were siblings aged older than 18 and younger than 30 years. The researchers identified three processes: (a) experiencing the pain; (b) hiding the pain; and (c) healing from the pain. Researchers discovered that anger, particularly toward the deceased and other family members for their actions toward the deceased, was the most common theme. One sibling described how she felt anger toward her brother for being "such a schmuck" (p. 351). While primarily children (as opposed to siblings) of completed suicide victims often experienced feelings of family disintegration, most of the siblings longed for re-creation of their lost family identity and traditions even as they aged into adulthood (Demi & Howell, 1991).

The long-term effects of the sibling suicide were substantial. Most of the sibling survivors experienced feelings of stigma and often expressed feeling ashamed or tainted by the suicide. Siblings often tried to conceal the suicide when moving to a new environment, as described by a sister who lied and claimed that her brother was still alive when a family friend asked how he was doing. Blaming was also a common theme, especially when directed toward other family members. Almost all of the siblings expressed feelings of sadness and loneliness that subsided over time. Feelings of lowered self-esteem expressed by a majority of the respondents caused problems in social relationships, and eventually carried over into the workplace as the siblings entered the workforce. Many siblings felt inadequate after becoming parents themselves and were distressed by poor relationships with their children. Some of the siblings could not become socially involved, while others participated in very destructive relationships. Some siblings feared the effects of the suicide upon their mental health. Many siblings experienced suicidal thoughts, including a sister who explained how she had always been afraid that she would commit suicide because "it's so familiar" (p. 352). Several respondents worried about their mental health and feared the genetic foundation of the suicide victim's mental illness (Demi & Howell, 1991).

For the sibling survivors, hiding the pain required energy and effort (Demi & Howell, 1991). Many families kept the suicide a secret in order to cope with the pain. Several survivors fled from their families and reminders of the deceased. A majority of survivors became extremely involved in school or work to escape their pain and recognized "working" as a socially acceptable coping mechanism. However, a few participants admitted to engaging in socially unacceptable and unhealthy conduct, including addictive behavior like overeating, drinking, or using illicit drugs. Most explained that there was no shared expression of grief within their families. Siblings frequently used denial to hide feelings of pain and grief, and many subjects did not recognize that their pain could be attributed to distorted or unresolved grief. Many survivors who used the coping mechanism of "avoiding" consciously pushed thoughts of suicide and death out of their immediate awareness (Demi & Howell, 1991).

In a similar and more recent Norwegian study focusing primarily on adolescents who had lost a sibling to suicide 6 to 23 months prior to the interviews, Dyregrov and Dyregrov (2005) found that these surviving siblings, particularly younger ones, suffered from posttraumatic and grief reactions, anxiety, and depression. Suffering from disenfranchised grief, the siblings were isolated from the parental grief community and circles of friends. Noting a lack of assistance for the surviving siblings, the researchers suggested a systematic outreach help program to aid them in their grief (Dyregrov & Dyregrov, 2005).

Most of the siblings reported that their hidden feelings included the following: stigmatization, blame, guilt, and a strong sense of rejection (Dyregrov & Dyregrov, 2005). Siblings living at home expressed the most anger, as well as subsequent guilt, about their deceased loved one choosing suicide as the method for death and problem solving. Guilt often resulted when the sibling knew information that could have prevented the suicide. Almost one third of the younger siblings were aware of previous suicide attempts and suicidal ideation of their deceased sibling. The siblings were also burdened by guilt when they kept secret from their parents knowledge of serious problems that triggered the suicide. Bowman, Alvarez-Jimenez, Wade, Howie, and McGorry (2014), in a study of first episode psychosis on sibling quality of life, had similar findings, although their study included brothers and sisters with siblings who attempted, not completed, suicide. Profound guilt accompanied the intense sadness and longing experienced by most surviving siblings. Although parents usually asked "why," the siblings could often explain the world of their deceased sibling that was completely unknown to their parents (Dyregrov & Dyregrov, 2005).

Dyregrov and Dyregrov (2005) also discovered that siblings generally felt alone in their grieving, as their parents often experienced difficulty caring for themselves. The siblings living at home at the time of the suicide often reported feeling "lost in the chaos" (p. 719), and the parents confirmed forgetting the siblings in the hours and days after the suicide. The siblings' experiences of feeling "forgotten" were very painful, even when the siblings believed that their parents were more affected by the death than the rest of the family. In the initial period following the suicide, older siblings often supported their parents, rather than getting support from their parents. Many of the older siblings expressed the need for someone outside of the core family to support the surviving siblings. The surviving siblings desperately needed to express their struggles with someone who would not expect anything back and could manage hearing about their pain (Dyregrov & Dyregrov, 2005).

Many of the siblings felt they could not seek support from their parents due to their parents' panic that something critical would happen to the surviving siblings (Dyregrov & Dyregrov, 2005). Such excessive worrying frequently resulted in overprotection of the siblings. Meanwhile, many of the young siblings worried about protecting their grief-stricken parents. In order to protect their parents, the siblings living at home often remained quiet in regard to their deceased sibling. The guilt of burdening their parents and the siblings' yearning to protect their parents caused them not to rely on parental care, but rather support from other family members, friends, and community members (Dyregrov & Dyregrov, 2005).

In a study regarding the psychosocial consequences of suicide among families, Lindqvist, Johansson, and Karlsson (2008) gathered data through a grounded theory model and unstructured interviews, as well as collecting data through official documents and records from the Department of Forensic Medicine in Umea, Sweden. In the retrospective study of the families of completed suicide victims, 10 families (parents and siblings) were interviewed, and the average time span between the adolescent suicide and first interview was 17 months. Researchers found out the age and sex of the completed suicide victims, as well as the method of suicide before the interviews were conducted as a sign of respect to the families (Lindqvist et al., 2008).

Lindqvist et al. (2008) found that the families involved with teenage suicides (victims aged 13 to 19) attempted to make sense of the event with premonitory signs and clues. The social stigma of suicide and ultimate lack of prevention of suicide by the family, especially parents, further complicated the tragedy. Prolonged reactions of grief and loneliness, overwhelming feelings of shame, and the search for motives behind the suicide caused qualitative differences in the bereavement process for suicide as opposed to other losses (Lindqvist et al., 2008).

Lindqvist et al. (2008) identified the search for "why" as a common theme among the families after death of a teenager by suicide. Surviving family members reported how the deceased teenagers often successfully disguised their suicidal ideation from families, peers, and other adults, therefore denying parents and siblings from providing support and the opportunity to help. A sense of forbidden anger permeated the interviews, as family members reported feeling guilty for being angry with a loved one who was so desperate and lonely. Surviving family members also experienced confusion resulting from their deceased teenager's former active social life, high achievement in school, or leadership of peers. Ironically, directly before the suicide, often much of the teenager's emotional turmoil appeared to diminish, and the families were at ease. Families faced difficulty understanding how common teenage problems could transform into suicide and suicidal ideation. Suicide letters held few answers and did not serve to enlighten or soothe the family members. In two of the cases, the letters included instructions for passing personal belongings to siblings, who primarily felt uncomfortable in accepting such belongings (Lindqvist et al., 2008).

Lindqvist et al. (2008) discovered that regardless of how much time had passed between the interview and suicide, families struggled to move on. After returning to everyday life activities, survivors faced anguish and anxiety that was slow to fade. Not one day could pass without family members thinking of their deceased loved one. Some family members considered committing suicide themselves, but decided not to after experiencing the consequences others face after a suicide. All families felt somewhat indifferent to the social consequences of losing someone to suicide in the family. Feelings of guilt, shame, and self-reproach were stronger than fears of social stigmatization (Lindqvist et al., 2008).

Lindqvist et al. (2008) reported that all but one parent described the outrage, shock, confusion, and disbelief that followed the suicide for months. Extended family, friends, and close members of their church served as a supportive presence, for which parents were appreciative; however, most families felt alone in their grief immediately after the suicide. Families were dissatisfied with close community members and friends who, the parents felt, expected the families to forget and move on with their lives. If younger siblings were present at the parent's interview, the parents were satisfied mostly with the siblings' silent participation. The researchers explained how few adults or professionals had previously succeeded in involving the younger siblings with sharing thoughts about the suicide. However, after follow-up interviews, these siblings experienced emotional/psychological benefits from participating in the interviews (Lindqvist et al., 2008).

Even after returning to normal activities, families remained preoccupied with the loss and often withdrew from casual socializing (Lindqvist et al., 2008). Some families felt low self-esteem, shame, and inferiority resulting from being deceived by their deceased loved one. Others experienced guilt caused by aggressive feelings toward the deceased adolescent for deciding to terminate their relationship with one another. Societal blame and decreased social support from prejudiced peers exacerbated the psychological distress of the surviving families. Suicide rates in families of suicide victims were twice as high as those among unaffected families (Lindqvist et al., 2008).

The researchers emphasized that grief therapy must address the survivors' struggle with finding meaning and significance in the suicide and their own lives (Lindqvist et al., 2008). Many of the families not only dwelled on the question of why their adolescent child or sibling could complete suicide, but also asked "what for?," suggesting a significant search for meaning as opposed to determining the rationality of the suicide, implied in the question of why. Helplessness and disempowerment were evidence of the families' altered psychological states (Lindqvist et al., 2008).

Depression and PTSD

In a longitudinal study spanning 3 years, Brent et al. (1996) evaluated parents and siblings of adolescent suicide victims for psychiatric sequelae. Although this study is over 17 years old, Brent et al. (1996) conducted two insightful, longitudinal studies in 1993 and 1996 addressing the psychiatric responses of suicide survivors that considered the different reactions of parents and siblings over 6 months and 3 years. The researchers explained that while adolescent siblings were at a sevenfold increased risk for developing major depression after 6 months of their teenage sibling's suicide, they did not show an increased risk of depression, PTSD, or other psychiatric conditions after 3 years. However, the grief symptomatology of the siblings remained elevated for a prolonged period of time compared to other family members (Brent et al., 1996).

In a sample consisting of 25 siblings of 20 adolescent suicide victims residing at home, Brent et al. (1996) evaluated PTSD using the PTSD Reaction Index, while the Texas Grief Inventory tested for grief symptoms. Researchers used the Kiddie Schedule for Affective Disorders and Schizophrenia-Present Episode (K-SADS-PE) to assess for current, past, and incident psychopathology in siblings and unexposed controls. The mean duration of depression was 6.3 months, while the median duration was 4 months. Rates of incident disorder over time were the same between siblings and controls, starkly contrasting findings of the impact of suicide upon friends. Siblings expressed more severe grief symptomatology persisting over 3 years than friends and acquaintances of the suicide victim. After approximately 1 year, mothers showed a significantly higher rate of new-onset major depression compared to mothers of controls. Although there were few long-term sequelae for the siblings, more long-lasting and marked psychiatric effects occurred in the mothers of adolescent suicide victims that would impact their ability to care for and support surviving siblings (Brent et al., 1996).

Although the siblings showed a high rate of incident depression, siblings in this longitudinal study experienced lower rates of psychiatric sequelae than controls (Brent et al., 1996). These findings markedly contrasted the increased risk of recurrent depression reported in unrelated friends of suicide victims. Interestingly, grief was not a risk factor for depression in siblings as it was for unrelated friends of suicide victims; however, compared to unrelated friends, siblings showed more severe grief. While the study needs to be replicated, younger siblings suffered more difficulties than older siblings of suicide victims. The researchers suggested that the reason for the difference in reaction between younger and older siblings of suicide victims could be the "family burden" of younger siblings, who could suffer more by living at home and remaining more dependent upon their parents.

This study resulted in the surprising finding of resiliency among siblings of suicide victims compared to their mothers, who suffered prolonged and profound psychiatric sequelae. The study strengthened the argument of the importance of family-based approaches for survivors of suicide (Brent et al., 1996).

In a consecutive study of 25 siblings of 20 adolescent suicide victims in Western Pennsylvania 3 years earlier, Brent et al. (1993) utilized K-SADS-PE to test the group for past, present, and new-onset psychopathology. Compared to controls, siblings showed a higher rate of previous psychiatric disorders, including previous suicide attempts, substance abuse, and conduct disorder (not affective disorder), prior to exposure. Even after the exclusion of the suicide victim, siblings had higher rates of lifetime psychiatric disorder in first-degree relatives compared to the unexposed control group. In particular, siblings experienced significantly higher familial rates of suicidal behavior, substance abuse, major depression, and unipolar depression disorder (Brent et al., 1993).

Brent et al. (1993) obtained family histories through use of the Family History-RDC and *DSM-III*; in addition, the researchers used the Texas Grief Inventory to assess grief symptoms. The siblings and control group experienced similar rates of the number and types of life events excluding the sibling suicide. When the interviews were conducted 6 months after the suicide, approximately twice as many siblings than controls showed evidence of psychiatric disorders. Significantly more siblings than controls experienced new-onset affective illness. A majority of the illnesses were classified as major depression beginning within 1 month of death, with a mean duration of 5 months. One sibling made a suicide attempt subsequent to exposure to sibling suicide compared with none in the control group.

Over half of the siblings experienced new-onset or exacerbated psychiatric disorders after exposure to sibling suicide (Brent et al., 1993). In general, siblings suffered from a greater severity of depressive symptoms than the control group. Depressed siblings suffered from a greater prevalence of clinically significant depressive symptoms, including suicidal ideation, psychomotor agitation, worthlessness, social withdrawal, guilt, concentration problems, and appetite/weight change (Brent et al., 1993).

Researchers directly interviewed the siblings and used the Adolescent Relationship Inventory and Circumstances of Exposure to Death to evaluate their closeness to the suicide victims and exposure to suicide (Brent et al., 1993). Researchers found that none of the exposure variables tested for, including seeing the scene of death, knowing the victim's plans before death, feeling that he or she could prevent the suicide, or having a conversation within 24 hours of the suicide, impacted rates of new-onset depression in the siblings (Brent et al., 1993).

Researchers concluded that sibling suicide had a "devastating" psychiatric impact upon the surviving siblings and other family members (Brent et al., 1993). Specifically, researchers considered the sevenfold increase in incidence of major depression in siblings and mothers of suicide victims over community controls to be very significant. The findings suggested that suicidal behavior in the adolescent siblings was more prevalent only with coexistent past or new-onset affective illness. The researchers discussed how, with a larger sample, siblings could be expected to show a higher rate of suicidal behavior compared to friends and acquaintances of the suicide victim due to a possible genetic component to suicidal behavior. Despite the study's small sample size, the results were consistent with other studies of youthful bereavement finding high rates of depression symptomatology and disorder accompanying serious loss. Depressive symptoms, such as suicidal ideation and previously reported risk factors for major depression, suggested the true depression (versus bereavement symptoms) of siblings and mothers of adolescent suicide victims. Based on the findings, siblings and mothers were at high risk of developing a depressive disorder subsequent to the sibling or child's suicide. Fathers of completed suicide victims were more likely than controls to experience depression and anxiety, but not at a statistically significant level. Researchers suggested family-based interventions for the siblings and parents of adolescent suicide victims (Brent et al., 1993).

Dyregrov and Dyregrov (2005) noted that despite warning signs or previous suicide attempts, all siblings in the study reported feeling completely unprepared for the realization that their brother or sister could actually complete suicide. Immediately after the suicide, the siblings described feelings of shock, confusion, and disbelief. The siblings then reported posttraumatic stress responses, including grief, depression, anxiety, and other "strange and scary" reactions following those initial feelings (Dyregrov & Dyregrov, 2005, p. 718).

While the siblings experienced severe levels of posttraumatic psychological distress, siblings living at home with their parents scored higher on standardized PTSD tests than their parents, while siblings living outside of the home scored lower than both groups (Dyregrov & Dyregrov, 2005). Severe/high levels of posttraumatic reactions as measured by the Impact of Event Scale were evident among 73% of younger siblings and 39% of older siblings. Younger siblings scored higher than older siblings and parents in the area of event-related avoidance. Lack of energy, sleeping problems, and trouble with concentration often led to social withdrawal among the siblings. The siblings reported that they experienced the loss of their assumptive worlds, and they were challenged by the significant demands to confront and manage the traumatic loss cognitively and emotionally (Dyregrov & Dyregrov, 2005).

Suicidality and Mortality

Rostila (2012) discussed how although the loss of a sibling often caused serious health and psychological sequelae, sibling loss remained the least-studied familial relationship in the bereavement literature. An increased mortality risk was associated with sibling loss in all age groups. The mortality risk was most significant for siblings at younger ages (18 to 39 years), especially when the sibling death was "unnatural," such as suicide, homicide, or an accident. Rostila (2012) discussed how this younger age group was often exposed to higher levels of immediate stress, more intense feelings of grief, greater difficulty coping with and accepting the death, and had limited resources for coping. Grieving parents were frequently unprepared to care for their surviving children. Unnatural deaths, including suicide, could cause PTSD and a consequently higher mortality risk in siblings. Suicide was associated with higher suicide rates among the siblings, with risk ratios of 3.72 for women and 2.42 for men losing a sibling to suicide (Rostila, 2012).

Researchers also discovered that genetics significantly influenced suicide risk (Tidemalm et al., 2011). By connecting three national population registers in Sweden, researchers examined familial clustering of suicide risk among 11.4 individuals. Despite the same environmental exposure, full siblings, with an odds ratio of 3.1, 95% CIs [2.8, 3.5], and 50% genetic similarity, were at a higher suicide risk than maternal half-siblings. Researchers could also conclude that genetics played a significant role in suicide risk after discovering that monozygotic twins were at a significantly higher risk of suicide than dizygotic twins. However, despite the same genetic similarity of 50%, full siblings also had a significantly higher suicide risk when compared to the offspring of the suicide decedent, so researchers concluded that shared environment also impacted suicide risk (Tidemalm et al., 2011).

Social Problems and Parental Circumstances

Home environments and parental circumstances after the suicide served as important contexts for the surviving siblings' grief (Dyregrov & Dyregrov, 2005). Parents tended to become isolated and withdrawn in accordance with their loss of energy and feelings of guilt and self-blame. High levels of psychosocial distress, reflected by somatic symptoms, anxiety, insomnia, social dysfunction, and severe depression, often led to permanently damaged qualities of life. Over half of the parents in the study experienced posttraumatic distress as indicated by the Impact of Event Scale, and 78% suffered from complicated grief reactions as identified by the Inventory of Complicated Grief (Dyregrov & Dyregrov, 2005).

Although most of the siblings received support and empathy from their friends before and immediately after the funeral, they felt that the quality of their friendships tended to decrease as time passed (Dyregrov & Dyregrov, 2005). Many of the adolescent siblings considered their friends to be immature as the siblings developed new values, philosophies of life, and changed identities after their siblings' completed suicide. The completed suicide resulted in the surviving siblings' perceived increased maturity and insight, as well as changes in identity, social roles, life expectations, and routine activities. However, the surviving siblings often noticed that their social networks would sometimes withdraw from the bereaved, and they frequently lacked understanding that grief took time. However, the siblings themselves often withdrew from friends and acquaintances who showed the least amount of empathy (Dyregrov & Dyregrov, 2005).

INTERVENTIONS

Sharing Thoughts With Empathetic Others

Healing the pain often occurred years after the suicide and was precipitated by work or interpersonal problems that inspired survivors to seek counseling (Demi & Howell, 1991). Survivors often expressed thoughts and feelings either privately and/or through emotional release, visits to the gravesite, or diaries and poems. Survivors often shared thoughts and feelings with others perceived as empathetic. Importantly, none of the survivors reported sharing thoughts and feelings with a parent, but instead with spouses and fiancées or friends and coworkers also experiencing a significant loss. Early in the bereavement period, none of the respondents reported receiving any therapy or attending self-help groups like Survivors of Suicide. All of the respondents who eventually sought therapy reported that it was "extremely helpful" (p. 354). Most of the survivors who obtained therapy said that they wished that they had received therapy earlier. Several of the respondents expressed that their advice for other suicide survivors was to talk about the suicide and obtain therapy (Demi & Howell, 1991).

The suicide of a parent or sibling often had extensive and long-term impact on survivors (Demi & Howell, 1991). The healing process for these survivors was complicated by efforts to hide pain. Since this study was performed, more outreach programs have been developed to provide crisis intervention for families experiencing suicide. Demi and Howell (1991) noted that further research was necessary to address the experiences of survivors of suicide. Early identification of unresolved grief by health care providers and appropriate referrals for counseling were necessary to care for the suicide survivors. Educational efforts should have focused on destigmatizing suicide, introducing healthy coping mechanisms for grief, and mobilizing support systems for survivors of parental or sibling suicide (Demi & Howell, 1991).

Lindqvist et al. (2008) reported how bereaved parents often requested care for surviving children, as well as immediate outreach and assistance from trained individuals. However, support was often poorly timed and sporadically provided. During the first phases of shock, confusion, and denial, families sought familiarity, comfort, and assistance with basic needs. Sometimes, these needs were left unmet and substituted by psychotherapeutic interference and anxiety of friends and community members. Clergy, mental health professionals, and others who have lost family members to suicide provided sufficient support for families who "need to talk." However, of those support systems, mental health professionals often underestimated the need for long-term support and did not provide enough extended care for the families (Lindqvist et al., 2008).

Going "Outside the Family" for Care

Younger siblings of completed suicide victims received primarily insufficient crisis care (Lindqvist et al., 2008). These siblings tended to feel more burdened than older siblings, and they required more time, persistence, and uncompromising readiness from adult supports to grapple with difficult questions and thoughts. After losing a child to suicide, parents of the siblings often lacked enough capacity to care for siblings. Therefore, these siblings required attention from support systems outside of the family. Direct care should have been provided not only to the parents and siblings individually, but also to the family as a whole. Group or family therapy, including parents, appeared to remain an appropriate treatment option for siblings coping with traumatic grief. The families' primary health care providers were responsible for providing support and organizing space for other community support systems to provide care. Families' needs change over time from "doing" activities associated with a death to simply "being"—that is, experiencing the sadness of grief (Lindqvist et al., 2008).

The absence of sufficient explanations of an adolescent suicide served as the chief issue in the grief process for surviving family members (Lindqvist et al., 2008). Health care providers, community members, and other support systems needed to prevent prolonged psychological and social isolation of the surviving families in grief. Better treatment and understanding for families who have lost an adolescent to suicide were also necessary, especially for the younger siblings who were often "forgotten" (Lindqvist et al., 2008).

Dyregrov and Dyregrov (2005) found that only 40% of the siblings in their study received community assistance after the suicide. Moreover, the assistance was very limited, and many parents lacked the energy or initiative to ask for help for their children. A majority of the interviewed parents sought additional and alternative methods of help for the younger siblings. Merely 6% of the younger siblings received help for more than 3 months, and the younger siblings were more reluctant than the parents to ask for help. While only 13% of the parents reported receiving help from a psychologist, nearly half of them reported not seeking help for their children (Dyregrov & Dyregrov, 2005).

Dyregrov and Dyregrov (2005) also identified an overwhelming need for family-based help and advice after a completed suicide. The first step in a family's healing was improved family communication that was supplemented by family-based interventions emphasizing affective problems and grief. The surviving siblings required complete information about the suicide, as well as opportunities to talk through their experiences and ask questions. The siblings were often relieved by information they received in a clear, slow, and careful manner. Schools and families needed to work together so that the school provided a caring and supportive environment where the surviving siblings could express their feelings and grief and receive help with educational challenges posed by the loss. Systematic help offered in a proactive and outreach manner was vital because social and emotional withdrawal resulting from suicide could prevent surviving family members from seeking or accepting assistance (Dyregrov & Dyregrov, 2005). In another Norwegian study, young people aged 13 to 24 years who lost a close relative or friend to suicide completed questionnaires and participated in focus group interviews regarding preferred psychologist interventions (Dyregrov, 2009). Among the group of suicide survivors in the study, 69% lost a brother or sister to suicide, and a majority of the participants expressed how the survivors needed help and support from outside of their families. Those in contact with public health professionals, such as psychologists, teachers, public health nurses, and clergymen, often received better follow-up to their needs compared to those lacking such connections. However, while psychologists played one of the most significant roles in supporting the young suicide survivors, the survivors tended to feel dissatisfied or frustrated with their care, which was often discontinued far too early. Participants described how barriers to receiving psychological support included difficulty initially establishing contact and a lack of assistance that occurs automatically after a sibling's completed suicide. The young survivors also often did not know who to approach or how to find appropriate care. Disappointing experiences and a lack of motivation frequently prevented the survivors from seeking additional care even if they needed the support. The most important barrier identified by the survivors was the lack of any system to recognize their need for help and support. Most parents failed to provide adequate support for their surviving children and did not encourage them to seek help. The survivors discussed the difficulty they encountered when seeking help as adolescents, when they considered receiving help as personal failure and felt concerned with what others thought of them. Discontinuation of contact with a psychologist resulted from stress and disappointment in the style or content of previous therapy (Dyregrov, 2009).

"Early, Automatic, and Stand-By Help": What Siblings Needed From Care Providers

The young survivors expressed feeling dissatisfied with their psychologists for several reasons. Many of the survivors' psychologists failed to address the survivors' significant problems, displayed professional and emotional uncertainty, trivialized the survivors' issues, and lacked true compassion, empathy, and consequent trustworthiness (Dyregrov, 2009). Several participants expressed how the psychologists were more concerned with the survivors' pasts, while never recognizing the following very important issues: feelings of guilt, anger, and anxiety; asking "why"; terrifying nightmares and dreams about suicide; and problems handling daily life due to a lack of coping skills for managing their pain. The siblings desired psychologists and other health care professionals to "push [them] a bit more" (p. 231) because they would often hide their problems and reject help. The survivors struggled with accepting reality immediately after the suicide, and repeated sensitive offers of help would often have been the solution. The participants desired advice regarding how to support parents and siblings, how they could cope with their personal difficulties, and what reactions to anticipate. Follow-up and therapy over time, as well as a routine, professional offer of help, were vital in the success of their interactions with psychologists and other health care professionals (Dyregrov, 2009).

The survivors desired therapists who would act as teammates and proactively help and advise the survivors in how to cope with their unique situations (Dyregrov, 2009). The survivors identified good care from psychologists and health care professionals as including the following: early, automatic, and stand-by offers of help, flexible, interested, and empathetic helpers, therapists knowledgeable about suicide and crisis psychology, and individualized help (Dyregrov, 2009).

TOWARD NO LONGER SHEDDING TEARS ALONE

Although the research is limited, findings are consistent regarding psychiatric and social sequelae of the "forgotten bereaved," as well as necessary interventions to help this population. Siblings of completed suicide victims, particularly younger siblings and siblings living at home with their parents, must receive automatic, early, and repeated offers of help from health care providers and community members, even after initial refusal. Health care providers must follow up with the care of the siblings and offer long-term interventions to ensure that they are not "forgotten" or suffering alone. Nurses, physicians, psychologists, and other health care professionals can offer treatment for the siblings' psychiatric sequelae and help with coping mechanisms and social problems in order to prevent early mortality and suicidality. The siblings should receive interventions from health care professionals outside of the family who are knowledgeable about crisis and suicide psychology. With family counseling, parents can learn about how to support their surviving sons and daughters.

CONCLUSION

Further research is required to ensure that siblings are no longer one of the least-studied familial relationships in the bereavement literature. Research should address the issue of why psychologists and other health care professionals are not succeeding in treating young suicide survivors. In addition, further research should address interventions for prevention of early discontinuation care. Health care providers need to understand how to prevent the markedly increased mortality and suicide risks in siblings, as well as how to improve the systems already in place for approaching families about care after completed suicide.

Nurses and other health care professionals have a significant role in supporting siblings who have lost a brother or sister to suicide. Helping siblings through their grief, psychiatric, familial, and social struggles can prevent the suicide or early death of the sibling. With proper care and treatment, siblings and parents of completed suicide victims can receive the help and support they desperately need and no longer bear the devastating pressure to shed their tears alone.

ACKNOWLEDGMENT

This chapter was written in loving memory of my big brother who took his own life but always supported and believed in me with a deeply caring heart, warm smile, brilliant mind, and unconditional love.—RK

CASE STUDY

Ted is an 18-year-old who attends college 200 miles away from home. His sister, Brenna, completed suicide 6 months ago. This semester, his grades have declined and he is experiencing difficulty with his peers: he is moody and often drinks to excess, despite being under age. He feels that no one understands his grief and he avoids talking about Brenna's death. His parents are in touch with him but he limits his conversation to topics other than Brenna's death and his feelings. He wants to protect them because he feels they are still overwhelmed by their own grief.

FOCUS QUESTIONS

1. What are the expected sequelae of sibling bereavement after completed suicide?
2. Describe how sibling suicide leads to disenfranchised grief.
3. How might Brenna's death affect Ted's emotional health further into adulthood?
4. What supportive interventions would be most helpful for Ted?

REFERENCES

Barrera, M., Alam, R., D'Agostino, N. M., Nicholas, D. B., & Schneiderman, G. (2013). Parental perceptions of siblings' grieving after a childhood cancer death: A longitudinal study. *Death Studies, 37,* 25–46.

Bowman, S., Alverez-Jimenez, M., Wade, D., Howie, L., & McGorry, P. (2014). The impact of first episode psychosis on sibling quality of life. *Social Psychiatry and Psychiatric Epidemiology, 49,* 1071–1081.

Brent, D. A., Moritz, G., Bridge, J., Perper, J., & Canobbio, R. (1996). The impact of adolescent suicide on siblings and parents: A longitudinal follow-up. *Suicide and Life-Threatening Behavior, 26*(3), 253–259.

Brent, D. A., Perper, J. A., Moritz, G., Liotus, L., Schweers, J., Roth, C., . . . Allman, C. (1993). Psychiatric impact of the loss of an adolescent sibling to suicide. *Journal of Affective Disorders, 28*(4), 249–256. doi:10.1016/0165-0327(93)90060-W

CDC—Definitions - Suicide—Violence Prevention—Injury. (2012). Centers for Disease Control and Prevention. Retrieved from http://www.cdc.gov/violenceprevention/suicide

CDC—National Violent Death Reporting System. (2015). Centers for Disease Control and Prevention. Retrieved from www.cdc.gov/violenceprevention/national violentdeathreportingsystem

CDC—Suicide Facts at a Glance. (2012). Centers for Disease Control and Prevention. Retrieved from www.cdc.gov/ViolencePrevention/pdf/Suicide_DataSheet_2012-a.pdf

Church, E. J. (2015). Examining suicide: Imaging's contributions. *Radiologic Technology, 86*(3), 275–298.

Demi, A., & Howell, C. (1991). Hiding and healing: Resolving the suicide of a parent or sibling. *Archives of Psychiatric Nursing, 5*(6), 350–356.

Dickens, N. (2014). Prevalence of complicated grief and posttraumatic stress disorder in children and adolescents following sibling death. *The Family Journal: Counseling and Therapy for Couples and Families, 22,* 119–126.

Dyregrov, K. (2009). How do the young suicide survivors wish to be met by psychologists? A user study. *OMEGA—Journal of Death and Dying, 59*(3), 221–238.

Dyregrov, K., & Dyregrov, A. (2005). Siblings after suicide—"The forgotten bereaved." *Suicide and Life-Threatening Behavior, 35*(6), 714–724. doi:10.1521/suli.2005.35.6.714

Hunt, Q. A., & Hertlein, K. M. (2015). Conceptualizing suicide bereavement from an attachment lens. *The American Journal of Family Therapy, 43,* 16–25.

Lindqvist, P., Johansson, L., & Karlsson, U. (2008). In the aftermath of teenage suicide: A qualitative study of the psychosocial consequences for the surviving family members. *BMC Psychiatry, 8*(1), 26.doi:10.1186/1471-244X-8-26

McIntosh, J., & Wrobleski, A. (1998). Grief reactions among suicide survivors. *Death Studies, 12,* 21–39.

Rostila, M. (2012). The forgotten griever: A nationwide follow-up study of mortality subsequent to the death of a sibling. *American Journal of Epidemiology, 176*(4), 338–346. doi:10.1093/aje/kws163

Shneidman, E. (1972). Foreword. In A. C. Cain (Ed.), *Survivors of suicide.* Springfield, IL: Charles C. Thomas.

Tidemalm, D. D., Runeson, B. B., Waern, M. M., Frisell, T. T., Carlström, E. E., Lichtenstein, P. P., & Långström, N. (2011). Familial clustering of suicide risk: A total population study of 11.4 million individuals. *Psychological Medicine, 41*(12), 2527–2534. doi:10.1017/S0033291711000833

White, P. G. (2006). *Sibling grief: Healing after the death of a sister or brother.* Lincoln, NB: iUniverse.

CHAPTER 16

Bereavement in Young Children With Siblings in Pediatric Palliative Care

Betty Davies, Camara van Breemen, Susan Poitras, and Eric Stephanson

During the past two decades, definitions of pediatric palliative care (PPC) have become increasingly clear and comprehensive (ACT, 2009; WHO, 2006), capturing the idea that PPC is both a philosophy and a type of care. Using a broad multidisciplinary approach that includes the family, PPC provides compassionate and nonjudgmental care to address physical, emotional, social, spiritual, and existential elements; enhance quality of life; and relieve suffering of the child and family. PPC begins at the time of recognition or diagnosis of disease, even in some cases before birth, and continues throughout the illness to the time of death and beyond for family members. Keeping the focus on the family and its members and providing bereavement support are central to this chapter; both imply that nurses and other PPC professionals must pay attention to the grief of siblings, particularly young siblings, that occurs in response to numerous losses during the course of a long illness trajectory and following the ill child's death.

Studies that have focused on children's experiences of the death of a brother or sister indicate that young siblings are greatly impacted by the loss. Problematic behavior in the siblings of deceased children seemed to be most common in preschool and school-age children, with the majority of problematic behaviors declining with age (McCown & Davies, 1995). Similarly, Gerhardt and coworkers (Gerhardt et al., 2012) studied social behavior and peer acceptance among cancer bereaved siblings 3 to 12 months after their loss and found that, according to their teachers ($n = 105$) and classmates ($n = 311$), the bereaved siblings in elementary school did seem more vulnerable and at risk for difficulties. However, even before the death of a brother or sister with cancer or other life-threatening conditions, young siblings are affected by witnessing the deterioration of health in the ill child and experiencing changes and disruptions in family life (Barrera et al., 2013) during the course of what is often a long-term condition requiring PPC.

THE LONG-TERM NATURE OF PPC

A common perception is that PPC programs are just for children dying of cancer, but only a small proportion of children admitted to palliative care programs have cancer. Although most research has focused on children with cancer, due to the development in recent decades of newer medications and technologies, the diagnoses of genetic, neurodegenerative, and metabolic conditions comprise the majority of life-threatening conditions of children requiring PPC (ACT, 2009). For example, among the number of children in the program at Canuck Place Children's Hospice in Vancouver, Canada, over a 15-year period, cancer comprised 29.9% of the children receiving clinical care, whereas the combined diagnoses of neurological disease, metabolic disease, or genetic multiorgan conditions comprised 42.5%. Of note, cancer made up 44.6% of deaths in that same period, while the combined diagnoses of neurological disease, metabolic disease, or genetic multiorgan conditions were 39.7% of deaths (Siden, Chavoshi, Harvey, Parker, & Miller, 2014; manuscript in submission).

These diagnoses result in an extended period of illness that follows a trajectory of stepwise decline (Steele, 2002) and may be followed by PPC teams for long periods of time. Consequently, all family members, siblings included, face numerous losses throughout the duration of the illness and grieve for loss of the child's intact body, mental function, or ability to talk as well as their own dreams and "normal" ways of being in the world, as illustrated by Jonah (age 10). (Note: Name and other details have been changed to protect the anonymity of all stories.):

> My big brother has [Duchenne muscular dystrophy]. A disease that by some chance of fate affected him, not me and I wonder why? I see him watch me sometimes. How I can walk, move, decide and do without a second thought or need to plan. He has learned to keep his feelings inside to cope. I guess so have I? I can think about the future and about my life. My brother also dreams about his life but also prepares for his dying. He is my hero. His courage and strength is demonstrated every day in every moment. This living grief hurts. A journey with a long road, many forks, bumps and turns never knowing which stretch of the road will be the last stop.

Though painful, the losses and grief along the way may present an opportunity for families to begin to think about their future without the child; however, anticipatory grieving can also take its toll, especially when the child's illness endures. In fact, Rando (1986) suggests there is an optimal length of anticipatory grief of 6 to 18 months. A shorter time does not give parents enough time to prepare for the loss, and a longer period has a debilitating effect on them.

ANTICIPATORY GRIEF

A common perception is that anticipatory grief somehow makes grief "easier" for the families of these children and implies that the surviving children have had the opportunity to learn about the disease and to prepare for the child's eventual death. However, this is not always true. Many parents hope that their child will be the miracle child who will recover at the last moment; they may attempt to put aside their fears of death rather than talking about it with their other children. In addition, any threat to the attachment between parent and child triggers a visceral, primitive response for survival and protection. When depression, anxiety, and grief of a mother caring for a dying child exceed her ability to cope, even though she may understand and try, she cannot change the overwhelming experience that dictates her responses. Moreover, parents are burdened with dual responsibilities; in one Australian study, parents acknowledged that they had not provided the usual amount of attention to the siblings during their deceased child's treatment. They expressed feelings of regret but felt they had to concentrate time and effort on their ill child's care, which left the other children feeling neglected: ". . .you don't mean to but that's the way it happens" (De Cinque et al., 2006, p. 74).

Such was the experience for Vicky and Alex's mother: Vicky (aged 7 years) and Alex (aged 5 years) had an older brother, Jon, who was diagnosed with an aggressive brain tumor that presented suddenly. Within 3 months of his first symptom, Jon was totally dependent on others to move his body and was losing his hearing, sight, and his ability to talk and eat. His parents were devastated and tortured by his losses and his emotional reactions to the situation. His mother was emotionally entwined with her son's experience and devoted her time and energy to supporting him. The siblings were bright and energetic children who were very loving of their brother and to their parents. They were confused and missed their own home, which the family had suddenly left for the urban-located children's hospital. Their mother was responsive to their requests but found it difficult to leave Jon and she was rarely separated from him even though Vicky and Alex were eager for time and attention.

Throughout the illness trajectory, with the ill child as the parents' main focus, increasingly siblings tend to feel almost invisible, resulting in feelings of fear, anger, anxiety, or depression (Eilegård, Steineck, Nyberg, & Kreicbergs, 2013). Unacknowledged grief before the death inhibits communication and preparation for death which, in turn, influences responses following the death when parents, in the midst of their own grief, may not be able to provide ongoing support to the bereaved siblings. Consequently, young siblings may come to the death with a "backlog" of unmet needs and misunderstandings. For young children for whom the need for parental support is great, this problem may be acute (Wender & the Committee on Psychosocial Aspects of Child and Family Health, 2012).

Moreover, when focusing on young siblings, common misconceptions about children come into play and sometimes interfere with how parents, extended family members, and other adults may treat youngsters during situations involving death. Myths include the idea that children do not grieve because they are "too young" to know what is going on, they "will not remember," or they will "get over it easily." Parents admit to "not having the words" or fear the children "can't handle it." For such reasons, adults may not explain what is happening to young children and exclude them from death-related events. In addition, well-intentioned adults believe they are "protecting" the children from sadness—but in fact, they are missing an opportunity to teach significant life lessons about how to deal with death and the emotions that accompany it.

PPC clinicians can play a key role in directly supporting and educating grieving parents and thereby also in indirectly supporting and educating the siblings. Nurses can support parents by listening to their fears and engaging them in discussion about child development and children's need for information and support so that they do not feel abandoned. Nurses can enhance healing by facilitating activities between the parent, the sibling, and the dying child so that those times can be remembered and honored over time. Providing opportunities for the sibling to "help" care for the ill sibling by holding his or her hand, singing a song (can be done remotely), drawing a picture, or having photos taken together gives tangible expression to the sibling relationship and to the identity of each child within the family. Having a conceptual map or a guide can help nurses and other health care providers remember and respond to the many factors influencing young siblings who are experiencing loss during the illness trajectory or after the death.

THE MODEL: SHADOWS IN THE SUN

Derived from research and clinical work with bereaved siblings, Davies's (1999) model uses the metaphor of "Shadows in the Sun" to guide the understanding of and interventions with bereaved siblings. The death of a brother or sister, like any significant life-altering event in a young child's life, has a lifelong impact—like shadows in the sun—perpetually influencing his or her ways of being in the world. Children have a natural propensity to grow and develop; they often struggle to find the sun even in the darkest of circumstances. The death of a brother or sister introduces dark shadows into siblings' lives. Attempting to prevent the pain and suffering of bereavement is like trying to stop the sun from casting shadows during the course of a day. Instead, significant adults in the child's life, when equipped with knowledge and compassion, journey with the child through the shadows. Through their interactions with one another, the shadows lengthen and shorten, darken and fade, come and go, and the child learns to travel with the shadows.

Davies's model consists of four major categories of sibling responses, described in the siblings' own words as "I hurt inside," "I don't understand," "I don't belong," and "I'm not enough." These responses occur within the context of three categories of influencing factors (individual, situational, and environmental). However, the most significant factor affecting bereaved siblings is how significant adults interact with them. Although derived from the experiences of bereaved siblings, the model applies also to helping siblings with the grief resulting from numerous losses that occur during a child's illness.

Sibling Responses

I Hurt Inside

This response includes all the reactions typically associated with grief that arise from the vulnerability of being human, from loving others and missing them when they are no longer with us: sadness, anger, frustration, loneliness, fear, and irritability. Unlike adults who often talk about their emotional responses, children are often unable or inexperienced at identifying what they are feeling and typically express emotions through behavior. For example, some children are hesitant to return to the familiar activities of playing, of wanting to be with friends, of walking to school, and of wanting to do new things. Others act out by not listening to their parents or by becoming irritable and belligerent. Some may complain of headaches, general aches and pains, stomach cramps, or disruptions in eating or sleeping patterns, or in school performance. Bereaved siblings will frequently complain of loneliness. Some bereaved children also feel guilty for the death of their sibling even when they held no responsibility for the death.

These are manifestations of normal grief, and unless they occur with severe intensity or for long periods of time, they are not necessarily indicators of maladjustment. Rather than assessing children's response to a death by identifying the presence or absence of any one reaction, it is more important to look for persistent changes, a pattern of problems, and the intrusiveness created by the grieving in the child's life (Webb, 2010). Moreover, the absence of a typical grieving reaction is not necessarily a cause for alarm; not all children are affected in the same way or to the same degree by a sibling's death. Parents, in fact, need to be advised that each child in the family will react differently, as did Vicky and Alex. They were busy and the energy of their grief was big and restless. They both found it hard to sit still or stay focused for very long but they reacted to their grief in different ways. Alex interacted intermittently with his brother but gravitated to distraction and fun. Vicky was very nurturing toward Alex and attempted to care for her mom. Both children were conscious not to burden their mom with their feelings. It was difficult for Alex to express his feelings verbally but he communicated his emotions and stress with meltdowns and low frustration tolerance. In play, he expressed chaos and anger toward health professionals. His sleep and appetite were unsettled and he began to avoid going to his mom for things, choosing instead to go to his dad or any other adult available to him.

In contrast, Vicky showed only happy reactions and kept her hurt to herself. She attempted to nurture her mom and take care of her. She also began to discipline Alex, which often would lead to conflict. She would often openly share her love with her brother and mom with hugs and kisses, yet as Jon's condition changed her ability to offer comfort grew less.

For children who are "hurting inside," nurses can provide a listening forum where parents can explore how they feel their healthy children are doing, in general, and what concerns or fears they may have for their grieving child. How is the child doing physically (eating, sleeping, energy level?), emotionally, and socially (playing, engagement, withdrawal, outbursts?)? What strategies are the parents using to support the sibling's functioning and adaptation to the absence of the child and the grief in the household? Nurses can also reassure parents that the wish to have children "behave" may be from their own desire to meet external expectations of children rather than their own goal to comfort and console their child. Adults must accept the child's feelings and behaviors as normal manifestations of grief and validate the child's experience: "Yes, it is sad" rather than "No more tears now!" They must be patient in allowing children to express their own thoughts and feelings in their own time and in their own ways. Adults who endeavor to share their own thoughts and feelings with children "model" how to grieve, instilling a sense of being together with them and offering hope for feeling better in the future. Fortunately for Vicky and Alex, although they longed for connection with their mom, their dad was patient with them and provided the emotional attention and physical nurturance they needed. He shared his thoughts and feelings with them and with his wife, and they found moments of connection that enabled them to share in Jon's care with their mom. On the other hand, when adults limit expression of reactions, children may conclude that there is something wrong with their feelings and stifle them.

I Don't Understand

This response is greatly influenced by a child's level of cognitive develop-ment. Children of all ages may be confused by the array of powerful feelings that surge within them; they may be mystified by the activity and reactions of others. Younger children are easily confused and bewildered by all that is happening. They may not comprehend that their brother or sister is never coming back, that death is forever. As they grow and develop, their under-standing of death expands and with it, increased distress when they fully realize their sibling will never return; furthermore, their expanding under-standing triggers additional questions and a need to review what happened to their sibling. Five years after her brother's death, while looking back at photos of her family with him in the hospital, Mary (now age 9) exclaimed to her mom, "So that's why you weren't at my birthday party that year!" How to explain events to young children can be challenging for both clini-cians and parents, and even more so when a child has developmental limita-tions as well.

Sarita was 6 years old when her sister, Harjinder, age 2 years, died of cancer. Sarita had been born with a congenital disorder that affected her cognitive, physical, and social development. Her capacity for understand-ing was unclear though her receptive language was relatively good. But she was not able to verbally express her thoughts and feelings about the loss of her sister. She relied on pictures to communicate. How could her family and the hospice staff honor Sarita's loss, her need to understand, and the evolv-ing process of understanding in the future?

PPC nurses, along with parents, play a major role in helping children who "don't understand" by explaining and interpreting all that is happen-ing during the illness, at the time of death, and after the death. Confusion and ignorance contribute to additional hurt, so adults must provide honest information at the level of the child's comprehension. If adults simply and compassionately explain reactions and sensations and not just events, and help youngsters learn to interpret their own reactions, children learn that it is okay to ask questions. In the company of understanding adults, children learn to accept the uncertainties of life.

Using the only communication to which Sarita had access—pictures—the hospice staff worked with the family to create a picture book with simple language to reflect Sarita's family story of staying at the hospice. The book began with describing Sarita and her family and what she enjoyed playing and doing at the hospice. It talked about her sister being sick with cancer and that, although many people who have cancer get better, the nurses and doctors could not make Harjinder better. It talked about when Harjinder died and about her family's religious beliefs, about her spirit, and where her body was buried. It affirmed that Harjinder would always be her sister and that Sarita's love and memories of her sister would be with her always.

For months after Harjinder died, the book was available to her at home and at school, along with other reading options. On occasion, Sarita would choose to read the book, but she would only read half way and close the book right before the page that stated her sister died. This continued until about 6 months after the death. Sarita then began to read the book often, from beginning to end. She also had a picture of her sister on her picture board where "feeling faces" were posted (to help Sarita indicate her own feelings).

Sarita continues to come and visit the hospice. It is a ritual that provides her comfort. It was the last place she saw her sister alive, and it is as if Sarita wonders if her sister will return. This may account for her desire to visit the hospice—to affirm that she will not. At home, Sarita has moved into her sister's room and she has adopted certain routines and items that are connected to her sister, which were not important to her prior to the death. It is her way of understanding what happened to Harjinder as well as her way of keeping connected to Harjinder. Explanations to siblings who themselves have compromised cognitive development present an added challenge, but successful strategies for helping these children, such as art and play, can be used for all children.

I Don't Belong

When children feel left out of what is happening, they feel as if they "do not belong." During a child's illness, or in the aftermath of a child's death, siblings often want to help, but do not know how; or if they try to help, their efforts are not acknowledged or are even criticized. When children verbalize their natural curiosity in the form of questions and are ignored or told to be quiet, they get the message that they are inappropriate and they begin to feel as if they "do not belong." The reorganization of roles and responsibilities that accompany the death of any family member may leave the child feeling as if he or she has lost his or her place in the family. Furthermore, bereaved children often feel different from their nonbereaved peers and this too contributes to feelings of not belonging.

Claudette was a curious 4-year-old whose brother had been born a year earlier with severe neurological impairment. This had been a normal pregnancy with no indication that there were concerns about the fetus. The parents were devastated and it was very confusing to Claudette who could not understand why her baby brother was not like other babies: "Why can't Henri play with me? Why can't I feed Henri from a bottle?" She wanted to help care for him but struggled with his lack of interaction with her, which prompted her to intensify her interactions with him to get his attention or a reaction that became aggressive and dangerous. Henri's condition was progressively declining. Claudette's parents wanted to help her understand what was happening with her brother and prepare her for his impending death so that she would not feel left out.

The nurse engaged with the family in a play session where Claudette played "baby" with baby dolls, clothes, diapers, and crib. They talked about babies and their baby parts: nose, fingers, toes, belly button—all the parts we can see on the outside. They then talked about parts on the inside of the body: bones, stomach, lungs, heart, and brain and that Henri's body was made differently than ours. The nurse explained that Henri was born with a condition that affected how his brain worked. The brain is a body part inside your head that is in charge of our body and how it moves, thinks, and feels. Also, his lungs and his body were becoming tired and it was getting harder for Henri to breathe—that was why he needed the mask on his face and suctioning, sometimes, to help him breathe easier. Even though the nurses and doctors tried to find ways to help, they were not able to fix Henri's body. Most people who get sick get better, and nurses and doctors can help and fix many things, but Henri's body could not be fixed. One day, Henri's body would stop working and his body would die. To die meant that his heart inside his body would stop working and his lungs would no longer breathe. They told Claudette that when you die, you do not talk, eat, sleep, or breathe.

They talked about the family's belief in heaven: "There is a part of our self that is separate from the body called the spirit which does not die and the spirit goes to a place called heaven." Mom and Dad said, "When Henri died he would become an angel. When his body dies, Henri will be placed in a casket along with his special things, like his blanket, that make him feel safe. You could choose something special to put in the casket with Henri, too." They continued: "Then there will be a special service at church for Henri when all of us, including grandma and grandpa and many of our friends, will be there. Henri's body will be there in his casket. If you would like to, you can stay at the funeral—we will sing songs and pray, and people will talk about Henri. You might see that some people cry—because they are sad that Henri has died, but this will be okay. Mommy and Daddy might cry and if you feel like crying, you can. We will hold hands with each other. If you would rather stay with Auntie Marie at her house instead of going to the funeral, that would be okay, too. Or if you want to come, and then feel like going out for a while to play, Jeanne (mother's cousin) will go with you." Further, they explained that the casket will then be buried in the ground at a cemetery where the body changes over time and returns to the earth. The cemetery is a place families sometimes visit to remember the person who died. Many feelings happen when someone dies. And, the parents moved into talking about different feelings and what makes them feel safe and comforted.

Adults can do much to prevent bereaved siblings from feeling as though they "don't belong" if they include the children and welcome their contributions. When children are included in what is happening, when they have an active role to play in plans and activities, and when they are prepared in advance for what is happening, children can manage very well. They feel part of the family and have valuable contributions to make. On the other hand, when children are excluded from the plans and activities, when they are not given a choice about the nature of their involvement, or when they are not adequately prepared for what to expect, they feel as if they do not belong; their presence and contributions are invalidated. Such children often seek a place of attention through acting out, risk taking, avoiding home, or withdrawing into themselves or their schoolwork.

I Am Not Enough

Siblings' feelings of "I am not enough" arise from perceptions that they should have been the one to die since, in their view, the deceased child was the parents' favorite, or was the smartest, the prettiest, or the "best" in some way. Moreover, siblings see their parents' distress, and creatively attempt to lift their parents' spirits by "being good," caretaking, or overachieving in school, for example. It is difficult for parents to manage their own grief; their personal resources are stretched to the limit, and their other children want their parents to "get back to normal." When parents continue to grieve, siblings may feel as if their efforts are in vain. They can feel they are not enough to make their parents happy ever again, as was the case for Tracy, age 9, who wondered:

> How do you fill shoes that can never be filled? When your best friend, confident, brother dies? He has left such a huge hole in our family it feels impossible to patch. He was our peace keeper and supporter. With him gone my parents and I do not know how to communicate anymore. My dad is so angry and sad that it is hard to talk to him. He and I fight all the time. My mom is in the middle but she does not know how to keep the peace. She ends up taking sides and then I feel ganged up on.
>
> I know my dad really misses Erik. He loved doing father–son things with Erik which I don't do. I am a girl. He does not know how to relate with me. I feel so lonely and scared most of the time. I wish he loved me the way he loved Erik. My parents are both back at work and I feel so alone without him. School is not any easier. It's hard to concentrate and I am falling behind. Most days I don't want to go to school and am too tired to get to school on time. I am not sleeping well. It is hard to fall asleep and I need my mom to lie with me. I get scared at night and wake up often with nightmares. Will things ever feel right again? Will I ever be enough?

Helping siblings feel valued, loved, and considered special by the adults in their lives is the best way to help children avoid feeling "I am not enough." Validating their worth, not necessarily for their accomplishments, but for just being in the world, is integral to making children feel special in the lives of the adults who mean the most to them. One way is for parents to stress the sibling's strengths and avoid comparisons with the child who died; another is to ensure that photos of both children are on display in the family home, not just of the deceased child. If adults interact with bereaved siblings in ways that comfort their hurt, clarify their confusion, and involve them in what is happening, it is unlikely that bereaved siblings will feel as if they are "not enough."

Contextual Factors

The aforementioned children's responses to grief do not occur in isolation but within a context of many interrelated variables. No one factor accounts for the total experience of any individual child. Three categories of factors come into play: individual, situational, and environmental.

Characteristics of the individual siblings include the child's age and gender, health status, temperament or coping style, and previous experience with loss. For example, loss occurring at younger than 5 years of age (or during early adolescence) and the presence of pre-existing psychological difficulties are warning signs for children at risk.

Situational factors include characteristics of the situation itself, such as duration of illness, cause of death, location of death, and the degree to which children were involved in the events pertaining to their brother or sister's illness, death, and related events such as the funeral or memorial service. In PPC, for example, siblings who witness considerable pain and suffering in the ill child may be more troubled than siblings of children who die peacefully. Bereaved children who are actively involved in the care of their sibling, in planning or have a role to play in the funeral or other commemorative rituals, demonstrate fewer behavioral problems than children who are excluded from such activities. Of course, giving children a clearly informed choice about whether or not they want to be involved is key.

Finally, psychosocial environmental factors have an enormous impact upon sibling grief. The nature of the predeath relationship, for example, is critical. When children have shared many aspects of their lives, or share a particularly close or meaningful relationship, the loss of one child leaves a large empty space in the surviving sibling and often results in more internalizing behaviors. Emotional closeness between siblings exerts a stronger influence on bereavement outcome than closeness in age, length of illness, or number of surviving children in the family. Nurses, parents, and other adults, therefore, need to be particularly sensitive to the needs of the sibling whose brother or sister held special meaning, such as Tracy whose brother was "my hero."

The family environment, including the social climate and level of functioning, also plays a central role. For example, in families where communication is more open than closed; feelings, thoughts, and ideas are more freely expressed; and a sense of cohesion or closeness exists, bereaved siblings exhibit fewer behavioral problems—illustrated by Claudette's parents in how they talked with her about Henri's condition and impending death. Since families do not live in social vacuums, their culture and community values and priorities also impact sibling bereavement. But the central critical factor influencing sibling bereavement is the nature of the interactions between the siblings and the significant adults in their lives.

COMMUNITY BEREAVEMENT RESOURCES

The philosophy of PPC indicates that nurses and other palliative care providers and palliative care programs are professionally and morally obligated to assist grieving children by being sensitive to and knowledgeable about the impact of loss and bereavement. To carry out this role responsibly, they should be able to communicate about sensitive issues, understand the nature of normal and abnormal bereavement reactions, and be knowledgeable about community resources to which the bereaved can be referred. These include regional children's hospitals or hospices; organizations such as The Compassionate Friends (www.compassionatefriends .org) or SuperSibs! for siblings of children with cancer (www.change.org/ organizations/supersibs); bereavement centers such as The Dougy Center (www.dougy.org/grief-resources/how-to-help-grieving-child); and sources of books or activities, such as Compassion Books (www.compassionbooks .com) and Grieving as a Family: Finding Comfort Together (www .sesamestreet.org/parents/topicsandactivities/topics/grief).

Many bereaved siblings have described their experience of participating in a specialized bereavement support group as an important part of their experience. Many parents concur with the value of such participation for their children and for themselves as some programs also sponsor family-centered grief groups, camps, or programs. The number of children's grief groups has increased markedly in the past 25 years throughout North America, the United Kingdom, and Australia, offered by palliative care programs in hospitals, children's hospices, or grief centers. Groups are offered in a variety of forms with regard to being time-limited or open-ended; weekly, monthly, or on a weekend; structured or unstructured or a combination of both. Regardless of the format, the children value their participation. In an evaluation of one program, the children valued learning that they were "not alone" in their thoughts and feelings; they were reassured that they were not as different from "other kids" as they previously thought (Davies, et al., 2007). Such bereavement groups may be helpful for most bereaved siblings, particularly younger children whose skills of expression limit their responses to loss. The following and final story illustrates how a child's lack of understanding resulted in much hidden hurt and feelings of guilt that, over time, increasingly affected his behavior and way of being in his world, and how his grief responses were altered by his participation in a bereavement group within a hospice program.

Brad was about 6 years old when his parents first came to the children's hospice because of a cancer diagnosis in their younger son, Robin, aged 3. During Robin's admissions for respite care and symptom management, his family stayed in a suite upstairs. He was good-natured, wanting to be involved in the normal activities of a 3-year-old. Yet his condition and medical treatments left him weak, sometimes in pain with a severe headache or an upset stomach, and usually restricted to his bed.

Mom stayed with Robin, while Dad took Brad back and forth to their home where Dad would try to go to work and on those days, drop Brad off at school (he was in grade one at the time). At times, both parents stayed with Robin, while Brad was at home with relatives. Mom rarely left Robin's bedside, but would mention to nurses that she worried about Brad missing her. Dad was busy with many details of everyday life, juggling his concerns for Robin with his love for his wife and family, and his work.

Brad was a typical 6-year-old, curious, open-hearted, quick with his opinions. At times he seemed anxious, asking where his mom or dad was, or what was being planned for him when they stayed in the hospice. Because the care for Robin's cancer had been ongoing for 8 months of extended hospital visits before coming to the hospice, "normal" family patterns were gone. Brad was a "good boy," eager to please, happy to play, pay attention to his brother, or sit quietly with his parents. Periodically he was especially quiet, or withdrawn, but given the circumstances, this was understandable.

When Robin died, there was a convulsion of grief in both parents, with many tears shed and shared with Brad while holding him. With his parents, Brad spent time with Robin after his death, so together as a family and individually each said their own goodbyes to Robin.

Six months after he died, the family began to participate in the concurrent bereavement groups for parents and children that met every 2 weeks, supported by staff leaders and volunteers. Mom's grief seemed to engulf every aspect of her life, while her husband was coping as best as he could. But Brad was more and more emotionally impacted by the long illness and death of his brother, and now also by his parents' struggle with grief: He seemed depressed, almost absent.

Assessments affirmed that Brad lacked affect. He did not make trouble, but neither did he express excitement or anticipation about events that he used to enjoy. Now in grade two, his teacher reported that his behavior seemed "flat"; even his conversations lacked the variety of tone and expression that would be expected from a 7-year-old boy. The loss of his brother over the previous 2 years now framed his emotional and psychological world. Brad seemed to be adopting the stoic patterns of his father, shutting down memories, thoughts, and feelings.

In the bereavement program, Dad demonstrated a determined effort to keep things together, to fulfill family and work obligations. Yet at times, his grief overwhelmed him in the parent group. Mom, on the other hand, was articulate and passionate in venting her feelings of loss, her profound inertia, and the betrayal of her life hopes for her family. She was also self-critical of her "neglect" of Brad while Robin was sick and dying, and struggled to be a good mom now in her grief.

Leaders of the children's group often mentioned the curious monotone pattern of Brad's speech. His physical movements also seemed to be less agile and visibly awkward, as though he was a wooden puppet. With the grief responses of his parents after Robin's death, Brad's behavior seemed to reflect the struggles within his family, and the dysfunction of his parents.

In some ways it seemed Brad had jettisoned his sense of self, and was only going through the motions of what was expected of him, still trying to be a "good boy," yet with little commitment. Although he did not complain, neither did he seem to enjoy his life. Because of the curious pattern of his speech, one volunteer even coined the term "flat Brad" to describe him. When interacting with other children in the program who had also lost a brother or sister, he patiently listened to hear about their experience, but rarely offered any questions or other commentary. One staff member suggested he was "hiding inside himself, trying to do what was needed without drawing any more attention to himself than necessary."

Mom spent more time with Brad, to make up for her sense that she had not done enough to encourage him, and Dad took him in his truck on errands, but neither parent felt they could get beneath the cooperative acquiescing persona of their elder son, who seemed to have lost the spunk and sense of fun they described in him before Robin's illness.

The sibling bereavement program in the hospice is child-centered. Each week the children are individually given an opportunity to speak about their brother or sister in the group, while holding a "talking stick" carved with many animals. The only person who can speak is the one holding the stick—which is passed solemnly around the group, highlighting the importance of each child, and his or her own experience of the feelings and thoughts about the child who had died. With trained volunteers participating at each step of the 90-minute program, the children participate in a creative craft, storytelling, big-muscle games, and in one-on-one quiet time with an adult leader. At the close of the meeting, each child lights a candle in honor of his or her sibling who has died, with the opportunity again to voice his or her own thoughts, feelings, or memories. Snacks are offered before joining the parents for a large "closing circle" ritual in the central foyer of the hospice building.

With the group meeting every 2 weeks, children quickly adapt to opportunities for learning, play, engagement, sharing, and fun. As the group normally involves no more than a dozen children, with about the same number of staff and volunteers, there is a positive ratio for adult helpers to encourage, listen, affirm, play with, and enjoy the children in the different activities and elements of the evening program.

As a compliant "good boy," Brad went along with whatever was asked or expected of him each week, yet rarely demonstrated any divergence from his monotone speech, his toy-soldier movements, and his flat affect. Volunteers and staff leaders felt he was "present," listening and paying attention to the stories of other children, and telling the same version of his story, without much elaboration, week by week.

After about 7 months, several new children joined the group. At the close of one evening, a volunteer reported overhearing Brad respond to a number of questions from a persistent new girl who was very outgoing. As they were walking together following the other children from the opening circle, down a hall to the stairs leading to the rooms where the children's program would take place, she asked him his name, whether he had brothers or sisters, where he lived, whether both his parents were there, and what grade he was in school. With each wooden answer, she shared information about herself in relation to the same question, with one exception. When she pointedly asked, "What killed your brother, I mean, what did he die from?" Brad answered in his usual quiet monotone without flinching or hesitating, "I killed him, and he died from cancer." Without being aware of the volunteer paying close attention following just behind them, this precocious girl then asked emphatically, "How could you kill him if he died from cancer?" to which Brad again answered in his monotone, "I slammed the door on his finger, and he went to the hospital and that was the beginning of the cancer."

In the hubbub of children proceeding down the staircase, this was the end of the conversation between the two children. However, during the debriefing later that night, the leaders strategized ways to learn more of Brad's belief about his actions leading to his brother's death. Because they did not want to single him out, they invited a nurse and a doctor to subsequent meetings of the siblings' bereavement group to speak about the illnesses represented by each of the families, in order to offer some realistic understanding of these diseases. They would include discussion of possible causes of various diseases and interactive question and answer opportunities (with a few planted questions among the younger volunteers) to prompt answers to some of the children's questions.

During the following weeks, during the presentation about cancer, the nurse and doctor explained briefly the medical challenges in understanding the origins of cancer. They explained that cancer is a mysterious illness that cannot be "caught" or "caused" by one person in relation to another. Without addressing Brad individually, they made it clear that "while we all feel sad when someone gets cancer, we still don't know what causes it, but we don't want people to feel guilty when they wonder whether they made it happen to someone."

Although Brad did not respond verbally to what had been shared, when it was his turn to hold the "talking stick" a few weeks later, he mentioned in his monotone that he thought he "might have caused his brother's cancer, but now he wasn't sure." This provided the opportunity for some gentle one-on-one time with a leader, when Brad's story was explored between the two of them. Through questions and answers, the leader was able to elicit from Brad his earlier "knowing" that he had caused his brother's death, in contrast to his present "not being sure." Because of the relational trust that had been established between them over many months, the leader and Brad were able to agree that although Brad did slam the door on his brother (not wanting to be followed everywhere by his younger sibling when he was going out to play with a friend) he had not meant to really hurt him, and that, in any case, cancer is not caused by a hurt like that.

During this interchange, while Brad participated in the back-and-forth questions and affirmations, his emotional tone was fairly low. Yet when asked, he was able to give verbal agreement that he now understood that whatever it was that caused the cancer in Robin, that it was not Brad's action in trying to swing the door shut on him. By sharing the story of Brad's mistaken belief with his parents, they were able to listen for signs of his processing this new information, in order to offer affirmation, acceptance, encouragement, and share grief about Robin's death. Mom continued to spend one-on-one time with Brad two or three times each week, in a growing variety of activities. Similarly, Dad joined Brad in practicing soccer and baseball for special father–son times each week.

While there was no sudden change in Brad's deportment, over a period of months volunteers and staff were able to document how Brad was becoming more expressive; on one occasion he expressed sadness with tears, on another he yelled in exuberance with other children playing an outside game. Brad was beginning to leave "flat Brad" behind, reintegrating with his "normal" psychosocial trajectory from before Robin's illness and death. He now spoke about Robin with sadness and also remembered times of great fun between them. He even mentioned how sometimes it was a pain having a younger brother want to follow you everywhere, when you just wanted to be with your own friends.

His parents were also more resilient and able to weave the sadness and loss of their family life together with times of hope for the future and present enjoyment of each other. The leaders' attention to the nuanced details of the life of each child, in the context of a positive community of other children and parents experiencing loss, helped support Brad toward a new sense of self, in which sadness and grief are balanced with self-affirmation, under-standing, and encouragement for the future.

CONCLUSION

A child's death has lifelong implications for that child's brothers and sis-ters. When adults, particularly parents, comfort those siblings who are hurting, teach those who do not understand, include siblings so they feel as if they belong, and validate siblings' sense of worth, those children are more likely to have increased self-esteem and maturity, to be more sensitive and empathetic and better prepared to handle death. In con-trast, when adults belittle children's expressions of hurt, disregard their questions and level of cognitive development, exclude them from day-to-day events and activities and shame them for not understanding, or for not responding as the adults expect, then the siblings live with feelings of regret and remorse where they feel that nothing good came of their experience. A dark shadow is cast far into siblings' futures. Of course, the experience of any sibling is complex, influenced by many factors, and as for Brad, the experience can change over time. The goal of helping bereaved siblings is to assist them integrate their losses in ways that are regenerative rather than degenerative in the continual unfolding of their lives so that a comforting shadow gently accompanies them on their jour-ney through life.

CASE STUDY

Janelle is a 6-year-old whose younger brother died in a palliative care unit at a community hospital. Janelle knows that her brother was sick frequently and asks her parents to tell her what happened to him. She cries frequently and does not want to go to school anymore. Janelle tries to help her mother with housework and plays with her dolls so that she does not disturb her mother, who also cries quite frequently.

FOCUS QUESTIONS

1. How can the Shadows in the Sun model provide insight into Janelle's experience?
2. What interventions would be most helpful for Janelle?
3. Using a family-focused viewpoint, what resources would be beneficial for Janelle's family?
4. What role does hopefulness have in this case study?

REFERENCES

Association for Children With Life-Threatening or Terminal Conditions and Their Families (ACT), Royal College of Paediatrics and Child Health. (2009). *A guide to the development of children's palliative care services* (3rd ed). Bristol, CT: Author.

Barrera, M., Alam, R., D'Agostino, N. M., Nicholas, D. B., & Schneiderman, G. (2013). Parental perceptions of siblings' grieving after a childhood death. *Death Studies, 37*, 25–46.

Davies, B. (1999). *Shadows in the sun: The experience of sibling bereavement in childhood.* Philadelphia, PA: Brunner/Mazell.

Davies, B., Collins, J., Steele, R., Cook, K, Distler, V., & Brenner, A. (2007). Parents' and children's perspectives of a children's hospice bereavement program. *Journal of Palliative Care; 23*(1), 14–23.

De Cinque, N., Monterosso, L., Dadd, G., Sidhu, R., Macpherson, R., & Aoun, S. (2006). Bereavement support for families following the death of a child from cancer. *Journal of Psychosocial Oncology, 24*(2), 65–83.

Eilegård, A., Steineck, G., Nyberg, T., & Kreicbergs, U. (2013). Psychological health in siblings who lost a brother or sister to cancer 2 to 9 years earlier. *Psycho-Oncology, 22*(3), 683–691.

Gerhardt, C. A., Fairclough, D. L., Grossenbacher, J. C., Barrera, M., Gilmer, M. J., Foster, T. L., Compas, B. E., . . . Vannatta, K. (2012). Peer relationships of bereaved siblings and comparison classmates after a child's death from cancer. *Journal of Pediatric Psychology, 37*(2), 209–219.

McCown, D., & Davies, B. (1995). Patterns of grief in young children following the death of a sibling. *Death Studies, 19*(1), 41–53.

Rando, T. A. (1986). *Parental loss of a child.* Champaign, IL: Research Press.

Siden, H., Chavoshi, N., Harvey, B., Parker, A., & Miller, T. (2014). Characteristics of a pediatric hospice palliative care program over 15 years. *Pediatrics, 134*(3), e765–e772.

Steele, R. (2002). Experiences of families in which a child has a prolonged terminal illness: Modifying factors. *International Journal of Palliative Nursing, 8*(9), 418–437.

Webb, N. (2010). Assessment of the bereaved child. In N. Webb (Ed.), *Helping bereaved children* (3rd ed., pp. 22–47). New York, NY: Guilford Press.

Wender, E., & The Committee on Psychosocial Aspects of Child and Family Health. (2012). Supporting the family after the death of a child. *Pediatrics, 130*(6), 1164–1169.

World Health Organization. (2006). *WHO definition of palliative care*. Geneva, Switzerland: Author. Retrieved from http://www.who.int/cancer/palliative/definition/en

CHAPTER 17

Supporting Grieving Children

Andy McNiel and Donna L. Schuurman

*U*tilizing both evidence-based research and practice-based experience, in this chapter we address children's developmental processing of a family member's death; consider the impact death has on children's mental, emotional, and social selves; and expand on the needs they have for understanding, expression, and meaning making. Shared reactions and common beliefs among diverse cultures that impact children's evolving understanding of grief, death, and dying are incorporated, including recommendations regarding discussing with children the impending death of someone close to them, as well as their participation in funerals and family rituals. Myths and misconceptions are discussed, with suggestions on how to support grieving children in individual and group settings.

DEFINITION OF TERMS

The terms *bereavement*, *grief*, and *mourning* are often used interchangeably in the literature addressing issues related to dying and death. For the purposes here, the term *bereavement* is used to describe the state of losing someone to death. (After a death one is "bereaved," but may or may not be "grieving.") The term *grief* refers to a person's holistic experience of losing a loved one—or a not-so-loved one. Although deceased people commonly receive the descriptor of "loved one," we should not make assumptions about the relationship children had to the deceased. Grief encompasses the emotional, intellectual, physical, and spiritual experience and response to loss, and the expression of grief varies greatly from person to person. The term *mourning* is used here as the outward expression of grief, including displays of emotion, involvement in rituals, and other external behaviors. (In the context of this definition, a person may be grieving, but not necessarily mourning. That is, he or she may or may not be displaying outward signs of internal thoughts and feelings.)

HOW CHILDREN UNDERSTAND AND PROCESS DEATH

How children will respond to the death of a family member is dependent on numerous internal and external factors. Internal factors include their chronological age, their developmental age, and their intellectual capacity. External influences include previous experiences with death, family and cultural contexts, the relationship they had with the deceased, the circumstances of the death, and the child's proximity or exposure to the actual death. All of these factors will influence both their understanding, and their responses to, the death of a family member. In addition, as children age and mature, they will process and reprocess their understanding of the circumstances and implications of the loss. Making sense of and adapting to the death of a parent or sibling is a lifelong process as children grow up and reach milestones in their lives into adulthood.

Preschool-Age Children

Although babies and young children do not fully understand the permanence of death, they can sense and respond to the absence of people and things in their lives they have become accustomed to, from blankets and binkies to parents and puppies. We should not assume because of their verbal limitations that they do not experience "goneness" and loss when cherished objects and people disappear.

Because young children do not fully understand the finality of death, they often ask repetitive questions, and it takes time for them to fully comprehend what "dead" means, and that the deceased will not come back. Concrete explanations in age-appropriate terms will help them understand. For example, "When someone is dead, the body they are in dies. That means they can't move, or see us, or cry, or go potty, or sing, or anything." While it is acceptable and preferable for parents and caregivers to tell the child what happens to the body after death, it should be in keeping with one's beliefs. These will vary based on the cultural, religious, and/or spiritual beliefs of the family.

Four-year-old Jacob, upon being told his mother was now "up in heaven," responded to this news with a command to his father to "Get ladder!" Five-year-old Ke'Say told his brother that "I know daddy died, but will he be died all day?" They often long for the presence of the deceased, not understanding why they cannot go and be with the person, or why the deceased cannot come to visit them. Their egocentricity, and lack of understanding that other people operate independently of them, can lead to expressions of frustration over the absence of the deceased, and often regressive behaviors like bed-wetting, biting, and thumb-sucking.

Elementary School–Age Children

Elementary school–age children are beginning to more fully understand that death is permanent and that the deceased person cannot return. While they also start to realize that others have their own independent thoughts and experiences, they continue to be egocentric and magical in their thinking, sometimes assuming personal responsibility for someone's death. For example, children might imagine that had they been more obedient their parent would not have died. Children of this age are also developing a more complete vocabulary, but they continue to struggle with the right words to articulate their thoughts and feelings. As a result, their grief is often expressed in their play, artwork, and interaction with other children. They will move in and out of their grief as they participate in normal childhood activities, seemingly happy in one moment and agitated in the next. Because they continue to be concrete in their thinking, they are likely to be confused by euphemisms for death, such as "passed on" or "went to be with the Lord."

Middle School–Age Children

Middle school–age children are experiencing extreme changes, both physically and psychologically. The death of a family member becomes yet one more change among many. They may be uncharacteristically tired due to the added strain of their grief on top of the physical changes they are already experiencing. Middle schoolers are developing the ability to think about life and death in more abstract ways and are able to better understand the impact the death of a family member has on everyone in the family. Children this age often worry about how others in the family are doing. If it is their parent who has died, they will often take on the role of that parent, particularly the parent of the same gender. For example, 11-year-old Jason told his mother and aunt after his dad died, "Well, it was good while it lasted, I guess now I have to quit school and get a job." After her mother died, 10-year-old Tanisha told her teacher, "I might not be at school very much anymore now that my mom died, because someone has to take care of my baby brother." Other common reactions are withdrawal from normal activities and extreme mood swings.

High School–Age Adolescents

Teenagers find a sense of belonging among their peers and by high school they have established their preferred peer groups. Teenagers have more fully developed the ability to think logically about abstract concepts and can more clearly articulate their thoughts and feelings using a variety of modes of expression. Adolescence is also characterized by a sense of invincibility, resulting in more risky behaviors and stepping out of previously established rules or traditionally held family beliefs. Bereaved teens in support settings with other bereaved teens have expressed that they feel different around their peers since the death because they do not look at life in the same way as their peers. Some common reactions in teenagers are extreme mood swings, participating in more risky behaviors, a decreased sense of fulfillment in normal activities, and withdrawal from family or friends. It is important to note that teenagers who experience the death of a friend from among their peer group often express their grief within the context of that peer group, as teenagers in this circumstance are more likely to support one another.

UNDERSTANDING HOW DEATH IMPACTS CHILDREN'S LIVES

Early modern theories about children's ability to understand death, and their capacity to mourn, evolved from Sigmund Freud, his daughter Anna Freud, and John Bowlby, among others. In "Mourning and Melancholia," Freud asserted that the ultimate goal in grieving was to detach from the relationship with the deceased in order to shift focus and energy toward present, living relationships and activities (Freud, 1917/1957). From the psychoanalytic perspective, he believed that young children lacked the ego strength to complete this task, and viewed grief as an emerging ability for children, not fully realized until adolescence. Anna Freud shared this belief, although she did advance the understanding of children's capacity for mourning after observing hundreds of orphaned Jewish children at the Hampstead War Nursery. From clinical and nonclinical observations, it became evident that children do grieve and are capable of mourning the death of a family member or friend.

The British psychiatrist John Bowlby, highly influenced by the work of Anna Freud, conducted research on infant's and children's responses to separation from their primary caregiver (Bowlby, 1960). His pioneering work in the early 1950s highlighted the significance of early attachment, as well as the potential long-term adverse implications of unaddressed separation and loss. His work represented a fundamental shift in thought from the belief that children were not capable of mourning to the belief that they do have the psychological capacity to understand loss, grieve, and adapt to the absence of significant persons in their lives.

Over the ensuing decades, more attention was given to understanding the needs of children bereaved by early deaths in their lives. The pivotal Harvard Child Bereavement Study, which began in 1987, followed 125 parentally bereaved children (ages 6–17) from 70 families for 2 years, along with a matched nonbereaved sample control group. Coprincipal investigators of the study, Phyllis Silverman and J. William Worden, found that the strongest variable affecting the functioning of a child after the death of a parent is the mental health of the surviving parent. Children whose surviving parent has high levels of depression and/or anxiety are at higher risk for negative outcomes, for example. Investigators at Arizona State University's Family Bereavement Program concluded that "positive parenting by the surviving parent is the single most consistently supported malleable mediator of the adjustment of parentally bereaved children" (Haine, Ayers, et al., 2008, p. 5). An obvious implication for successful outreach services for grieving children and teens is the inclusion of services and resources for their parent or parents, whenever possible.

For many bereaved children, the negative consequences following their parent's death did not appear until 2 years after the death, highlighting the long-term nature of coping with bereavement (Silverman, 2000; Worden, 1996).

Another significant finding from the Harvard Child Bereavement Study was that children who maintained an ongoing connection with the deceased parent did not show adverse outcomes. The ongoing connections included ongoing rituals of remembrance (not simply the societally sanctioned funeral rituals), speaking to photos, writing letters to the deceased, as well as conversing in dreams, for example. Hogan and DeSantis (1994) developed a taxonomy of what helped and what hindered adolescent's bereavement after the death of a sibling, using the term *ongoing attachment*. Worden and Silverman's study led to Klass, Silverman, and Nickman's (1996) theory of "continuing bonds" and the value and importance of maintaining a connection with the deceased, contrary to Freud's earlier posit.

Margaret Stroebe and Henk Schut's "Dual Process Model" of grief points out that "children shift back and forth between grief and engagement—a dual process of 'loss orientation' dealing with and processing various aspects of the loss experience, and 'restoration orientation' of adapting to the demanding changes triggered by the loss while trying to cope with the many activities of daily life" (Stroebe & Schut, 1999, p. 216).

Factors Impacting a Child's Grief

Each child has unique circumstances and factors that impact his or her grief experiences. Two of these have been addressed: (a) their age and maturity level and (b) their relationship to the surviving parent (for parentally bereaved children/teens, or parents, for sibling/friend bereaved children/teens). Other influential factors include: (c) their personality and personal preferences; (d) the relationship they had to the deceased person; (e) past experiences of loss; and (f) the circumstances of the death.

Personality and Personal Preferences

Children are individuals with budding personalities and specific preferences about how they wish to interact with the world around them. They express their individual personalities and preferences through their play, which includes activities ranging from arts and crafts to games and athletics. Grief too will be reflected in the personality and in the preferred activities of children. Because of this, expressions of grief will vary among children of the same age. Some children will talk openly about the deceased person, while others will not. Silence about a deceased person is not an indication that children are not grieving, but is most likely a normal response in children with a reserved disposition. Children who are more extroverted might talk openly about the deceased or ask many clarifying questions about the death, funeral, and related topics.

Relationship to the Deceased Person

Worden (1996) observed differences in children who characterized their predeath relationship with the deceased as "very good" and children who saw the predeath relationship as "less than good." Children who viewed the relationship as very good "were likely to have shared interests with the dead parent, and were more likely to have stayed attached to the parent. . .[they] found it easier to talk about their feelings, they cried more, and they more frequently visited the gravesite" (Worden, 1996). Children with a pre-existing relationship that was less than good described more anger and anxiety associated with their grief (Worden, 1996). Further, if the last interaction with the deceased before they died was one of contention (i.e., being reprimanded for inappropriate behavior, arguing with a sibling) or if the last interaction was a loving, fond memory (i.e., they said, "I love you," or spent time together doing something fun) it plays an important role in children's grief after a death. When someone dies who was abusive, unkind, or contributed to an environment of chaos, it is not unusual for children to react with a sense of relief after his or her death, particularly when the deceased person's absence improves a child's living environment. This can also be true of deaths that were the result of long-term illnesses.

Past Experiences of Loss

Children experiencing the death of someone for the first time are encountering a new experience for which they have no prior context. In this regard, children are incorporating the reality of death into their understanding of how the world works. Children struggle with specific aspects about the concept of death itself. Speece and Brent (1984) in their literary review identified three concepts about death with which children often struggle: irreversibility, nonfunctionality, and universality. They suggested that it is common for children to not fully understand that when someone dies that person cannot come back to life, that his or her bodily functions stop working, and that death is something that happens to people of all ages. One bereaved child asked his mother after attending the graveside service, "How will we be able to get food to dad so he can eat if he is buried under the ground?" Another child asked her father, "When will mommy be coming back from heaven? I really miss her." Because children struggle with these concepts, it is normal for children to ask questions related to the death as they formulate their ideas about death, conceptualize how death fits with the natural laws of life, and understand what it means to their individual lives.

Children who have experienced the death of a family member, friend, or even a favorite pet are more likely to have a more fully developed concept of death, though each loss will have its own implications on children's daily lives. For some, this means that less energy is required to adapt to certain ideas about death. At the same time, multiple death experiences present another set of possible challenges. Children who have experienced the death of multiple significant persons might also experience a heightened preoccupation with death or live with a fear of who will be the next person to die. Along the same lines, children living with multiple sudden or violent death loss experiences might struggle with a sense of hopelessness for their own future that could lead them to act out or exhibit other problem behaviors.

Circumstances of the Death

Sudden violent death can further complicate the already difficult experience of grief. Children grieving the sudden violent death of someone not only grieve the absence of the deceased, but often struggle with intense feelings of anger and fear. Children often direct these powerful feelings toward those closest to them, though it can manifest itself in problem behaviors at school and other social settings.

Children grieving the death of someone from suicide often experience additional challenges further complicated by social stigma and a lack of understanding about causes of suicide. They may feel abandoned, or that the deceased did not love them. They may feel anger toward self or others, for contributing to the person's hopelessness, or for not preventing the death. While these same responses may also occur after deaths from disease or accidents, families who have experienced a suicide death often receive less social support than those whose family member died from illness or accidents.

Common Reactions to Loss

The way children experience and express their grief varies for each person. Some children need to talk about the person who died and others might not talk about the person at all. Many express their grief through art, play, music, or writing. In whatever ways children experience and respond to their losses, their behaviors are expressions of how they adapt to life without the physical presence of the person. This section highlights some common reactions to loss. It is essential to keep in mind that these are generalizations and that it is important to listen to children, meet them on their terms, and come to understand their unique grief reactions when providing support and encouragement.

Children who are grieving may experience a range of common emotions such as anger, sadness, fear, guilt, and regret. Children often move in and out of their grief, as they experience normal childhood activities. Many children lack the language or understanding to articulate what they are feeling through words. As a result, children often "act out" or experience mood swings throughout the day, seemingly unrelated to their loss. Children will incorporate their grief into their play. From Piaget to Adler, research and literature on childhood has long substantiated that play is important to children and a necessary tool as they incorporate new experiences, ideas, and emotions into their lives.

Bereaved children become keenly aware that people in their life can die. For example, if a parent dies, children are likely to worry about the safety of the other parent. They might also worry about what will happen to them if their other parent dies—who will care for them or how they will live without their parents. This can make bedtime particularly difficult for grieving children. Thoughts about the deceased and the heightened emotional energy can make it challenging to fall to sleep. Quiet moments like bedtime may play host to an array of fearful thoughts associated with grief.

Feelings of guilt are also a common challenge for bereaved children. Children tend to be egocentric and often believe that something they said, did not say, or did or did not do caused the person to die—often referred to as "magical thinking." They might believe that if they had told their dad they loved him more, he would still be alive, or if they had not talked back to their mother, she would not have died.

Bereaved children often feel misunderstood by those around them, including their peers. Many children grieving the death of a parent or sibling may not know anyone among their peer group dealing with the same experience. Well-meaning adults sometimes say hurtful things in an attempt to provide comfort, but frequently only reinforce children's feelings of not being understood. Others do not acknowledge the loss at all, adding to children's sense of isolation and alienation.

It is also important to consider that grief is long-lasting and children will experience their grief at different times on varying levels throughout their life into adulthood. Adults, whose parent died when they were children, express that, although their grief had changed in duration and intensity, they still have grief over their parent's death.

WHAT GRIEVING CHILDREN NEED

The death of someone close is a life-changing transitional experience for children. How it is handled has the potential to either heighten the risk of problem behaviors, or promote an individual's health extending into adolescence and adulthood. There are many factors that support healthy outcomes in the life of bereaved children. Children who experience adversity, like the death of someone in their life, can, with the right support, grow through the experience, but this "posttraumatic growth" does not occur in a vacuum. What are the factors that support these healthy outcomes and make it more likely that bereaved children will thrive and grow?

Children Need the Truth

Many adults would prefer their children not having to deal with the difficult realities that accompany death. Because of this, adults often use euphemisms like "passed away" to describe death. Using terms that represent other things to children, however, can cause confusion around the truth of what really happened. As discussed earlier, children struggle with concepts of irreversibility, nonfunctionality, and universality (Speece & Brent, 1984). The use of accurate language to describe death provides a context to understanding the reality of what has taken place: (a) people of all ages die; (b) a deceased person's body functions no longer work; and (c) they cannot come back from being dead.

It is also challenging for adults to tell children the truth about *how* a person died, particularly in the case of homicide or suicide. Although it may not be easy to share the truth about how someone died with children, honest answers build trust, help provide understanding, and allow children to feel comfortable approaching the adults in their lives with questions because they know they can trust them to tell the truth. Children know more than we think they do and by not telling the truth, we risk leaving children to process complicated information on their own, rather than with loving adults. While telling the truth is important, it is also important to not overshare. Providing unnecessary or gruesome information about a death can be as harmful as offering children false information. Truthful information should be provided to children considering their age of development and maturity level. It is best when the individual sharing information with children is someone with whom they have a trusting, loving relationship, so questions and ongoing dialogue can persist beyond the initial conversation.

Children Need Healthy Relationships With the Adults in Their Lives

Children take cues from the adults in their lives. They are observing, interpreting, mimicking, and testing the behaviors of these adults. When someone dies, children watch the reactions of their parents and other adults. It is not unusual for children whose parent is not functioning well after a death to also struggle. Children need the adults in their lives to model healthy behavior while grieving. Bereaved children who have a loving relationship with their caregiver(s), characterized by understanding and openness, are less likely to experience problem behaviors because of their grief (Worden, 1996).

Children Need Acknowledgment

An adult whose mother died when he was 9 recalled that during the funeral and the weeks following, he felt invisible to everyone around him. He said that his dad and other adults in his life consoled one another, shared stories, socialized, but never acknowledged him. This example continues to be a common experience among children. Consumed by their own grief or unaware that their children are grieving, adults often do not acknowledge their children's grief experiences. Yet, it is helpful to children when the adults in their lives acknowledge their presence. When children feel understood by family and friends and when they have the opportunity to express their grief in their own unique way, they feel less alone, which normalizes children's feelings. Children will move toward adults who appropriately acknowledge their presence at a funeral, family event, or when they are expressing their grief.

Children Need Respect

At the same time that children need to be acknowledged, they also need adults to respect their personal space. Children do not thrive in an environment that attempts to force them to talk about their grief. This is a common mistake among parents and professionals attempting to support bereaved children. As Silverman (2000) expressed, grief is not an illness that requires treatment. Grief is an internal, personal, transitional process, which is integral to children's development into the person they will become. Children fare better in an environment that allows them to express their grief in their own way and in their own time. Adults should avoid bombarding children with questions, oversharing about their own grief, and dominating conversations.

Children Need Boundaries

Maintaining clear boundaries is a challenge in many homes following the death of a family member. When the adults in a family are grieving, boundaries are often blurred. Children living in an environment with a lack of boundaries are more likely to experience problem behaviors as a result of their loss. Clearly communicated and established boundaries provide a safe context for children to express their thoughts and feelings. For example, while it is normal for children to experience anger as part of their grief, it is important for children to be held accountable for problem behaviors that could result from that anger. It is never acceptable for children to express their anger in violent ways toward others or themselves, but those behaviors sometimes happen because their anger is not acknowledged or channeled. Establishing clear boundaries and holding children accountable to these boundaries help ensure their safety as they find healthy ways to express their full range of feelings, including anger.

Children Need Routines/Predictability

For many bereaved children, their sense of control over their world has been compromised. The death of someone in their life interrupts routines and the relative predictability of their lives. Just as boundaries can be blurred when adults in their lives are grieving, so too can long established routines be impacted. The combination of a loss of perceived control and blurring of established routines creates a stressful environment for children. Though it might be challenging after a tragic event, maintaining routines for children will help them to avoid some of the stress that comes as they adapt to the absence of the deceased person. Routines help children feel a certain level of predictability about their environment, providing them with a safe space to express their feelings.

Children Need Choices

Established routines and boundaries must provide children with a variety of options in their play and other daily activities. Children are able to better express their grief in their own way and in their own time when they are given choices within the context of established routines and structured boundaries, whether at home, school, or other group environments. The ways children express their feelings of grief are varied; so, too, should their options for expression be varied. This will offer an opportunity for children to move toward preferred activities and heighten their ability to process their grief in a way that feels safe to them. When establishing a formal setting for providing support to children, that setting should include as many activities and options as the setting will allow.

TALKING TO CHILDREN ABOUT DEATH

As mentioned previously, discussing death with children can be challenging for adults. Children are commonly shielded from conversations about death and dying in the family setting, but this does not mean that children are not encountering the subject on a regular basis. Many popular children's movies contain images of death and explore the challenges of living with grief. Many of the main characters in popular kids' movies are dealing with the death of at least one, if not both parents. Their loss is often an integral part of the plot and related to the challenges presented through the main story. Children also see images of death in popular television cartoons, many of which further perpetuate confusion related to irreversibility and nonfunctionality. Because of this, avoiding discussions about death does little to keep children from thinking about death and formulating ideas about it. On the contrary, talking to children about death and other important life concepts can provide a context for them to better adapt to the changes brought about by the death of someone in their own life.

TALKING TO CHILDREN ABOUT THE IMPENDING DEATH OF SOMEONE CLOSE TO THEM

Discussion about the impending death of someone in children's lives is an evolving conversation. When someone is diagnosed with a life-altering, possibly terminal illness, it is important to begin the conversation with children from the beginning of the illness. Share with the children the name of the illness and seek age-appropriate ways to explain what the illness is and how it might impact the person with the illness and normal family routines. For example, it is helpful for children to understand the difference between cancer and having an upset stomach or a cold. This will decrease the likelihood that children associate these less threatening illnesses with more serious life-limiting ones.

Children experience time differently than adults, in that periods of time often seem lengthier for children. Because of advances in treatment today, it can be difficult to predict the duration and intensity of an illness. Instead, information should be shared as it becomes part of the reality. For example, it is advisable to share about the treatment or medication and possible side effects. This will give children a context for changes they may see in the person or that they might experience in their relationship with the person (i.e., mom's hair is falling out, or dad is tired and doesn't play with me as much now). If there have been significant changes in the appearance or personality of a person with an illness since the last time children saw him or her, it is helpful to have someone children trust to prepare them for the visit by describing what the children are likely to see and experience.

Children might have questions about the illness or even ask about the possibility of death. Answering children's questions openly and honestly provides the context for dialogue about the reality of the situation and strengthens a trusting relationship between parents and their children. As the illness progresses to a terminal diagnosis, conversations can begin to evolve to include discussions of death. Children ought to be given informed choice about their participation in planning for funerals and rituals, being mindful of their age, maturity level, and personality.

SHARING THE NEWS OF DEATH WITH CHILDREN

It is important to share with children accurate, age-appropriate information about the death of someone close to them. It is also best when the person sharing the information is a loving adult who the children trust and with whom the children have an ongoing relationship. Avoid euphemisms that can be confusing; instead use language like "dead" or "die" that provides an accurate context for children to process the reality of what has happened. Be prepared for any number of reactions, from intense emotional expression, silence, avoidance, and even laughter or seemingly inappropriate use of humor. Children might also ask to go play or want to go back to the activity they were engaged in prior to being interrupted with the news. All of these reactions are normal as children will move in and out of their grief in their own way and in their own time. Expect that some children will not talk about the death or the deceased person at all, while others will talk openly about their feelings. Be prepared for questions, expecting that children might ask the same question multiple times as they seek the information they need as they need it. Be patient with them as they explore what this death means to their lives.

CHILDREN'S INVOLVEMENT IN FUNERALS AND RITUALS

Professionals are often asked by parents and caregivers whether children should attend funerals or what exactly should be their involvement in these memorial rituals. Attending or participating in funerals, visitations, or other rituals is not harmful to children, but there are some considerations that will help guide adults as they seek to be supportive and understanding to children about this issue. Children function best when they are told what to expect and are given choices about their level of participation.

Using age-appropriate examples and language, explain to children what they are likely to see and experience when attending the memorial activity. Explain about the casket and if the body will be viewed, and what that might look like. Share that the child is likely to see many different emotional reactions, from sadness and anger to humor and laughter, based on what is normal in their particular cultural context. Tell them that there are going to be many people there, some who they know and see often, or have not seen in some time, or even people they do not know. Allow opportunity for children to react to what you are telling them and be patient with their questions about what you are describing.

When you have shared, listened to their responses, and answered their questions, give them an option to attend. Some children will want to attend the services and activities associated with the death, while others will not. Children should never be forced to attend funerals or to view the deceased person's body. If children choose to attend a funeral it is helpful to establish a plan in case they change their mind or need a break. Designate a trusted adult who is willing to companion the children during the event. Let the children know that they can participate as long as they want but that if they are ready to leave or need a break, they can let this person know. Preparing children, providing options, and having a plan will help ensure a healthy experience for children.

CULTURAL ISSUES IMPACTING GRIEVING CHILDREN, TEENS, AND FAMILIES

Although death (that of others as well as one's own eventual demise) is a universal experience shared by all, cultural differences are relevant and should be factored into how best to respond to children, teens, and their families who are bereaved. One of the dangers, however, is cultural stereotyping, whether related to gender (females turn outward/males turn inward, or females express through emotion/males express through action), ethnicity (any blanket statements about what any specific ethnic group does or does not do, and does or does not believe), religious affiliation, country of origin, and so on. There is a sense in which every family—nuclear and extended—impacted by the death of a family member is a culture in and of itself.

Cultural competence, the ability to function effectively in the context of cultural differences, is a critical component of successful support for children and their families. The following recommendations, adapted from the Substance Abuse and Mental Health Services (SAMHSA) publication on building cultural awareness among American Indian and Alaska Native populations, apply across other cultures as well.

1. Learn how the family or community refers to itself and use its terminology.
2. Honestly and clearly explain your role and show respect by being open to other ways of thinking and behaving.
3. Listen and invite people to educate you about specific cultural protocols in their community.
4. Avoid stereotyping based on looks, language, dress, and other outward appearances (SAMHSA, 2009).

These recommendations apply to every child, and every family, regardless of which cultural, ethnic, or religious background they belong to (or appear to belong to).

Supporting Grieving Children in Individual and Group Settings

Just as each child or teen is unique, no "one size fits all" program, therapy, or therapeutic intervention will fit the needs of everyone. Not all children or teens who are bereaved need professional help. Some may flourish in group settings that help normalize their experience, but groups are not for everyone. There are many approaches to providing support to bereaved children, in both individual and group settings. No matter which approach one chooses to employ, a supportive environment for bereaved children takes into consideration the needs of bereaved children, provides a flexible environment with a variety of play options, makes room for kids to freely express their own thoughts and feelings, and establishes predictable expectations and shared routines.

Establishing routines and setting clear expectations for behavior are key components to a healthy supportive environment for children. Children function better when they know what behavior is expected of them and when they are aware of the schedule. Providing routines that are predictable is helpful to bereaved children who have experienced interruptions to their daily routines due to the death of someone in their life and/or the grief everyone around them is experiencing.

Providing a variety of possible choices along with expectations and routines will help ensure that an environment is indeed supportive to a broad range of personalities and personal preferences. While there are formal times of sharing introductions and checking in with one another, the ideal setting will provide the opportunity for children to choose activities with which they are most comfortable. Through their play, children are able to express their thoughts and feelings. Children thrive when they are allowed to set the tone and take the lead in their chosen play or activity. When adults join them in their play and follow their lead, they validate children's feelings and respect their individual space.

CONCLUSION

In this chapter, we have addressed how children process the death of a loved one. Developmental theory has been used to explain how children understand death. Knowing how children's developmental levels affect their understanding of loss is crucial in determining clinical approaches to bereavement care for children. For example, how one shares the news of a death with a child should be determined by the child's age and development because cognitive processing of the permanence of death changes as children mature. Emotional responses to loss also manifest differently according to age and clinicians must be aware of how grief affects children and teenagers differently, avoiding a "one-size-fits-all" approach to care and support. Involvement of children in funerals and death rituals can be controversial and may be a source of conflict within families at the time of loss. In this chapter, we have discussed ways to approach this issue and have offered practical advice that can be shared with families when a death occurs.

For older children and teens, youth culture influences the expression of grief, as do the cultural, ethnic, and religious preferences of the family. However, it is crucial to avoid assumptions about how the child or teen may respond to loss. Individual or group support interventions for youth provide the means to explore a child or teenager's understanding of the death, emotional response, progress through processes of grief, and the effect of the loss on other areas of the child's life. This information can help clinicians to implement effective interventions that are developmentally and culturally appropriate.

CASE STUDY

Nine-year-old Mary experienced the death of her 12-year-old brother 6 months ago. Mary describes her brother as her "best friend." Mary's mother, Henna, states that Mary and her brother were very close and that Mary seems lost without him. Henna expresses concern that Mary did not want to attend the funeral, but hid behind her at the funeral home and hid her face during the services. Now, Mary plays with her brother's toys and asks if she can sleep in his room.

FOCUS QUESTIONS

1. Based on the information in the chapter, are Mary's expressions of grief to be expected for her age?
2. Would you have any concerns about Mary's manifestations of grief? Why or why not?

3. How can Henna's concerns be addressed?
4. What interventions would be helpful for this family?
5. Which resources offered in the chapter would be most appropriate for this family?

REFERENCES

Bowlby, J. (1960). Grief and mourning in infancy and early childhood. *Psychoanalytic Study of the Child, 15*, 9–52.

Freud, S. (1957). Mourning and melancholia. In J. Strachey (Ed.), *The standard edition of the complete psychological works of Sigmund Freud* (Vol. 14, pp. 237–260). London, England: Hogarth Press and Institute for Psychoanalysis. (Original work published in 1917.)

Haine, R. A., Ayers, T. S., Sandler, I. N., & Wolchik, S. A. (2008). Evidence-based practices for parentally bereaved children and their families. *Professional Psychology: Research and Practice, 39*(2), 113–121.

Hogan, N. S., & DeSantis, L. (1994). Things that help and hinder adolescent bereavement. *Western Journal of Nursing Research, 16*(2), 132–153.

Klass, D., Silverman, S., & Nickman, S. (Eds.). (1996). *Continuing bonds: New understandings of grief.* Washington, DC: Taylor and Francis.

SAMHSA. (2009). *Culture card: A guide to build cultural awareness: American Indian and Alaska native.* Washington, DC: Author.

Silverman, P. R. (2000). *Never too young to know: Death in children's lives.* New York, NY: Oxford University Press.

Speece, M. W., & Brent, S. B. (1984). Children's understanding of death: A review of three components of a death concept. *Child Development, 55*(5), 1671–1686.

Stroebe, M., & Schut, H. (1999). The dual process model of coping with bereavement: Rationale and description. *Death Studies, 23*, 197–224.

Worden, J. W. (1996). *Children and grief: When a parent dies.* New York, NY: Guilford Press.

CHAPTER 18

Moments Matter: Exploring the Evidence of Caring for Grieving Families and Self

Rana Limbo and Kathie Kobler

The room was so filled with people who loved the small child that the only space left for me was to kneel at the foot of his bed, positioning myself so I could watch for signs of dyspnea or pain. All I saw though, was a 2-year-old gently transitioning from life to death, snuggled between his parents who were lying in bed with him. My eyes caught the parents' shoes, which were jumbled on the floor under the bed, not far from where I was kneeling. My first thought, "I can never fit in those shoes," because I wear a size 5 shoe, and their feet were much larger. Then a humbling realization struck me to the core, "I can never fit in those shoes," because these dear people will eventually arise from the bed after their son's death, put their shoes back on, and walk out into a world that I can never fully comprehend. I remember praying, "Yet may wisdom and discernment meet me with ways to best support this family as they grieve."
(Kathie Kobler)

*P*atient- and family-centered care began in the late 1940s, yet a half-century later, professionals must still advocate for family-centered bereavement care when a baby or child dies. In this chapter, we provide an overview of both perinatal and pediatric bereavement care by summarizing an array of current research and practice topics. Bereavement care exemplifies an area of practice for parents, families, and care providers where *moments matter.* Much of the chapter's content highlights the significance of moments, moments in which relationships are made or dissolved, memories are created, transformation occurs, and hope shifts. Being in the moment means that one person connects with another in a way that each may hold in mind for a lifetime while pressures of time, crowded spaces, other voices, and deep heartache fade into the background.

In addition, we provide strategies that promote self-care for those who provide care to the bereaved. We also outline core concepts of gold standard education for staff to enhance the provision of evidence-based, family-centered bereavement care from competency development through certification and ongoing continuing competence activities. Importantly, we define "family" through a multicultural and nongender-specific lens, using this definition to frame clinical practice guidelines for integrating quality bereavement care for families experiencing a miscarriage, stillbirth, neonatal death, or pediatric death in a hospital setting.

BACKGROUND

The number of persons—parents, siblings, grandparents, friends and other loved ones, and professional care providers—affected by children's deaths is staggering. Children, no matter the age at which they die, embody hopes, dreams, and lifetimes of anticipated events—first words, first steps, first days of school, graduations, finding partners, and having children of their own. We live with the deeply held assumption that parents die before their children. When miscarriage, stillbirth, the prenatal diagnosis of a life-limiting congenital condition, the death of a newborn, or an older child's death occurs, life becomes less certain, challenging the core assumption that children outlive their parents. For parents, this was not just *any* child. This child was *my* child, *our* child, our legacy, born with the expectation of joy-filled days with family and friends. Births are celebrated and lives of children are valued in cultures across the world, making the death of a baby or older child a devastating event for the family and their entire community.

RELATIONSHIP-BASED CARE

In this chapter, we frame the care provided by an interprofessional team as *relationship-based* (Kobler, 2013a; Koloroutis, 2004; Limbo & Kobler, 2010; Lindsay, Cross, & Ives-Baine, 2012). We conceptualize relationship-based care as *the tie that binds,* a phrase we used in the title of a published paper on relationships in perinatal bereavement (Limbo & Kobler, 2010). Being connected or bound together through relationships is central to this chapter. We use *professional* in this chapter as a generic noun to indicate any of the wide variety of health care providers involved with families, including nurses, social workers, chaplains, genetic counselors, and physicians, among others, and whose work together comprises an interprofessional team. We identify relationships between and among parents, parents and child, parents and professionals, child and professionals, professionals and extended family members, and among various professionals. We emphasize initiating and maintaining relationships as central to the standard of care provided from the time of diagnosis through follow-up after death. Finally, we summarize recent research findings on several of these relationship dyads to provide ongoing evidence of the importance of relationship in perinatal and pediatric bereavement care.

Relationships of Parents With Their Children

Parents and Their Child Who Died or Is Dying

Professionals at the bedside, most notably nurses, have the opportunity to interact in an intimate way with parents, seeing their deepest pain and also sharing in small joys that are part of a bereavement experience. Final acts of caregiving—whether for a child who is dying or who has already died—can be created in the moment by simple questions such as: "What would you like to do before she dies?" or "What had you thought about doing and haven't been able to yet?" (Limbo & Lathrop, 2014). A parent may lie in bed with his or her child, singing a favorite song or reading from a favorite book, or hold the child and speak to him or her.

Many times, when facilitating such opportunities that honor the parent–child relationship, unexpected moments of meaning and peace unfold, bringing comfort to the child, parents, and care team, described in the following story.

> Our somber procession carefully made our way through the halls to the private patio garden. The parents' request: the warmth of sunshine on their 9-month-old baby as she was compassionately extubated and transitioned to dying. Led by the clinical nurse specialist, the mother cradling her dying baby and father pushing their wheelchair, a small army of nurses, respiratory therapists, and physicians followed alongside.
>
> One other joined the group: a mother robin, with her nest containing three babies precariously placed on a patio light fixture. What happened next amazed all who were present. We positioned the family in sunlight, watched as mother nestled her baby over her heart, father wrapped his arms around both. As we stepped back, the mother robin took our place, positioning herself on a ledge about 3 yards from the family.
>
> She began to sing, pause, watch, repeating the cycle numerous times, never changing her position. The mother robin even stayed when our team moved in to assess, administer medications, or offer words of comfort. It wasn't until after we pronounced the baby's death and the parents began weeping

loudly that mother robin left her vigil spot, and returned to her nest. All who were present that day still recall fondly the gifts of music and presence shared so freely by the mother bird with this family. (Kathie Kobler)

When their child dies, parents' greatest fear is that they will forget aspects of their child's physical appearance. Keepsakes ease these fears by providing them with tangible ways of remembering and connecting as the weeks and years go by. Photos are more accessible than in the past because of technology such as smartphones. Some hospitals use professional photographers who provide photos to families at no cost. Most hospitals also have cameras that staff can use for capturing meaningful moments of family members and their child.

Other examples of memorabilia include clothing the child wore, handprints, footprints, a baby ring, plaster molds of hands and feet, and ink tracings of the child's hands with siblings' hands (Boss, Kavanaugh, & Kobler, 2011; Limbo & Kobler, 2010). Tattoos, memory gardens, jewelry, and a handbuilt casket or cremation vessel are ways that parents may create keepsakes on their own, staying connected to their child in a tangible way. Some families also participate in community events such as a remembrance walk, memorial service, or holiday candlelighting.

The role of a professional when working with bereaved families is to serve as a guide and support development of relationships, helping families focus on what is most important to them. The following story, told through the voice of their nurse, illustrates relationships between two couples who shared mutual love for an expected baby, among the couples and the baby, and between each couple and the nurse.

> I had the privilege of meeting with two couples last night, bound by their mutual love for Jonathan, a baby boy yet to be born. One of these couples would be parenting Jonathan after his birth, the other couple was the "gestational carriers"—the woman was pregnant with the baby to be parented by the other couple. Also known as a "surrogate mother," she and her supportive partner had formed a relationship of respect and caring with Jonathan's parents.
>
> Jonathan was diagnosed with a severe heart defect that would limit his life and cause great suffering. These four persons were in agreement as to what was best for him, to induce labor early and let him die a comfortable death in the arms and presence of the many persons who loved him. As the meeting neared its end, the mother who would parent Jonathan, crying, thanked the woman pregnant with their son for loving and

holding him, physically, as she could not right now. She knelt down and kissed the pregnant woman's belly, cupping her unborn son in her hands as best she could.

In the spirit of supporting these couples in this heartbreaking situation, I offered a blessing or baptism. Although Jonathan's parents did not feel the need for such a ritual, they fully supported doing so if it would bring peace to the surrogate mother and her partner. My job here was to create space for these persons, joined in their commitment to Jonathan, to share in an intense moment of love and respect for each other and for their baby. (Emilie Lamberg-Jones)

Parents and Their Surviving Children

Health care professionals who work with families when a child dies may be well-positioned to assist parents with their other child or children, the deceased child's siblings. The nurse may be the first person parents ask, "How do we tell the children?" (Limbo & Kobler, 2009). Health care providers can begin helping parents understand and respond to their other children by encouraging them to listen to their child's concerns and fears. Young children need assurance that they did not cause the death and could not change the outcome (Hunter & Smith, 2008). Using simple explanatory language such as "The baby's body didn't work anymore" can avoid complexities that young children cannot understand (Schaeffer & Lyons, 2010).

Children, when prepared for what they will see or hear when their sibling is dying, are uniquely able to see past tubes, wires, and sickness to just see their brother or sister. For those siblings who are unable to be present at the time of the child's death, health care providers may offer suggestions for ways that siblings can be connected to the situation without being physically present. Older children can be included in planning and carrying out ritual. Recording a message or song, making a drawing, and sending a comforting item for the dying child are all ways younger siblings can be involved. A parent could ask (if the parent does not already know), "What will you miss the most?" or "What were you planning to do that was most important?" These questions may help a child reflect on actual time together or wished-for moments, either of which could create powerful ways for children to say good-bye.

Just like their parents, surviving siblings will experience a lifetime of living and growing with the knowledge of their sibling's death, revisiting the moments, and redeveloping their understanding of the event as they mature. The American Academy of Pediatrics acknowledges the importance of providing ongoing assessment and support for grieving siblings in their report on supporting the family after the death of a child (Wender et al., 2012).

Relationship Between Parents

Another relationship dyad of critical importance in perinatal bereavement care is that between parents. Grief is often examined as an individual phenomenon, which makes the idea of Stroebe and colleagues' (2013) research on couples particularly intriguing. In a study of 219 parent couples whose children died from illness, accident, or intentional injury, Stroebe and colleagues (2013) found an interpersonal pattern for both men and women of "partner-oriented self-regulation" (POSR; p. 395), a phenomenon in which each parent held in his or her own grief to spare the other parent from witnessing his or her individual suffering. Interestingly, POSR had the paradoxical effect of actually increasing grief for both partners.

A child's death is a potential threat to a couple's relationship stability, according to the findings of several contemporary researchers. In a study of a sample from a national database of over 3,000 women, Schreffler, Hill, and Cacciatore (2012) found that women who had experienced miscarriage or stillbirth were more likely to also report being divorced. Although some couples described the trauma of a child's death as bringing them closer, this study demonstrated that the opposite is more likely. Divorce rates differed significantly ($p < .001$) between women who had experienced a perinatal loss (32%–43% were divorced) and those who had not (27% were not divorced) (Schreffler, Hill, & Cacciatore, 2012). Gold and colleagues (2010) reported similar findings from an analysis of another national database. These findings have important implications for professionals working with couples after a miscarriage, stillbirth, or other child deaths, alerting these couples to seek out sympathetic others outside of their relationship for support, in addition to turning to each other.

Cacciatore and Raffo (2011) interviewed six lesbian couples who identified a more disenfranchised grief than that experienced by heterosexual couples when social stigma surrounded their same-sex relationship. Because the journey of getting pregnant is complex—socially, emotionally, medically, financially, and legally—the "experience of loss is amplified" (Peel, 2010, p. 724). Black and Fields (2014) noted that the decision to become *parents* may leave same-sex couples marginalized. State laws govern legal status of parents and for same-sex couples, the laws may serve as barriers to their desired goals, creating another layer of grief when their baby dies. For additional research findings on lesbian couples, see Wojnar (Chapter 8, this text).

Professionals have the opportunity to thoughtfully consider ways they can support meaningful moments between parents. Providing time alone, assuring that each has had nourishment, and including both in conversations may help meet the needs of each parent, separately and together. Thinking of how to create a circle with each parent, their child, and the care provider can create an intimate space for closeness and emotional expression.

Relationship Between Nurse and Child

Parents identify the importance of the relationship that others form with their baby, whether the baby dies during pregnancy, is stillborn, or dies after birth (Gold, 2007). In recalling the moments after her daughter's stillbirth, a mother remarked in an interview about her experience, "I remember the nurse rocking her back and forth, patting her butt." The mother smiled as she recalled the moment, realizing that the nurse responded no differently than if her daughter had been born alive. Now I Lay Me Down To Sleep (www.nilmdts.org), a volunteer bereavement photography service, published a photo on a social media site of three grieving nurses who had cared for a mother and her newly delivered stillborn baby. The photo received millions of views, was shared around the world, and captured a scene that resonated with anyone who has been at the bedside supporting parents when their child of any age died.

A pattern of "essential engagement" highlights the unique relationship between neonates and neonatal intensive care nurses (Lindsay, Cross, & Ives-Baine, 2012, p. 246). The nurses experienced a "call-to-presence" (p. 246) from the baby, bringing the two into relationship, leading to profound effects on the nurse when the baby died (Lindsay et al., 2012). Those at a dying baby's bedside may experience brief moments of joy while bearing witness to their tiny patient's struggles. Black (1993) described one of these moments in this way: "As I talked that silly adult talk . . . [Shawndra] smiled . . . ! Her face was beautiful and whole and healthy, filled with a baby smile that meant she could hear me, see me, and respond to the world with joy" (p. 138).

As health care professionals enter into relationship with children of all ages, they open their mind and hearts to being present throughout the child's trajectory of care, including at the end of life. The poem at the conclusion of this chapter, *On Rocking Arthur*, describes author Kathie Kobler's "call to presence" and what it meant to her to be in relationship with a baby who died and his mother. The mother was able to say good-bye one last time via telephone, a uniquely meaningful final moment. We discuss the unique aspects of what it means for professionals to be witness to a woman's loss after miscarriage, parents' experience after the birth of their baby still born, a patient's dying, and the suffering and grief that may follow in the latter portion of this chapter.

PROFESSIONALS CARING FOR BEREAVED PARENTS

Honoring Relationship

Moments matter for professionals who care for families when a child dies, as these moments are key elements in developing and maintaining relationships. Being engaged in a meaningful relationship with patients and families helps to honor their experiences and may also limit professional burnout. For example, Perry (2008) reported that oncology nurses revealed a key condition to avoiding professional emotional and spiritual fatigue: They made the most of moments to remain engaged in the care of their patients. Nurses identified three categories of moments: (a) moments of connection; (b) making moments matter; and (c) energizing moments. Care providers may view end-of-life or bereavement care as requiring time, which is at a premium in busy hospital environments.

Watching for, making the most of, and reflecting on those brief periods of time in which something profound occurs offer a way of finding meaning, value, and memories in the relationship with those cared for. In recounting her care of a drug-addicted mother in labor with her eighth baby, Van Damme (2009) recalled the moment she heard the mother plead, "Please don't go" (p. 446). In that moment of connection between the patient and the nurse, and in the nurse's decision to stay with the laboring mother past the end of her shift, both experienced what it means to be in relationship.

Price, Jordan, and Prior (2013) studied parent- and professional-identified issues during end-of-life care for a child diagnosed earlier with a life-threatening condition. The researchers looked for convergence, topics that both parents and professionals agreed provided opportunities for improvement. Two of the three are highly relevant to this chapter: structured bereavement services and support of the child's siblings. One solution for structured bereavement support was to identify someone trained in bereavement to establish a relationship with families and provide relevant guidance and emotional support. Both professionals and parents identified the need for sibling-focused interventions that helped families know what to do and increased competence in those providing care.

Gold (2007) summarized research that included the same difficulties between parents and professionals after a baby died. For example, in numerous studies she reviewed, one or both parents were distressed at a lack of emotional support from professionals. These behaviors included insensitivity such as a nurse failing to mention the second twin who died when caring for the mother and the living twin, avoiding the parents, or avoiding the subject of their baby's death. In these emotion-filled, yet tender moments of end-of-life care, it is imperative that providers strive to bridge communication or relationship gaps with parents. Just as Van Damme (2009) elected to "be with" the woman who was laboring by staying with her, we now describe how touch, compassionate silence, and ritual can provide effective ways of being with patients.

Touch

Touching another person is a form of intimacy and a way to connect in relationship. Regarding the appropriateness of touch, Cacciatore and Flint (2012a) wrote, "There is no more appropriate time for intimacy than when a family is facing traumatic death" (p. 66). Therefore, in any clinical encounter, care providers need to consider both the appropriateness and potential response of using touch. Its purpose may be to create connection, provide comfort or, at times, to gain one's attention when he or she is lost in intense emotion.

One form of touch that can be particularly supportive for those who are grieving a death of a loved one (e.g., a mother who has recently given birth to a baby who was stillborn) or, in the context of this chapter, a child nearing the end of life is rubbing of the back, arms, hands, legs, or feet. Unless medically contraindicated, massage can even be used on infants. Massage may calm emotions, reduce pain, or serve as a reminder between parent and child or care provider and patient of a relationship that is communicated without words. One mother's final act of caregiving with her 8-year-old son in his last minutes of life was to crawl in bed with him, silently holding him next to her as he took his final breaths. The mother of a preterm newborn who died within a few hours of birth recounted several years later the meaningful memory of her nurse giving her a nighttime backrub in a dark room with no words exchanged between them. When 10-year-old James, dying of cancer and too weak to get out of bed, looked at his nurse, she instinctively reached for his feet. She watched him close his eyes, relaxing to the gentle massage she provided as death approached.

Promoting opportunities for touch or skin-to-skin contact between parent and child is a way to honor their relationship while cocreating moments that will remain with parents forever. Health care professionals often wonder how they may best reach out in touch to grieving parents, family members, or staff. One approach is to watch how the family is interacting physically with each other, and adjusting their care to model their interactions. Otherwise, when moved to do so, the professional may choose to gently touch the other between elbow and shoulder, the body range that is most culturally respectful to offer compassionate touch to another.

Silence

Silence is a practice used by many health care professionals as a means to foster communication. Back, Bauer-Wu, Rushton, and Halifax (2009) noted that silence comes from the deepest place in human interaction, rather than as a simple communication strategy. The idea that silence lies *within* and *between* the practitioner and patient is profoundly different from using silence as a strategy during a conversation, essentially waiting to see what will happen next. Compassionate silence is anchored by the practitioner's breath, a mindful awareness of the qualities of one's own breathing (Back et al., 2009).

Compassionate silence is part of one's *quality of mind* (Back et al., 2009), to which one pays attention without any undue expectations as to what will happen. Instead, the practitioner simply lets the relationship unfold. Generally this type of silence has a *moment-by-moment quality* (p. 1115), offering a strong sense of presence. It is neither awkward (as silences often can be) nor invitational. Rather, compassionate silence results in moments that naturally unfold.

We suggest a means of practicing compassionate silence in a patient encounter, using these steps (Back et al., 2009):

1. Pause at a moment during which you imagine that something deeper may come out of your shift from a narrative, storytelling mode to one of silence.
2. Pay attention to your breath as you breathe in and out.
3. Note what your body is doing, how you feel, and what responses you are having.

The patient may notice the difference in what you are doing and mirror it. Or perhaps the patient will at first seem uncomfortable and then relax when he or she recognizes that nothing is expected. This is a contemplative practice, one that is consistent with Cacciatore's ATTEND model (Chapter 6, this text). By honoring moments of silence that unfold during relationship, professionals allow parents to gather their thoughts, reflect on emotions, or consider the next actions as they experience their child's death.

Engaging in Ritual

We define ritual as growing out of relationship (Limbo & Kobler, 2013). As care provider and parent work together or as the care provider serves as a nonintrusive guide, ritual can be cocreated, or jointly created. "Through co-creation, care providers can acknowledge family members' ability to ascertain what is most important in the moments ahead" (Limbo & Kobler, 2013, p. 7). We identify ritual as having three relational components: participation, intention, and meaning making (Kobler, Limbo, & Kavanaugh, 2007). *Participation* implies that parents and care providers are jointly engaged in the process of creating ritual; *intention* signifies implied action, meaning ritual in the context of bereavement has a purpose; and *meaning-making* refers to outcomes of ritual, what parents or others involved make of the ritual, and how it is integrated into their grief and their memories.

Cacciatore and Flint (2012b) reported that bereaved parents participated in ritual to maintain and extend the existing bond they have with their child, that ritual helped them feel more in control, and allowed for meaning reconstruction, which may transform their grief. Ritual can be planned actions that reflect a family's religious or cultural beliefs, such as a welcome blessing or baptism. Or ritual can emerge from unplanned moments that unfold through relationship, such as pausing to signify the moment when a mother enfolds into her arms the child near death.

The opportunity for care provider and parent to cocreate ritual can present itself in many ways. Photos may also document ritual. Photography can also be considered a type of ritual when parents are involved in the creation of the photos. Photographer Todd Hochberg (n.d.; toddhochberg .com), known for his extraordinary photography of dying or deceased children and their families, advocates for remaining in the background, taking photos or not, but carefully watching for what those in the room are saying and doing (Limbo & Kobler, 2013). His photos include an older sibling reading his favorite book to his dying sister and parents bathing their baby, carefully and gently examining every part of their son's body. In describing his mindset for bereavement photography, Hochberg stated, "I aim to be fully present and mindful of the moment" (Limbo & Kobler, 2013, p. 26). Ample evidence exists to support photography as a standard of practice for families when a baby or older child dies. Blood and Cacciatore (2014) reported that 92 of 93 parents endorsed having photos of their deceased child.

Matt Mooney, father of Eliot who lived 99 days with trisomy 18, created a film *99 Balloons* to document Eliot's short life, one filled with ritual. Here is how Matt described the transformative role of ritual for his family:

> . . . there is no map, the smallest anchor to that present moment and now to a former reality—indeed, to a person that we love beyond measure—this tether becomes a means to bind you to what you will never forget. Ritual has served as a way to remind us and others that what we see is not all there is or was or, I believe, will be. (Limbo & Kobler, 2013, p. viii)

Mindfulness of Setting

Health care professionals must be mindful of creating a safe setting for families to interact with their child, in ways that are meaningful to them. Parents receiving palliative care support report appreciating the opportunity to discuss possible choices of where their child's death may occur (Dussel et al., 2009). Home is the preferred location for death by both parents and health care professionals caring for a child with cancer (Kassam, Skiadaresis, Alexander, & Wolfe, 2014). Hospital deaths, especially those in the emergency department (ED), tend to be unplanned and more sudden, leaving parents potentially experiencing a high level of shock as part of their grief.

While death in the ED is common, it occurs within an environment geared toward quick thinking and efficient actions (O'Malley, Barata, & Snow, 2014). Care providers and their senior leaders may not focus on family-centered bereavement care or meaningful moments in this fast-paced environment dedicated to saving lives. Professionals working in an ED who provide care to those experiencing a miscarriage, or death of an infant or older child, need skills in responding to the sudden, often unplanned, nature of the loss, whenever it occurs. For that reason, we highlight care in the ED using two case studies of unexpected death: miscarriage and pediatric death.

Miscarriage

Women who come to the ED with a potential miscarriage typically experience bleeding and/or cramping. With the large majority of miscarriages occurring in the first trimester, these women are likely to be between 4 and 12 weeks pregnant. In a longitudinal study of 60 women who were followed for 1 year after a miscarriage, Limbo and Wheeler (1986) reported that approximately 75% of the women felt they had "lost" something, which they referred to as a pregnancy or a baby. The other 25% of women considered the miscarriage to be a life experience, but not an event that created a sense of loss or grief. Côté-Arsenault and Dombeck (2001) also reported variation in how women perceived the meaning of a miscarriage: no loss, pregnancy, baby, a baby with a name, or a child who would now be a certain age. These studies and others related to the care of pregnant women with symptoms or signs of miscarriage underscore the importance of determining what this experience means to a woman who presents in the ED with a possible miscarriage.

Case Study: Inevitable Miscarriage

Deanna came to the ED alone, 10 weeks pregnant, and "not feeling right." After an ultrasonogram, the ED physician said that he wished he had different news, but there was no heartbeat. Deanna began to cry, saying "I can't believe this. Are you sure? I felt pregnant until about 2 days ago." After expressing that he wished he had different news, the physician left and the perinatal bereavement social worker, based in the ED, came to see Deanna. The social worker sat beside Deanna, sometimes in silence, to learn how Deanna viewed her miscarriage (i.e., as a life event, pregnancy loss, death of a baby); provided written material on miscarriage; and after the social worker's visit was complete, asked the nurse to see Deanna. During the conversation with Deanna, the social worker heard Deanna use the term *baby* to refer to her pregnancy and miscarriage. She shared this information with the nurse. The nurse provided supplies to Deanna, helping her prepare for the eventuality of having a miscarriage at home. The supplies included a container to place on the toilet seat, pads, and a container for the miscarriage remains. Deanna's partner came to take her home and she told him, "I'm so glad that they prepared me for what to do if I have a miscarriage at home. I might have a D&C [dilation and curettage to empty the uterus] in a few days, but in the meantime, I know what to do."

Death of a Child in the ED

In a systematic review of the literature, Garstang, Griffiths, and Sidebotham (2014) noted that in the event of a child's sudden death, parents want privacy, the ability to see and hold their child, and full details of the death. If barriers exist that prevent them from achieving their goals, they are likely to experience bitter regret and feel that they were "deliberately evaded" (p. 269).

Case Study: Death of a Child

An ambulance and paramedics arrived at the emergency entrance of a hospital with Darren, followed closely by several police cars. Darren was 19 and had been involved in a knife fight in which he was mortally wounded. Emergency personnel were unable to resuscitate Darren. The police, who were present in the ED, did not allow his parents to see their son because he was involved in a crime. His mother remained distraught for months afterward, mourning not only her son but her lack of opportunity to say good-bye. A bereavement nurse and chaplain provided two opportunities as part of follow-up care that eased Darren's mother's suffering. First, the nurse and chaplain offered to accompany her on a visit to the room in which Darren died. Darren's mother wanted to do this, but it took a number of appointments before she was able to actually visit the room. While there, the bereavement nurse placed a rose on the bed. Knowing this mother's strong religious faith, the chaplain sang one of her favorite hymns.

Darren's family also wanted a grief conference after his death (see Box 18.1). They asked that the chaplain, the paramedic who cared for Darren at the scene and in the ambulance, and his ED nurse be part of the conference. The parents expressed relief when the paramedic explained that although they administered cardiopulmonary resuscitation (CPR) from the time they arrived until he was declared dead in the ED, he had not breathed or moved. The paramedic also told the parents that his colleague whispered encouraging words to Darren in the ambulance, a point during which the parents and Darren's sister were visibly moved. The nurse explained how carefully they transferred Darren to the bed in the ED and described the care with which they handled his body. At the end of the grief conference, the professional staff and Darren's family shared hugs. Everyone in the room was tearful.

BOX 18.1 GRIEF CONFERENCE GUIDELINES

A grief conference can be set up as part of follow up to help parents resolve any unanswered questions they have concerning their baby's death. If an autopsy or genetic studies were done, the conference can be scheduled when the report is available so it can be reviewed at the same time. When coordinating a time for the grief conference, check to see how long it usually takes for autopsy or genetic study reports to be completed. If no autopsy or genetic studies were done, the conference can be scheduled at any time, with a general guideline of 6 weeks post-loss.

As facilitator, the professional care provider makes arrangements with the pathologist's office to have the autopsy reports sent to the appropriate physician and the facilitator.

Upon receiving an autopsy or genetic study report, the facilitator contacts the offices of the obstetrician and the pediatrician or neonatologist to arrange for a 1-hour grief conference. If feasible, arrange several different dates and times from which the family can choose.

Once potential dates have been arranged, the facilitator telephones the family to schedule the grief conference. At that time, the family is asked who they would like to have present at the conference. They may choose any health care professionals, as well as family members or friends. The facilitator then notifies the health care professionals as to time and date.

A letter of confirmation on the grief conference—including date, time, and place—is sent to the family. The grief conference may be a time to again offer parent support group information to the family.

Source: Wilke and Limbo (2012). Copyright 2012 by Gundersen Lutheran Medical Foundation, Inc. Reprinted with permission.

Evidence That Supports Professional-Led and Parent-Led Aftercare

There is eventually a transition in relationship between parents and health care professionals following the moments and events immediately surrounding a baby or older child's death. Families may experience deep longing for the familiar faces of those who became part of their child's daily life after leaving the hospital where their child died, or when their child's hospice nurse will no longer need to visit. Continuing to see the family with specific therapeutic goals can help fill the void. Being able to talk about their child with someone who knew him or her reminds the parents of the relationships that helped sustain them during their life's most heartbreaking times. They take comfort that their child was known by others. Follow-up care can take many forms. Follow-up care as we are using the term in this chapter does not involve formal psychotherapy or other forms of care requiring a professional counselor; rather, we are referring to the personal follow-up contacts generally made by a member of the interprofessional team who cared for the patient and family.

With the Internet becoming an increasingly indispensible resource, those who have experienced a death or severe fetal diagnosis during pregnancy, a stillbirth, death of a newborn, infant, or older child may use an online resource as their first form of support. Blogs, online chat groups (both closed and open), scheduled online support group meetings, in-person support groups, and peer volunteers are a few electronic resources available to bereaved parents. Carlson, Lammert, and O'Leary (2012) reviewed the evolution of group and online support in the past 35 years. They noted that in-person support (self-help groups and telephone follow-up from a health care provider) prevailed early on. However, in the past few decades specialized online groups (e.g., pregnancy after loss, prenatal support when the baby has a life-threatening condition) have provided additional options. In a Finnish study of mothers whose child died at age 3 or younger (Nikkola, Kaunonen, & Aho, 2013), women reported that the intervention (support materials, peer contact, and professional contact) helped them cope with their grief. They expressed positive responses to support that included both health care providers and peers or other community-based opportunities. The study was not designed with a comparison group, however.

Resolve Through Sharing® (RTS) developed a grief conference model (see Box 18.1) over 30 years ago that provided an opportunity for parents and others they chose to meet together some time after a child's death to review whatever was on the parents' minds (Wilke & Limbo, 2012). Such meetings should be guided by the parents' wishes and preferences, not the health care team's agenda. Similarly, Meert and colleagues have created a framework for follow-up support with parents who have experienced the death of a child in a pediatric intensive care setting. These meetings offer an opportunity for parents to both gain information and give feedback about their pediatric intensive care unit (PICU) experience (Meert et al., 2014). Health care professionals are encouraged to offer whatever follow-up model they provide with commitment and consistency.

CAREGIVER SUFFERING

Most health care professionals would likely embrace the idea that they experience their own grief when their patients die. Bearing witness to suffering is a part of professional practice for all those involved in end-of-life and bereavement care. Ferrell and Coyle (2008) wrote that nurses and many other professionals bear witness to suffering routinely.

Grief and Moral Distress

Bearing witness to grief and death can create a traumatic stress response. Those who manage their feelings of helplessness, loss of control, and loss do so by a process of oscillating (Stroebe & Schut, 1999), shifting between grief and restoration, or grief-oriented and healing- or restoration-oriented coping (Papadatou, 2009; Stroebe & Schut, 1999). For example, a neonatal intensive care nurse may care for a baby for several months, perhaps watching the baby grow and begin to overcome the effects of extreme prematurity. Then one day, the baby suffers an intracranial hemorrhage, her condition rapidly deteriorates, and in a few days, she dies. The nurse, chaplain, social worker, physician, and others who provided care for the baby may feel sad, helpless, or profound grief. Those feelings, however, may alternate with times of restoration that are filled with hope, awareness of other babies who need the person's care, and optimism that the support given to the baby's parents helped them weather their tragedy.

Rushton, Kasniak, and Halifax (2013) define moral distress as "a reality of clinical practice" (p. 1). Moral distress indicates that the care provider perceives that a moral line has been crossed—that what is happening is in some way wrong—and the care provider feels helpless to change it. Results can include moral outrage, anger, and burnout (Rushton et al., 2013). In a narrative on moral distress (Ferrell & Coyle, 2008), a nurse stated, "Our technology has surpassed our humanity" (p. 94), summarizing the conflict a professional may experience when treatment or other intervention surpasses what could have been a natural—and presumably more peaceful—death.

Being unable to affect futile treatment, patient pain and suffering, and potential long-term negative outcomes (e.g., lowered cognitive functioning) may cause moral distress in professionals (Ferrell, 2006).

An intervention designed for pediatric palliative care providers lessened the intensity of moral distress among interprofessional team members (Brandon et al., 2014). Designed to provide support and education, the Pediatric Quality of Life Program consists of two major components. These include education on principles of palliative care for all pediatric staff and consultation delivered by two physicians and a pediatric nurse practitioner (PNP). The physicians and PNP met with unit-based end-of-life care teams for care planning, family conference planning, and debriefing. Using pre-intervention and post-intervention moral distress surveys, researchers found that the respondents reported significantly fewer instances of situations causing moral distress (e.g., those that prolonged suffering or death) after the program was implemented ($p = .01$; Brandon et al., 2014).

The need for some form of support or recognition of professional suffering (grief and moral distress) is a common, perhaps universal, need. Kobler (2014) summarized the various strategies proposed in the literature (see Table 18.1) that aid professional caregivers in both the grief-focused and restorative-focused phases of their own responses to a patient death.

Table 18.1 summarizes strategies that may offer support, provide opportunity for reflection, and ultimately aid in processing the repetitive nature of work that is connected with suffering. A distinguishing feature of these types of self-care activities is that attendance is optional and those present are not required to discuss feelings or situations with which they are not comfortable.

The role of the facilitator of such staff support events is one that requires skill in group process; high emotional intelligence; an understanding of what is involved in maintaining consistent group and individual safety; and understands the meaning of moments, both as part of the situation that each person describes and as part of the group debriefing. Facilitators should study the research on each method, become familiar with the underlying theoretical frameworks, and become knowledgeable about aspects of quality and how to measure a strategy's success. Good information on the success of the strategy can be collected during a voluntary wrap-up time at the end of the session, in which attendees are asked, "Please identify one thing that happened today that you value and will remember and another example of one thing you wish would have happened differently."

TABLE 18.1 Synthesis of the Literature: Strategies to Support Caregivers Following a Patient Death

STRATEGY	PRIMARY AUTHOR	STRATEGY
Structured peer or mentor support	Baverstock, 2006 Eagle, 2012 Ewing, 2004	Mentor approach used in hospices to navigate experience after patient death Peer review and support Partners in caring for NICU peer support
Facilitated team processing	Bateman et al., 2012 Baverstock, 2006 Blacklock, 2012 Hill, 2012 Keene, 2010 Maloney, 2012 Roesler, 2009 Rushton, 2006	Wrap-up model: Facilitated team processing after every pediatric death Hospice team meetings with debriefing Modified critical incident stress model Informal and facilitated debriefing after critical incident resulting in death Structured team bereavement debriefing process after pediatric deaths Critical incident stress model for pediatric teams following death Supportive debriefings & team root cause analysis after critical event Facilitated team bereavement debriefing after all pediatric deaths
Reflective practice activities	Ihlenfeld, 2004 Kearney, 2009 Kearney, 2010 Rashotte, 2005	Reflective writing and journal sharing for health care teams Listing of reflective questions for caregiver processing of events Reflective video to reconnect caregivers with meaning of their work Caregiver storytelling and reflection after "haunting" deaths
Promoting staff self-care	Baverstock, 2006 Kearney, 2009	Hospice organization dedicating time for caregiver self-care activities Self-care and self-awareness strategies for use in the workplace
Co-creating ritual	Limbo, 2013 Papadatou, 2002	Touchstones and creative ideas for co-creating ritual for caregivers Importance of ritual for honoring caregivers' experiences with patient death

NICU, neonatal intensive care unit.

From Kobler (2014). Copyright 2014 by Wolters Kluwer Health. Reprinted with permission.

The following examples are ways in which these strategies may be implemented.

1. The chaplain who provides chaplaincy services for the birthing center facilitates a meeting for labor and delivery staff who wish to come together to talk about the recent death of a mother in labor with twins at 37 weeks gestation. The twins survived after an emergency cesarean birth. Both are in the neonatal intensive care unit (NICU) and will likely be discharged in about 2 days. The chaplain knows this is the first maternal death on this unit in more than 5 years. An OB/GYN physician and two nurses involved in the birth told the chaplain that there is a feeling of sadness and guilt that pervades the unit.
2. The clinical nurse specialist (CNS) lets PICU staff know that together they will talk about what they need, some sort of tangible way of acknowledging their own grief and their love for a child who died 4 months after a car accident, with her entire hospitalization occurring in the PICU. Several staff members told the CNS that one of the residents has been deeply affected because he was especially close to the child's parents, and that a child life specialist "can't stop crying." The CNS believes a ritual could help the staff.
3. The social worker assigned to the NICU was asked by one of the NICU respiratory therapists to help the staff process a recent death of triplets, born at 23 weeks gestation. One baby was stillborn, another lived for approximately 2 hours, and the third for 3 days. The social worker learned that several staff members are upset about the efforts made to save the third baby, believing that the invasive procedures were unnecessary, futile, and caused the baby to suffer.

We invite you to review each of these scenarios based on the chapter's content. They may serve as discussion questions for your next class, staff meeting, or interprofessional rounds, and enhance the chapter's case study.

Pause, reflect, acknowledge, and be mindful (PRAM) (Limbo & Kobler, 2013), a framework for professional practice, provides another self-care strategy appropriate for those who bear witness to others' suffering. The PRAM framework, designed to create a reflective practice, reminds those using the framework to take time, to be in the moment, and to reflect on the here and now. We offer three examples of how the PRAM framework may be incorporated into professional practice on a daily basis.

1. A chaplain may pause before entering the room of a mother whose baby was stillborn only hours before, knowing the baby is in the room, actively framing this first meeting of bereaved parent and her baby.
2. A neonatologist thinks about how she will learn what advance care plans the parents of a baby diagnosed prenatally with trisomy 18 and hypoplastic left heart will choose.

3. The pediatric ethicist pauses at the conference room door as he considers the potential strong emotions he will hear as the interprofessional team meets to discuss the long-dying of a baby born at 23 weeks who has had numerous postnatal complications.

The Role of Education

Relational Learning

To have a meaningful impact on the lives of children with life-threatening conditions and their families, educational initiatives need to be guided by pedagogy tied to the everyday relationships in which practitioners, children, and families are engaged (Browning & Solomon, 2006). Nurses experienced their highest anxiety when required to provide support for the dying or bereaved (Peters et al., 2013). Research studies conducted with those who provide bereavement and/or end-of-life care reflect that professional education makes a difference in reducing anxiety, and increasing comfort and competence (Feudtner et al., 2007). The content of education for those involved in death and dying needs to include skill-building activities that engage the learner and enhance relational communication strategies (Browning, Meyer, Truog, & Solomon, 2007), ultimately forming an "emotional standard of care" (p. 905). Empathy, regarded as taking the other's perspective, "walking in their shoes," can be learned (Back & Arnold, 2014). Kelley and Kelley (2013) summarize strategies for teaching empathy: modeling, comfort skills, compassion, active listening, and practice.

Relational learning involves educational opportunities that include the importance of *being,* in addition to what and how to communicate (Browning & Solomon, 2006). The authors provide specific suggestions for how organizations (e.g., a health system) can create and support relational learning. These include (a) creating an interprofessional team of leaders committed to a standard of care (e.g., bereavement) or a population of patients and families (those experiencing perinatal or pediatric death); (b) formal learning with appropriate faculty, including patients and families; (c) a culture that supports ethical behavior; and (d) educational initiatives tied to overall organizational learning and mission.

Interprofessional certification is available through the Hospice and Palliative Credentialing Center (HPCC) to the numerous disciplines providing perinatal and pediatric bereavement care (see Resources, www .advancingexpertcare.org). The Certified in Perinatal Loss Care (CPLC) credential and the Certified in Hospice and Palliative Care Pediatric Nursing (CHPPN) credential provide opportunities for recognition as experts in providing bereavement support and end-of-life care to child-bearing families.

CONCLUSION

These words link key concepts of this chapter: "Ritual flows from relationship. Relationship forms a bridge from suffering to hope. Hope transforms" (Limbo & Kobler, 2013, p. 13). Bereavement care providers are often asked: "How can you do that? It must be so hard." The answer: because experiencing and witnessing the suffering of deep personal loss is transformative. We end with a poem that brings nurse, mother, and baby into relationship and provides an example of the deep meaning this work has to those who are engaged in it.

On Rocking Arthur

The room seems so empty now,
I am left holding you.
Your family has gone,
But traces of their tears are evident
in the dampness of your clothes.
Their whispers of love
still hang in the air.

I sink into the rocking chair,
cradling your motionless body
in my arms.
Together we rock.

You are so beautiful,
your face and body perfectly formed.
It is hard to believe that inside
you were too broken and sick
to remain long on this earth.
Tears fall as I think of all
your poor body has suffered & endured
in the fight to live.

Minutes pass, and then an hour.
For some unknown reason,
I am unable to stop rocking you.

I have sung to you,
prayed for you,
thanked you for allowing me
to have a small part in
your short life.

But still, I am unable to put you down.

Friends peek around the curtain,
their worried looks convey
the unspoken words of concern. . .

The rhythm of our rocking is broken
by the familiar ring of the telephone.
It is your Mother.
Crying,
wishing she could tell you
of her love just one more time.

She thinks you are already far away. . .

Smiling through tears, I gently reply,
"We've been waiting, shall I put the receiver close to him?"

Faint strains of a lullaby drifted upwards. . .
We had arrived.

From Kobler (2013b). Used with author's permission.

CASE STUDY

Alex is a 25-year-old patient who has been admitted to the mother/baby unit after her son, born at 22 weeks gestation, lived for approximately 15 minutes and then died. She is devastated, cries most of the time while awake, and asks that her husband, Samir, not enter her room. Alex feels that her husband is very disappointed because "the baby was our first son." They have three daughters, aged 1, 3, and 5. Samir sits in the lounge most of the day and asks the nurse, Nola, to please let Alex know that he is not upset with her at all. Nola delivers the message but Alex still refuses to allow Samir in her room. Alex and Samir's parents visit often and Alex's mother, Tanya, describes Alex as "inconsolable." Samir and his parents explain that they feel helpless and do not know what to say or do for Alex. Samir also shares with Nola that he is struggling with how to explain the loss to their daughters who were very excited about their new sibling.

FOCUS QUESTIONS

1. Based on the case study, how does Alex seem to interpret personhood in relation to her son?
2. What interventions cited in the chapter would be most helpful for Alex? For Samir? For their children? For the grandparents?
3. How might various members of the interprofessional team guide family members and Nola?
4. What support would be most helpful for nurses like Nola who face difficult circumstances like these on a daily basis?

RESOURCES

Websites

- advancingexpertcare.org
- perinatalhospice.org
- plida.org
- www.resolvethroughsharing.org

Standards and Guidelines

SOURCE	PERTINENT RESOURCE	WEBSITE
Healthychildren.org	"Helping children cope with death." An online resource for understanding children's reactions to various types of losses (e.g., death of a grandparent or sibling)	http://www.healthychildren.org/English/healthy-living/emotional-wellness/Pages/Helping-Children-Cope-with-Death.aspx
American Academy of Pediatrics	Policy statement pediatric palliative care and hospice care commitments, guidelines, and recommendations guidelines for support of the family after a child's death	http://pediatrics.aappublications.org/content/132/5/966.full
National Hospice & Palliative Care Organization	CHiPPs newsletters	http://www.nhpco.org/childrenspediatricschipps/professional-resources

(continued)

(continued)

SOURCE	PERTINENT RESOURCE	WEBSITE
Hospice and Palliative Credentialing Center	Information regarding certification of pediatric palliative care and perinatal loss care	http://hpcc.advancingexpertcare.org/competence/rn-peds-chppn/
Hospice & Palliative Nurses Association	Numerous resources regarding palliative care in various specialties, grief and loss, role delineation, current research, continuing education, and certification, and perinatal loss	http://hpna.advancingexpertcare.org/
The Joint Commission	Resources on advanced certification for palliative care programs, including standards and process; standards on education for staff providing end-of-life care	http://www.jointcommission.org/certification/palliative_care.aspx
World Health Organization	Recommendations for end-of-life and palliative care	WHO Global Atlas on palliative care at the end of life: http://www.thewhpca.org/resources/global-atlas-on-end-of-life-care Symptom management at the end of life: http://www.who.int/3by5/capacity/palliative/en/ Mental health care after trauma (including bereavement): http://www.who.int/mediacentre/news/releases/2013/trauma_mental_health_20130806/en/ Guidelines for the management of conditions specifically related to stress (including bereavement): http://apps.who.int/iris/bitstream/10665/85119/1/9789241505406_eng.pdf?ua=1
British Columbia Ministry of Health	Guidelines & protocols: palliative care for the patient with incurable cancer or advanced disease part 3: Grief and bereavement	http://www.bcguidelines.ca/pdf/palliative3.pdf
Society of Obstetricians and Gynaecologists of Canada	Stillbirth and bereavement: guidelines for stillbirth investigation	http://sogc.org/guidelines/stillbirth-and-bereavement-guidelines-for-stillbirth-investigation/
Sands: Stillbirth & Neonatal Death Charity	The Sands Guidelines	https://www.uk-sands.org/professionals/resources-for-health-professionals/the-sands-guidelines

REFERENCES

Back, A. L., & Arnold, R. M. (2014). "Yes, it's sad but what should I do?" Moving from empathy to action. *Journal of Palliative Medicine, 17,* 141–144.

Back, A. L., Bauer-Wu, S. M., Rushton, C. M., & Halifax, J. (2009). Compassionate silence in the patient-clinician encounter: A contemplative approach. *Journal of Palliative Medicine, 12*(12), 1113–1117.

Bateman, S. T., Dixon, R., & Trozzi, M. (2012). The Wrap-Up: A unique forum to support pediatric residents when faced with the death of a child. *Journal of Palliative Medicine, 15*(12), 1329–1334. doi:10.1089/jpm.2012.0253

Baverstock, A. C., & O'Finlay, F. (2006). A study of staff support mechanisms within children's hospices. *International Journal of Palliative Nursing, 12*(11), 506–508.

Black, B. P. (1993) Caring in hellish places. In M. M. Styles & P. Moccia (Eds.), *On nursing: A literary celebration: An anthology* (pp. 131–143). New York, NY: Jones & Bartlett Publishing.

Black, B. P., & Fields, W. S. (2014). Contexts of reproductive loss in lesbian couples. *MCN, The American Journal of Maternal/Child Nursing, 39*(3), 157–162.

Blacklock, E. (2012). Interventions following a critical incident: Developing a critical incident stress management team. *Archives of Psychiatric Nursing, 26*(1), 2–8. doi:10.1016/j.apnu.2011.04.006

Blood, C., & Cacciatore, J. (2014). Best practice in bereavement photography after perinatal death: Qualitative analysis with 104 parents. *BMC Psychology, 2,* 15–25.

Boss, P., Kavanaugh, K., & Kobler, K. (2011). Prenatal and neonatal palliative care. In J. Wolfe, P. Hinds, & B. Sourkes (Eds.), *Textbook of interdisciplinary pediatric palliative care* (pp. 387–401). Philadelphia, PA: Saunders.

Brandon, D., Ryan, D., Sloane, R., & Docherty, S. L. (2014). Impact of a pediatric quality of life program on providers' moral distress. *MCN, The American Journal of Maternal/Child Nursing, 39*(3), 189–197.

Browning, D. M., Meyer, E. C., Truog, R. D., & Solomon, M. Z. (2007). Difficult conversations in health care: Cultivating relational learning to address the hidden curriculum. *Academic Medicine, 82*(9), 905–913.

Browning, D. M., & Solomon, M. Z. (2006). Relational learning in pediatric palliative care: Transformative education and the culture of medicine. *Child and Adolescent Psychiatric Clinics of North America, 15*(3), 795–815.

Cacciatore, J., & Flint, M. (2012a). ATTEND: Toward a mindfulness-based bereavement care model. *Death Studies, 36,* 61–82.

Cacciatore, J., & Flint, M. (2012b). Mediating grief: Postmortem ritualization after child death. *Journal of Loss and Trauma: International perspectives on stress & coping, 17*(2), 158–172.

Cacciatore, J., & Raffo, Z. (2011). An exploration of lesbian maternal bereavement. *Social Work, 56*(2), 169–177.

Carlson, R., Lammert, C., & O'Leary, J. M. (2012). The evolution of group and online support for families who have experienced perinatal or neonatal loss. *Illness, Crisis, & Loss, 20,* 275–293.

Côté-Arsenault, D., & Dombeck, M. B. (2001). Maternal assignment of fetal personhood to a previous pregnancy loss: Relationship to anxiety in the current pregnancy. *Health Care for Women International, 22*(7), 649–665.

Dussel, V., Kreicbergs, U., Hilden, J. M., Watterson, J., Moore, C., Turner, B. G. . ., & Wolfe, J. (2009). Looking beyond where children die: Determinants and effects of planning a child's location of death. *Journal of Pain and Symptom Management, 37*(1), 33–43.

Eagle, S., Creel, A., & Alexandrov, A. (2012). The effect of facilitated peer support sessions on burnout and grief management among health care providers in pediatric intensive care units: A pilot study. *Journal of Palliative Medicine, 15*(11), 1178–1180. doi: 10.1089/jpm.2012.0231

Ewing, A., & Carter, B. S. (2004). Once again, Vanderbilt NICU in Nashville leads the way in nurses' emotional support. *Pediatric Nursing, 30*(6), 471–472.

Ferrell, B. R. (2006). Understanding the moral distress of nurses witnessing medically futile care. *Oncology Nursing Forum, 33*, 922–930.

Ferrell, B. R., & Coyle, N. (2008). *The nature of suffering and the goals of nursing.* New York, NY: Oxford.

Feudtner, C., Santucci, G., Feinstein, J. A., Snyder, C. R., Rourke, M. T., & Kang, T. I. (2007). Hopeful thinking and level of comfort regarding providing pediatric palliative care: A survey of hospital nurses. *Pediatrics, 119*(1), e186–e192.

Garstang, J., Griffiths, F., & Sidebotham, P. (2014). What do bereaved parents want from professionals after the death of their child: A systematic review of the literature. *BMC Pediatrics, 14*, 269.

Gold, K. J. (2007) Navigating care after a baby dies: A systematic review of parent experiences with health providers. *Journal of Perinatology, 27*(4), 230–237.

Gold, K. J., Sen, A., & Hayward, R. A. (2010). Marriage and cohabitation outcomes after pregnancy loss. *Pediatrics, 125*, e1202–e1207.

Hill, P. E. (2012). Support and counseling after maternal death. *Seminars in Perinatology, 36*, 84–88. doi:10.1053/j.semperi.2011.09.016

Hochberg, T. (n.d.). *Touching souls: Healing with bereavement photography.* Retrieved from http://toddhochberg.com/main.html

Hunter, S. B., & Smith, D. E. (2008). Predictors of children's understandings of death: Age, cognitive ability, death experience and maternal communicative competence. *Omega, 57*(2), 143–162.

Ihlenfeld, J. T. (2004). Applying personal reflective critical incident reviews in critical care. *Dimensions in Critical Care Nursing, 23*(1), 1–3.

Kassam, A., Skiadaresis, J., Alexander, S., & Wolfe, J. (2014). Parent and clinician preferences for location of end-of-life care: Home, hospital or freestanding hospice? *Pediatric Blood Cancer, 61*, 859–864.

Kearney, G. (2010). We must not forget what we once knew: An exemplar for helping nurses reconnect with their history and rediscover their passion for nursing. *Journal of Holistic Nursing, 28*(4), 260–262. doi:10.1177/0898010110376322

Kearney, M. K., Weininger, R. B., Vachon, M. L., Harrison, R. L., & Mount, B. M. (2009). Self-care of physicians caring for patients at the end of life "Being connected. . .a key to my survival." *JAMA, 301*(1), 1155–1164. doi:10.1001/jama.2009.352

Keene, E. A., Hutton, N., Hall, B. & Rushton, C. (2010). Bereavement debriefing sessions: An intervention to support health care professionals in managing their grief after the death of a patient. *Pediatric Nursing, 36*(4), 185–189.

Kelley, K. J., & Kelley, M. F. (2013). Teaching empathy and other compassion-based communication skills. *Journal for Nurses in Professional Development, 29*(6), 321–324.

Kobler, K. (2013a). Honoring relationship in pediatric palliative care. In G. R. Cox & R. G. Stevenson (Eds.), *Final acts: The end of life: Hospice and palliative care.* Amityville, NY: Baywood Publishing Company, Inc.

Kobler, K. (2013b). On rocking Arthur. In R. Limbo & K. Kobler, *Meaningful moments: Ritual and reflection when a child dies* (p. 65). La Crosse, WI: Gundersen Medical Foundation, Inc.

Kobler, K. (2014). Leaning in and holding on: Team support with unexpected death. *MCN, The American Journal of Maternal/Child Nursing, 39*(3), 148–154.

Kobler, K., Limbo, R., & Kavanaugh, K. (2007). Meaningful moments: The use of ritual in perinatal and pediatric death. *MCN, The American Journal of Maternal/Child Nursing, 32*(5), 288–295.

Koloroutis, M. (Ed.). (2004). *Relationship-based care: A model for transforming practice.* New York, NY: Springer.

Limbo, R., & Kobler, K. (2009). Will our baby be alive again? Supporting parents of young children when a baby dies. *Nursing for Women's Health, 13*, 302–311.

Limbo, R., & Kobler, K. (2010). The tie that binds: Relationships in perinatal bereavement. *MCN, The American Journal of Maternal Child/Nursing, 35*(6), 316–321.

Limbo, R., & Kobler, K. (2013). *Meaningful moments: Ritual and reflection when a child dies.* La Crosse, WI: Gundersen Medical Foundation, Inc.

Limbo, R., & Lathrop, A. (2014). Caregiving in mothers' narratives of perinatal hospice. *Illness, Crisis, & Loss, 22*(1), 43–65.

Limbo, R. K., & Wheeler, S. R. (1986). Women's response to the loss of their pregnancy through miscarriage: a longitudinal study. *The Forum: Newsletter of the American Association for Death Education and Counseling, 10*(4), 1–2, 4–6. Retrieved from http://www.adec.org/adec/ADEC_Main/Publications/The_Forum/Forum-Homepage.aspx

Lindsay, G., Cross, N., & Ives-Baine, L. (2012). Narratives of neonatal intensive care unit nurses: Experience with end-of-life care. *Illness, Crisis, & Loss, 20*, 239–253.

Maloney, C. (2012). Critical incident stress debriefing and pediatric nurses: An approach to support the work environment and mitigate negative circumstances. *Pediatric Nursing, 38*(2), 110–113.

Meert, K. L., Eggly, S., Berg, R. A., Wessel, D. L., Newth, C. J. L., Shanley, T. P.,. . .& Nicholson, C. E. (2014). Feasibility and perceived benefits of a framework for physician-parent follow-up meetings after a child's death in the PICU. *Critical Care Medicine, 42*(1), 148–157.

Nikkola, I., Kaunonen, M., & Aho, A. L. (2013). Mother's report of a bereavement follow-up intervention after the death of a child. *Journal of Clinical Nursing, 22*, 1151–1162.

Now I Lay Me Down to Sleep. (n.d.). Retrieved from https://www.nowilaymedowntosleep.org/

O'Malley, P., Barata, I., & Snow, S. (2014). Death of a child in the emergency department. *Pediatrics, 134*(1), e313–e330.

Papadatou, D., Bellali, T., Papazoglou, I., & Petraki, D. (2002). Greek nurse and physician grief as a result of caring for children dying of cancer. *Pediatric Nursing, 28*(4), 345–353.

Papadatou, D. (2009). *In the face of death: Professionals who care for the dying and bereaved.* New York, NY: Springer.

Peel, E. (2010). Pregnancy loss in lesbian and bisexual women: An online survey of experiences. *Human Reproduction, 25*(3), 721–727.

Perry, B. (2008). Why exemplary oncology nurses seem to avoid compassion fatigue. *Canadian Oncology Nursing Journal, 18*(2), 87–99.

Peters, L., Cant, R., Payne, S., O'Connor, M., McDermott, F., Hood, K., . . . Shimoinaba, K. (2013). How death anxiety impacts nurses' caring for patients at the end of life: A review of literature. *The Open Nursing Journal, 7*, 14–21.

Price, J., Jordan, J., & Prior, L. (2013). A consensus for change: Parent and professional perspectives on care for children at the end-of-life. *Issues in Comprehensive Pediatric Nursing, 36*(1), 70–87.

Rashotte, J. (2005). Dwelling with stories that haunt us: Building a meaningful nursing practice. *Nursing Inquiry, 12*(1), 34–42.

Resolve Through Sharing® bereavement services. (n.d.). Retrieved from http://www.bereavementservices.org

Roesler, R., Ward, D., & Short, M. (2009). Supporting staff recovery and reintegration after a critical incident resulting in infant death. *Advances in Neonatal Care, 9*(4), 163–171. doi:10.1097/ANC.0b013e3181afab5b

Rushton, C. H., Reder, E., Hall, B., Comello, K., Sellers, D. E., & Hutton, N. (2006). Interdisciplinary interventions to improve pediatric palliative care and reduce health care professional suffering. *Journal of Palliative Medicine, 9*(4), 922–933. doi:10.1089/jpm.2006.9.922

Rushton, C. H., Kasniak, A. W., & Halifax, J. S. (2013). A framework for understanding moral distress among palliative care physicians. *Journal of Palliative Medicine, 16,* 1074–1079.

Schaeffer, D., & Lyons, C. (2010). *How do we tell the children? A step-by-step guide for helping children and teens cope when someone dies* (4th ed). New York, NY: Newmarket Press.

Schreffler, K. M., Hill, P. W., & Cacciatore, J. (2012). Exploring the increased odds of divorce following miscarriage or stillbirth. *Journal of Divorce & Remarriage, 53,* 91–107.

Stroebe, M., Finkenauer, C., Wijngaards-DeMeij, L., Shut, H., van den bout, J., & Stroebe, W., (2013). Partner-oriented self regulation among bereaved parents: The costs of holding in grief for the partner's sake. *Psychological Science, 24,* 395–402.

Stroebe, M. S., & Schut, H. (1999). The dual process model of coping with bereavement: Rationale and description. *Death Studies, 23,* 197–224.

Van Damme, L. (2009). Moments like this. *Nursing for Women's Health, 13*(5), 446–448.

Wender, E., & The Committee on Psychosocial Aspects of Child and Family Health. (2012). Supporting the family after the death of a child. *Pediatrics, 130*(6), 1164–1169.

Wilke, J., & Limbo, R. (2012). *Resolve through sharing bereavement training: Perinatal death.* La Crosse, WI: Gundersen Lutheran Medical Foundation.

Index

Printed in the United States
By Bookmasters